Clinical Pathophysiology
Made Ridiculously Simple

Aaron Berkowitz

MedMaster Inc.
Miami, Florida

Made in the United States of America

Published by MedMaster, Inc.
P.O. Box 640028
Miami FL 33164

Cover by Richard March

Contents

Chapter Outlines

Preface

In retrospect, I wish someone had stood up on the first day of medical school and said, "Everything you will learn here has essentially two goals: how to diagnose disease and how to treat it. The goal is to teach you how to develop a differential diagnosis, how to evaluate a patient further to zero in on a diagnosis, and how to treat the disease diagnosed." Although it seems like a simple statement, if it were truly understood by students at the outset of medical school, and if an effort were made during all pre-clinical teaching to explain how material is relevant to these goals, a strong framework for the learning, understanding, and application of medical knowledge would develop in each student from day one. The move toward integration of the preclinical sciences has been a large step toward this goal, and a much-welcomed change from the previously artificial separation of anatomy from physiology from pathology from biochemistry...etc. However, at present, there is no book that provides the student with a clear and concise overview of the mechanisms, diagnosis, and treatment of diseases from this integrated perspective. The goal of this book is to fill that perceived void, linking the study of pathophysiology with its relationship to normal physiology on the one hand, and with clinical reasoning in diagnosis and treatment on the other.

The chapters may be read in any order and are linked via cross-references, where relevant. In the most prevalent curricular model at present, this book would ideally serve as a guide to the second year of medical school as well as a review for the USMLE Step 1. I essentially wrote it as the book I wish I had during second year to understand why I learned what I did in the first year, and why what I was learning in second year would be relevant to what followed. This book can help to serve as the "mental filing folders" for the deluge of information presented in the first two years of medical school. The book could also serve as a review for health professionals of any type at any level of training seeking a refresher on the basics.

This book uses simple anatomical and physiological concepts to create a framework for the understanding of disease processes and the symptoms, signs, and lab findings that they produce. Each chapter begins with a brief discussion of "how an organ system works" (anatomy/biochemistry/physiology), which is then followed by what logically could cause malfunction of the organ system (pathology/pathophysiology). Following the establishment of this framework, specific disease mechanisms are discussed in this context, and the symptoms, signs, diagnosis, and treatment of these diseases are elaborated upon. In a complementary approach, the accompanying CD-ROM, designed by Dr. Stephen Goldberg, allows the student to proceed in the opposite direction: one can select a symptom, sign, or lab finding and see all of the many diseases that could cause it, classified by pathophysiological mechanism.

Information on histopathology, epidemiology, diagnostic algorithms, treatment protocols, and psychosocial aspects of medicine can be found in many other sources, so none of these areas are treated in detail here. Rather, I try to present an aerial view of the "forest" of clinical pathophysiology, all the while pointing out the "trees." A section or even an entire chapter can be read in one or two sittings, thus providing an overview of the functioning of a given organ system, how it can malfunction, the disease entities that can cause such malfunction, and how, in principle, one can diagnose and treat such entities.

The goal of the chapter of cases is not just to ask you "what's the most likely diagnosis?", as many USMLE-type questions do, but also to help you think pathophysiologically through the symptoms/signs and diagnostic reasoning. Thus, the goal is not to "arrive at the answer" but rather to understand the possibilities and how to logically distinguish among them. This is a book that will certainly help to prepare you for your coursework and the USMLE, but more importantly, it will provide you with a logical framework and reasoning strategy with which to approach clinical medicine, and ultimately serve to enhance your ability to take care of your patients.

Aaron Berkowitz

Acknowledgments

This book could not have been completed without the mentorship, support, and advice of Dr. Stephen Goldberg, President of MedMaster Books. Dr. Goldberg has helped me bring this book from its initial conception to its present quality, and has generously provided the illustrations and programmed the accompanying CD-ROM. His insightful suggestions on pedagogy, prose, and making things ridiculously simple have been extraordinarily helpful in shaping this book at all stages of its conception and development.

I was also incredibly fortunate to have many phenomenal expert reviewers, to whom I express my deepest gratitude. Each of the following physicians generously offered extremely valuable advice, suggestions, clinical and scientific insights, and very helpful perspectives on pedagogical organization. I heartily thank Doctors Jay Adler, Todd Brown, Paul Dworkin, Derek Fine, John Flynn, H. Franklin Herlong, Steven Gittler, David Newman-Toker, Alison Moliterno, David Pearse, Richard Preston, and Joseph Shuman. I am also very grateful for the extraordinarily precise proofreading skills of Phyllis Goldenberg, whose suggestions were extremely helpful in making the flow of the text as clear as possible. The book gained much from the input of all of these individuals; I alone am responsible for whatever imperfections remain.

This book is dedicated to all of the wonderful teachers who have been responsible for my education up to the present from Hillview Nursery School, Russell Elementary School, Paxon Hollow Middle School, Marple Newtown High School, George Washington University, and Johns Hopkins School of Medicine, and to my first teachers, my parents and grandparents.

This book is also humbly dedicated to the memory of David Atkins, one of my first mentors in the sciences—and many other areas—at George Washington University. Though he was not known for making things 'ridiculously simple' by any means (his courses in neurobiology and comparative anatomy inspired both awe and fear among students), I was privileged to study with him for the entirety of my undergraduate education, enjoying many pearls of wisdom and many hearty laughs.

CHAPTER 1. THE CARDIOVASCULAR SYSTEM

ANATOMICAL OVERVIEW

Fig. 1-1. Basic circulatory circuit. Deoxygenated blood from the right side of the body travels to the right heart by way of the venous system. The right hearts pumps this blood to the lungs via the pulmonary artery. The lungs oxygenate this blood and send it to the left heart by way of the pulmonary veins. This oxygenated blood is pumped by the left heart through the aorta to the body.

Fig. 1-2. Heart chambers and valves. There are four heart valves. The two atrioventricular valves (mitral and tricuspid) lie between the atria and the ventricles, and the aortic and pulmonic valves lie between the ventricles and their outflow vessels (aorta and pulmonary artery). During *systole*, the ventricles contract, forcefully expelling blood into the outflow vessels; while this occurs, the atrioventricular valves prevent backflow of this blood from the ventricles to the atria. During *diastole*, the ventricles relax and fill with blood from the atria; while this occurs, the aortic and pulmonary valves prevent backflow of the blood that has just been ejected during systole. Mnemonic for the atrioventricular (AV) valves: The t*ri*cuspid is on the *ri*ght. The mitra*l* is on the *l*eft.

HEART FAILURE

We will first discuss the manifestations and treatment of heart failure as a means of reviewing cardiac physiology. Following this, we will examine the four

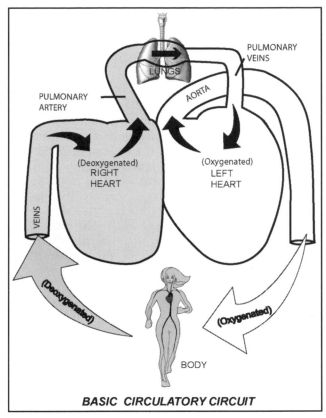

Figure 1-1

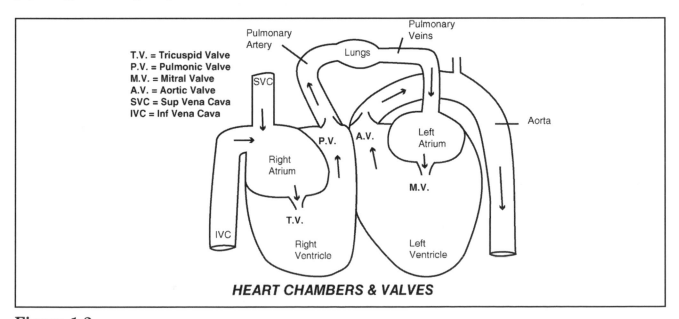

Figure 1-2

components of the heart (muscle, valves, electrical system, and blood supply), how each can be affected by disease, and the pathophysiological and clinical manifestations of such diseases.

Left Heart Failure

Fig. 1-3A. Left heart failure. Consider a patient who gets short of breath with activity. Shortness of breath means that the lungs are somehow affected. The lungs may be affected *directly* (by pulmonary disease) or *indirectly* (e.g., by cardiac disease). How could cardiac disease affect the lungs? Imagine that a patient's left ventricle cannot pump as well as it should (the causes of such pumping problems comprise the bulk of this chapter). This would decrease the flow from the left heart to the body, which in turn would cause blood to back up into the pulmonary vasculature (Fig. 1-3A). This backup increases pressure in the pulmonary veins, causing transudation of fluid into the lungs. This results in *pulmonary edema*, which causes shortness of breath (*dyspnea*).

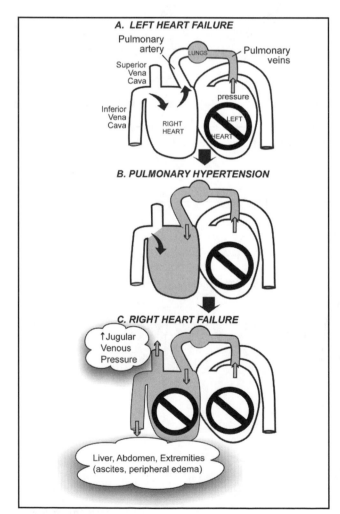

Figure 1-3

The name congestive heart failure comes from the congestion in the lungs caused by backup of flow from a failing left heart. On physical exam, you might hear crackles in the bases of the lungs as a result of this excess fluid. The worse the failure and the more fluid in the lungs, the higher up in the lung fields these crackles will be heard (as the lungs fill with fluid from the bottom up).

Right Heart Failure

Fig. 1-3B. Left heart failure as a cause of right heart failure. The right ventricle is not nearly as strong as the left ventricle, since it only squeezes into the low-pressure pulmonary system, whereas the left ventricle must squeeze into the higher-resistance systemic vasculature. The right ventricular walls are thus thinner than the walls of the more muscular left ventricle. Any disease process that increases resistance in the pulmonary vasculature (*pulmonary hypertension*) can cause the right heart's job to be increasingly difficult for this thinner-walled ventricle. Because backup of flow in left heart failure can increase pressure in the pulmonary vasculature, left heart failure can cause pulmonary hypertension and subsequent right heart failure.

Fig. 1-3C. Right heart failure. If the right heart fails, *now* where does the blood back up? Where does the blood in the right heart come from? The simple answer is the body; more specifically, the venous return from the body via the superior and inferior venae cavae. What would you expect to see on physical exam if the venous return backs up? An *elevated jugular venous pressure* (JVP). The jugular veins in the neck are a straight shot to the superior vena cava, which is a straight shot to the right heart. The JVP thus serves as a sort of barometer of right heart pressure. Where else would the blood back up? Backup can reach the liver, the abdomen, and the rest of the body via the inferior vena cava. Thus, *ascites* (fluid in the abdomen), *hepatic congestion*, and *peripheral edema* (fluid in the ankles, legs, etc.) can be signs of right heart failure.

Symptoms and Signs of Heart Failure

We have been discussing how a failing heart causes blood to *back up*. A failing heart *also has trouble maintaining forward flow* — this was the whole reason for this backup in the first place. What symptoms might be caused by decreased *forward* flow? Decreased blood flow to the muscles and the rest of the body can result in fatigue, weakness, and shortness of breath. Decreased blood flow to the brain may cause drowsiness or changes in mental status.

Fig. 1-4. Symptoms and signs of heart failure. Orthopnea and paroxysmal nocturnal dyspnea are two additional symptoms that can appear in heart failure. *Orthopnea*: The classic story is that a patient gets very short of breath upon lying down. Why? What *changes*

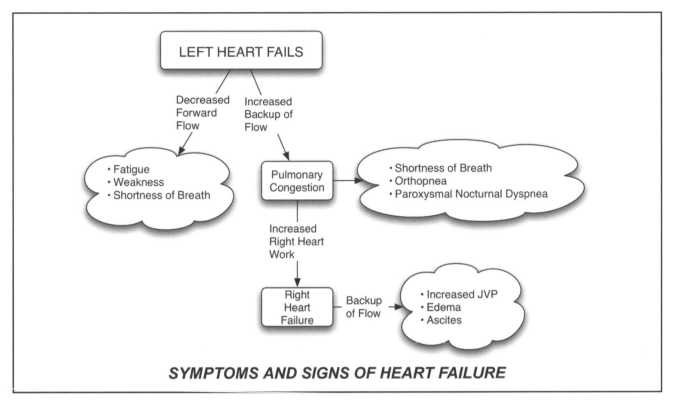

SYMPTOMS AND SIGNS OF HEART FAILURE

Figure 1-4

physiologically when one lies down? When one is standing, gravity causes venous blood to pool in the feet. When one lies down, all of this blood can find its way back to the heart more easily, suddenly increasing the heart's work. Normally, the heart can handle it, but a weak and failing heart cannot, and the blood backs up into the lungs, causing shortness of breath. You can ask the patient, "How many pillows do you sleep on?" Of course, some people just like to sleep on a lot of pillows, but if you ask, "What would happen if you were to lie flat?", a patient with heart failure may tell the classic story that s/he cannot breathe as easily when lying flat.

A related symptom is *paroxysmal nocturnal dyspnea*. The pathophysiology is the same, though the end result is that the patient wakes up in the middle of the night coughing and short of breath, classically resolving when the patient gets up and goes to the window for air.

Preload, Afterload, and Treatment of Heart Failure

Preload is the pressure that fills the ventricles during diastole, and *afterload* is the resistance that the heart faces during systole. More specifically, preload is the blood pressure in the left ventricle at the end of diastole, right before the ventricles contract. Where does

this come from? Originally, the preload comes to the heart from the *venous* system. Afterload is the systemic vascular resistance, or the resistance to flow in the arterial tree against which the heart must work (**a**fterload is created by the **a**rteries).

Fig. 1-5. Treatment of heart failure. In heart failure, there is decreased forward flow and increased backup of flow. The goals of therapies are thus to *increase forward flow* and *decrease backup of flow*. To increase forward flow, cardiac output must be increased. To decrease backup, the workload on the heart must be decreased.

- **Increasing forward flow by increasing cardiac output** can be accomplished by one of two basic mechanisms:
  - *Increase the force of ventricular contraction (**inotropes**, e.g., digoxin/digitalis, dopamine/dobutamine, amrinone/milrinone)*
  - *Decrease the rate of contraction to increase filling time (**beta-blockers**, e.g., propranolol, metoprolol). The increase in filling time allows more blood to accumulate in the ventricles before contraction, leading to a subsequent increase in cardiac output.*

- **Decreasing backup by decreasing the heart's work.** The heart's work is to pump the preload

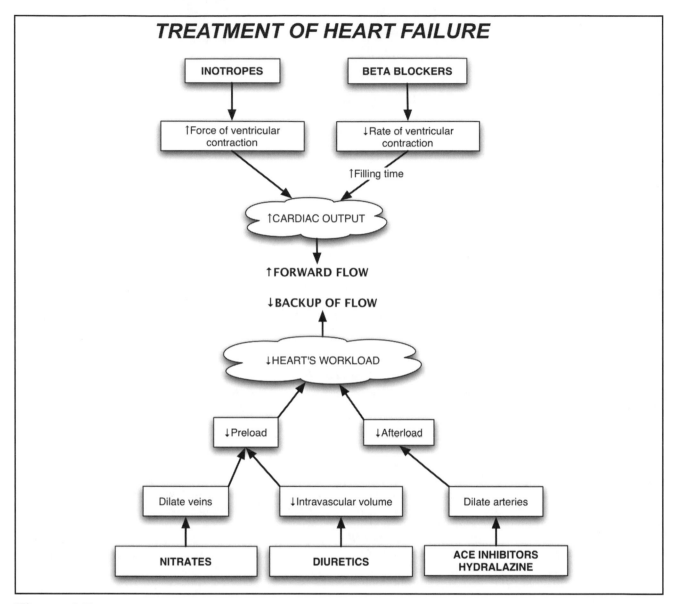

TREATMENT OF HEART FAILURE

Figure 1-5

against the afterload. In heart failure, what could be done to preload and afterload to make the heart's job easier? Therapies should *decrease* preload and *decrease* afterload. How can preload be reduced? One can decrease venous return by *dilating veins*, which slows the return of blood from the veins to the heart (*nitrates* have this action). Also, one can use *diuretics*, which cause the patient to urinate more, reducing the intravascular fluid volume. Success of diuretic therapy can be monitored by observing the decrease in symptoms/signs related to excess fluid, such as shortness of breath and edema. *Arterial dilators* decrease afterload (e.g., ACE inhibitors, hydralazine).

The Kidneys in Heart Failure

Fig. 1-6. The kidneys in heart failure. Since cardiac output is weak in heart failure, the perfusion pressure in the kidneys decreases. The blood volume itself is *not* changed, but the pressure at which this volume reaches the kidneys decreases, hence the term *effective blood volume* decrease. Effective volume depletion also occurs in cirrhosis.[1] When the kidneys sense de-

---

[1] Cirrhosis is scarring of the liver that can impede blood flow through the hepatic portal system, causing portal hypertension (see Fig. 4-12). Due to this blockage in the venous return, blood pools in the gut's venous system. Again, the *effective* blood volume that reaches the kidney decreases because a large volume of the body's blood supply stagnates in the mesenteric veins.

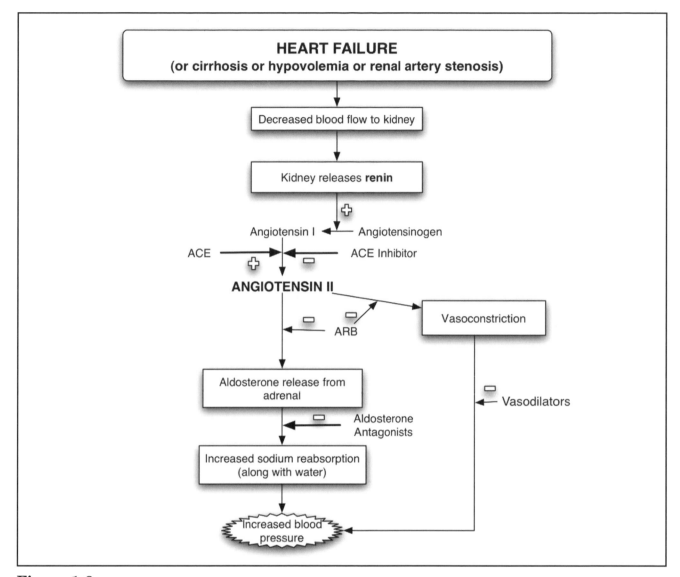

Figure 1-6

creased perfusion pressure, they try to increase this pressure by increasing blood volume. How can the kidneys increase blood volume in response to decreased perfusion pressure? Through the renin-angiotensin-aldosterone system. This system senses decreased renal perfusion and releases renin, which increases conversion of angiotensinogen to angiotensin I. Angiotensin I is in turn converted to angiotensin II by angiotensin converting enzyme (ACE). Angiotensin II causes vasoconstriction, which raises the blood pressure. Angiotensin II also stimulates aldosterone release from the adrenal gland. This leads to increased sodium reabsorption by the kidneys, which causes water to follow it, which increases intravascular volume. The increased vasoconstriction and increased blood volume raise the blood pressure. Additionally, the perceived low volume status causes release of antidi-

uretic hormone (ADH) from the posterior pituitary. ADH increases water reabsorption in the kidneys, further contributing to increased volume and increased blood pressure.

If the heart is already having trouble handling the existing blood volume, are the kidneys and ADH helping by increasing plasma volume in heart failure? No. This increased intravascular volume further aggravates the backup into the lungs and body as discussed above. ACE inhibitors (Fig.1-6) decrease the conversion of angiotensin I to angiotensin II. Reducing angiotensin II production decreases both aldosterone release and angiotensin II-induced vasoconstriction, thus inhibiting further increase in blood volume and blood pressure. Angiotensin II receptor blockers (ARBs) block the angiotensin II receptor, leading to a similar effect.

Aldosterone itself can be blocked at its receptor by aldosterone antagonists such as spironolactone.

THE FOUR COMPONENTS OF THE HEART AND THEIR DISEASES

We have just discussed the physiologic basis of the clinical manifestations of heart failure, but *why* does the heart fail? The heart has four components that help it to pump blood: *muscle*, *valves*, an *electrical conduction system*, and the heart's own *blood supply*. If any of these four elements is not working properly, this impedes the heart's ability to pump blood to the tissues, which can lead to both "decreased forward flow" symptoms/signs (fatigue, weakness, shortness of breath) and increased "backup of flow" symptoms/signs (shortness of breath, paroxysmal nocturnal dyspnea, orthopnea, edema, elevated JVP). Be it disease of the muscle, valves, electrical system, or coronary vasculature, if the heart is not functioning optimally, these are the sorts of symptoms that can occur. Ischemic heart disease (e.g., angina, myocardial infarction) and inflammation of the heart can also cause *chest pain* in addition to these symptoms. Although the above symptoms are characteristic of cardiac disease of some sort, they are certainly not exclusive to cardiac disease. For example, shortness of breath can also be due to pulmonary disease, anemia, or anxiety; chest pain can also arise from esophageal, musculoskeletal, or pulmonary disease.

Diseases of the Heart Muscle

The ventricular muscles relax during diastole, accepting blood; they contract during systole, ejecting this blood. If the musculature thickens (*hypertrophy*), the ventricle cannot relax as well, and the ventricle chamber size is reduced, decreasing how much blood it can

receive (*diastolic dysfunction*). If the musculature thins and weakens (*dilatation*), the strength of the ventricular muscle decreases, and it cannot contract as forcefully (*systolic dysfunction*).

Cardiac Hypertrophy

Fig. 1-7A. Cardiac Hypertrophy. Hypertrophy means increased growth. Hypertrophy of cardiac muscle can be caused by genetic disease (*hypertrophic cardiomyopathy*) or by certain pathophysiologic circumstances. What circumstances make any group of muscles grow big and strong? Hard work. What would cause the heart to have to work hard? Let's take it one side at a time. The left heart squeezes blood to the body, namely to the entire systemic vascular tree via the aorta. This resistance is the *afterload*: what the heart works against. Thus, one cause of increased strain on the left heart is increased blood pressure in the arteries (*hypertension*). What else might cause the left ventricle to have to work extra hard? Reviewing figure 1-2, note that blood goes from the left ventricle through the aortic valve to the aorta. In *aortic stenosis*, the left ventricle has to squeeze hard against the resistance posed by the stenotic aortic valve. Over time, this can cause left ventricular hypertrophy.

What causes *right* ventricular hypertrophy? Using the same logic, what site of increased resistance would cause the right heart to have to work harder? Since the right heart ejects into the lungs, any process that increases resistance in the pulmonary vasculature (*pulmonary hypertension*) can lead to right ventricular hypertrophy and eventual failure. Examples include left heart failure (Fig. 1-3B), pulmonic valve stenosis, and pulmonary causes (Fig. 2-5). Right heart failure secondary to a pulmonary cause is called *cor pulmonale*.

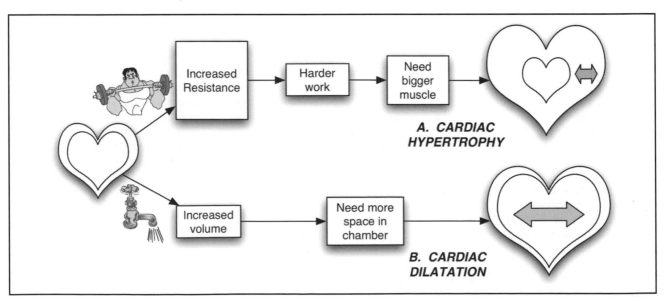

Figure 1-7

If any process increases the resistance that the heart must pump against, the heart will have to work harder to squeeze, and can eventually grow big and thick. Although this growth may initially be compensatory, it eventually reaches diminishing returns.

Consequences of Cardiac Hypertrophy. First, the increased thickness of the hypertrophied ventricular wall also makes it more difficult to adequately perfuse. As the cardiac muscle outgrows its blood supply, *ischemia* (decreased blood flow/oxygen supply) can occur, which can result in angina, and/or infarction. Second, what does the hypertrophied heart do *better* than the normal heart, and what does it do *worse*? The hypertrophy allows the heart to squeeze better, but its thick walls do not *relax* as well. In addition, the muscle can get so thick that the chamber becomes quite small. Poor relaxation and small chamber size lead to decreased filling of the ventricles, which results in decreased cardiac output. Ventricular relaxation occurs during *diastole*, so since the hypertrophied heart cannot relax as well, cardiac hypertrophy causes *diastolic* dysfunction. If the heart cannot relax optimally, it cannot *fill* optimally; thus, forward flow decreases and backup of flow occurs. Hypertrophy of the left ventricle can eventually lead to left heart failure symptoms and signs, and right ventricular hypertrophy can lead to right heart failure symptoms and signs (Fig. 1-4).

Treatment of Cardiac Hypertrophy. If the hypertrophied heart has a smaller chamber size, and does not fill optimally, the treatment(s) of choice should decrease heart rate and contractile force, allowing for increased filling and increased cardiac output. *Beta blockers* and *calcium channel blockers* accomplish these goals.

Restrictive Cardiomyopathy

In *infiltrative diseases*, substances can accumulate in the heart muscle, such as amyloid (which can occur from amyloidosis or multiple myeloma) or iron in hemochromatosis. Rarer diseases, such as sarcoid and Pompe's disease, can also lead to infiltration, causing a restrictive cardiomyopathy. The pathophysiology in restrictive heart disease is essentially the same as in cardiac hypertrophy: the heart is stiff and does not relax well (diastolic dysfunction).

Treatment of Restrictive Cardiomyopathy. One treats the underlying cause if possible. Otherwise, the treatment is the same as that for heart failure, aiming to increase forward flow and decrease backup of flow (Fig.1-5).

Cardiac Dilatation

Fig. 1-7B. Cardiac Dilatation. The dilated heart is big and baggy, not thick and strong like the hypertrophied heart. Genetic diseases, drugs, alcohol, and viral myocarditis can cause *dilated cardiomyopathy*. Pathophysiologic circumstances can also lead to cardiac dilatation. If hard work makes the heart get big and thick, in what pathophysiological situation would the heart become bigger and floppier? Dilatation occurs when the heart needs to handle *more* blood than usual. When would the left ventricle end up with extra blood? In *aortic regurgitation*, when the left ventricle contracts, instead of sending all of the blood out to the body, some of the ejected blood leaks back through the aortic valve into the ventricle. If there is aortic regurgitation, the heart can dilate over time to accommodate the extra blood leaking back into it across the aortic valve.

What is another reason that extra blood might leak back into the left ventricle? Hint: The aorta is one way out of the left ventricle— what's the only other way (assuming no holes)? The left atrium. What if instead of all of the blood going forward during systole, some of it squirted backward into the left atrium, then flowed back into the ventricle during diastole? This would have the same effect on the left ventricle as aortic regurgitation: the left ventricle would have to handle extra blood. What normally assures that blood flows forward from the left ventricle through the aorta and not back into the atria? The mitral valve. So a leaky mitral valve can lead to mitral regurgitation into the atrium. This will increase the amount of blood that the left ventricle receives, which can cause it to dilate.

What could cause the *right ventricle* to be overloaded with extra volume? Similar to their analogues on the left, pulmonic or tricuspid regurgitation can lead to right ventricular dilatation. Additionally, an atrial septal defect (ASD) or a ventricular septal defect (VSD) will lead to increased blood in the right heart. Though septal defects are often birth defects, a VSD can also occur as a complication of a myocardial infarction.

Consequences of Cardiac Dilatation. Since it is "baggy," a dilated ventricle should have no problem relaxing. However, a dilated ventricle is weakened and thus gives a weaker squeeze during systole. This is called *systolic* dysfunction. Let's compare this situation to cardiac hypertrophy. In hypertrophy, the ventricle gets stiff and squeezes well but does not adequately relax. *In contrast, in cardiac dilatation, the heart is too relaxed and does not give a good squeeze.* The loss of a good squeeze leads to both diminished forward flow and backup of flow.

Systolic dysfunction like that caused by cardiac dilatation can also occur from weakening of heart muscle secondary to *ischemia* (decreased blood flow/oxygen supply).

Treatment of Cardiac Dilatation. Treatment is the same as for heart failure, aiming to increase forward flow and decrease backup of flow (Fig.1-5).

Fig 1-8. Summary of diseases of the heart muscle.

The Valves and Their Diseases: Stenosis and Regurgitation

Review Fig. 1-2. The heart valves *allow* blood to flow forward and *prevent* blood from flowing backward. What could go wrong with a valve? Valvular pathology can cause a valve to be bad at allowing blood to flow forward through it (*stenotic*) or bad at preventing back flow (*regurgitant*). There are four valves and two possible pathologies for each (stenosis and regurgitation), so there are eight basic valvular pathologies. Definitive treatment for any valvular pathology is surgical repair or replacement. Criteria for valve surgery can involve symptoms, severity of valvular dysfunction, and/or findings on echocardiography, depending on the type of valve lesion, age of the patient, and other clinical factors.

Fig. 1-9A. The normal cardiac cycle. The active contraction that ejects blood from the ventricles is systole. As the ventricles contract, the mitral and tricuspid valves slam shut to prevent regurgitation into the atria. The sound produced by the closure of the atrioventricular valves is *S1*. During systole, blood flows across the aortic valve to the aorta and through the pulmonic valve to the pulmonary artery. Also during this time, blood fills the atria to prepare for the next cycle. When systole is complete,

the open vs. closed status of the valves reverses. Now, the mitral and tricuspid valves must open to allow blood to pass from the atria to the ventricles for the next systole, and the aortic and pulmonic valves slam shut to prevent regurgitation back to the ventricles. *S2* is the sound of the aortic and pulmonic valves slamming shut. S2 heralds the beginning of *diastole*, the relaxed phase of the cardiac cycle. During diastole, blood passes from the atria across the open mitral and tricuspid valves into the ventricles. The filled ventricles then contract (systole) again, and we are back where we began.

S3 and *S4* are extra heart sounds that can be heard in heart failure (S3 can also occur normally in young patients). If heard in the context of heart failure, S3 is associated with a dilated heart/systolic dysfunction, and S4 is more typical with a hypertrophied heart/diastolic dysfunction. Since S3 occurs right after S2 (but well before S1), what could this sound represent? What happens during this phase of the cardiac cycle? Blood flows across the atrioventricular valves into the ventricles. If there is still blood left in the ventricles (e.g., because it could not squeeze it all out due to its poor systolic function), a sound may be heard as blood flows in and splashes against the blood still left in the ventricle. Although this may not be exactly what produces the sound, it is a helpful way to remember that *an S3 occurs in a*

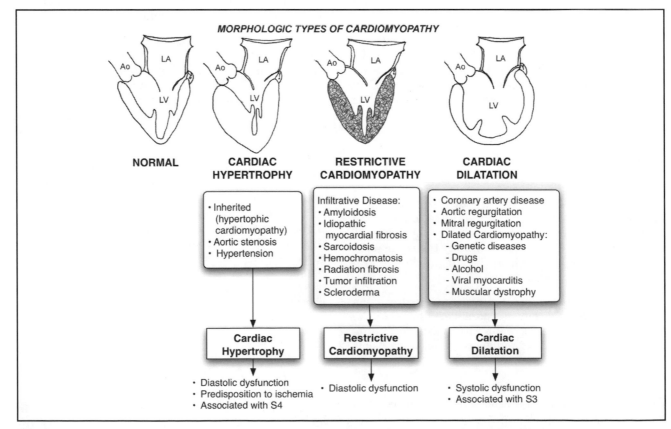

Figure 1-8. Modified from Chizner: *Clinical Cardiology Made Ridiculously Simple*, MedMaster, 2006

dilated heart. Since there is still blood left in the ventricle because of a weaker ventricular contraction than normal, the blood flowing in from the atria makes noise. S4 comes after S2 (and S3 if present), and just before S1. What could this sound represent? At the very end of diastole, the atria contract, squeezing the last of their blood to the ventricles. The S4 is a sound produced when the atria squeeze against a stiff ventricle (i.e., in a hypertrophied heart with diastolic dysfunction). Mnemonic:

The number 3 looks like a puffy dilated number, whereas the number 4 looks like a small chamber with rigid surroundings (hypertrophied ventricle).

Aortic Valve

Aortic Stenosis can cause cardiac hypertrophy because of the increased resistance it presents to left ventricular contraction. Causes of aortic stenosis include

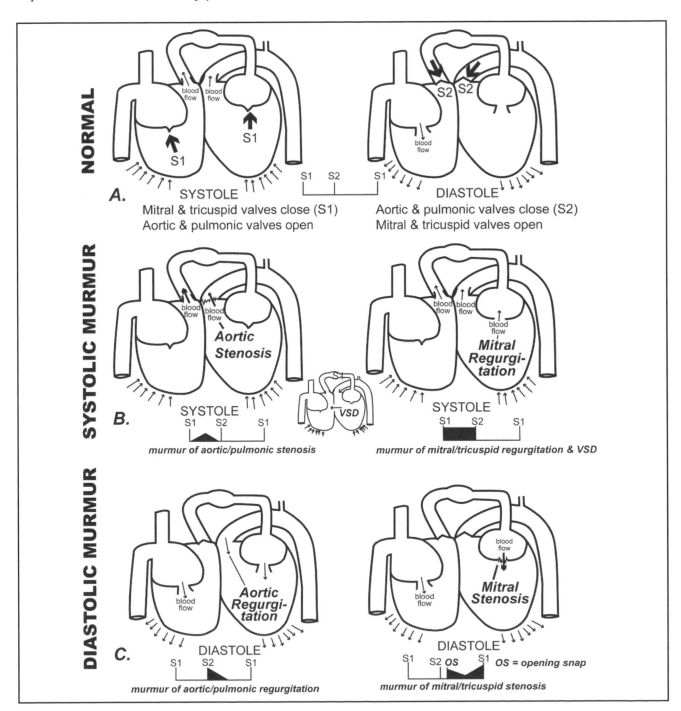

Figure 1-9

aging (also called senile calcification), congenitally bicuspid aortic valve, and rheumatic heart disease.

Fig. 1-9B. The murmur of aortic stenosis. To determine the murmur of any type of valvular dysfunction, ask yourself, "When does blood go across this valve?" Blood flows across the aortic valve when the left ventricle contracts, i.e., during systole, between S1 and S2. Therefore, if there is aortic stenosis, where the blood does not flow normally across the valve, a murmur will occur between S1 and S2. This is known as a systolic murmur. The murmur must stop at S2 since that sound signifies that the aortic valve is closed (i.e., no more blood can flow through it).

What would the shape of this murmur be? Imagine a stiff door with lots of screaming people behind it trying to push it open. At first it opens only slowly, letting in a few screaming people, but as the door opens more, more screaming people can get through. Still, although the door does not open completely, people are always squeezing through. This is a good image for aortic stenosis: The murmur starts off quietly since the valve is only slightly opened, allowing only some "murmuring" blood through. Gradually the valve opens more, but still not all the way. This allows more blood to flow through, but it is still "murmuring" blood due to the narrowed opening. Finally, as blood flow across the valve decreases, the volume of the murmur decreases. This is called a *crescendo-decrescendo* murmur, because it gets louder as it proceeds and then diminishes before S2. The murmur of aortic stenosis is also referred to as a *systolic ejection murmur*.

One final detail about the sound of aortic stenosis is that the *quality of S2 changes*. Why would this be? What does S2 signify? S2 signifies the closing of the aortic and pulmonic valves. If the aortic valve is stiff, it opens poorly and closes poorly (i.e., it does not snap shut, but weakly closes). So how would the S2 change? S2 would be *softer* since it is the sound of only one valve (the pulmonic) slamming shut instead of two.

Other manifestations of aortic stenosis. Another classic physical finding in aortic stenosis involves how the carotid artery pulse feels (*carotid upstroke*). Instead of blood slamming up against the carotids at high pressure, it is sent up more slowly and with less force because it is "held up" by the aortic stenosis. Thus, instead of brisk pulses, the pulses are called *parvus et tardus*, meaning weakened and delayed. What symptoms would be caused by reduced flow in the carotids? The carotids feed the brain, and when the brain does not get enough blood, syncope, lightheadedness, and/or dizziness can occur. Other manifestations of aortic stenosis are those that can occur as a result of the induced cardiac hypertrophy. To review, patients with cardiac hypertrophy can have angina and/or myocardial infarction (because the thicker ventricular wall cannot be adequately perfused). They can

also feel weak and fatigued because flow to the body is inadequate since the stenotic valve inhibits this flow.

Aortic Regurgitation can lead to a dilated left ventricle. Aortic regurgitation can occur because of weakening of the valves or dilatation of the aortic root. Dilatation of the root causes the valves to be farther apart from each other, leaving space through which backflow of blood can occur. Diseases that can lead to aortic root dilatation include Marfan's syndrome, Ehlers-Danlos syndrome, and syphilis.

Fig. 1-9C. The murmur of aortic regurgitation. When in the cardiac cycle could blood leak back through the aortic valve? S2 is the sound of the aortic valve closing. If there is aortic regurgitation, the valve allows regurgitation after closure, so the murmur occurs *after* S2, during diastole. Thus, the murmur of aortic regurgitation is a *diastolic murmur*.

Other manifestations of aortic regurgitation. Aortic regurgitation affects blood pressure and pulses. First, let's review what blood pressure actually measures. There are two numbers, systolic pressure and diastolic pressure (e.g., 120/80). The top number, systolic pressure, refers to the pressure during systole, i.e., when the heart is squeezing. The bottom number, diastolic pressure, refers to the pressure being maintained when the heart is relaxed. The squeezed-out blood is normally prevented from falling too much in pressure because the aortic valve shuts behind it. This helps maintain pressure during diastole. In aortic regurgitation, after a forceful squeeze, some of the blood falls back down into the left ventricle. Which pressure (systolic or diastolic) will be affected and why? Assuming the squeeze is normal, the systolic pressure should be unchanged. However, when the aortic valve allows regurgitation, the diastolic pressure is not maintained since instead of supporting the column of blood in the aorta, the valve collapses. Since the diastolic pressure falls and the systolic pressure stays the same, the distance between the two numbers increases (*widened pulse pressure*). How would this widened pulse pressure manifest on physical exam? Imagine this gush of blood coming from the heart and then falling back...gushing out, falling back. You can actually *feel* this in the pulses (*bounding pulses*). This can sometimes be so drastic that it can be visible, for example in the carotids (*Corrigan's pulse*), or with the patient's head actually bobbing with each pulse (*De Musset's sign*).

Due to decreased forward flow and increased backup of flow in aortic regurgitation, heart failure symptoms can occur (e.g., dyspnea on exertion, etc., see Fig. 1-4).

Mitral Valve

Mitral Stenosis. Nearly all cases of mitral stenosis are caused by rheumatic fever, a disease much less common in the U.S. since the introduction of antibiotics, but more common in developing countries. Despite decreased prevalence in the U.S., some patients who had rheumatic fever as children are still alive and can have resultant mitral stenosis. More rarely, mitral stenosis can occur congenitally or in endocarditis.

What are the roles of the mitral valve? First, to allow blood to pass from the left atrium to the left ventricle during diastole, and second, to prevent backflow into the left atrium when the left ventricle contracts during systole. If the valve is stenotic, it is the first of these functions that is impaired, and thus the upstream portion of the circuit is affected. What is upstream? Immediately upstream from the mitral valve is the left atrium. Mitral stenosis causes the left atrium to dilate. Because of the stretching of the electrical fibers induced by this dilatation, atrial fibrillation can develop. Further upstream, the pulmonary vasculature is also affected by this backup, which can lead to shortness of breath. Eventually, the chronically elevated left atrial pressure can cause pulmonary hypertension and even right heart failure.

Fig. 1-9C. The murmur of mitral stenosis. When does blood pass across the mitral valve? Between S2 and S1, during diastole. So this is a diastolic murmur.

Other manifestations of mitral stenosis. The sound of the stiff mitral valve snapping open can sometimes be heard (*opening snap*). When would you expect this to occur? Shortly after S2. The timing of this snap reflects the severity of the stenosis. If the mitral stenosis is *severe*, this leads to higher left atrial pressure than if the stenosis were less severe. What would this do to the opening of the valve? If the pressure is high, the valve will snap open quite quickly. If the stenosis is less severe and the left atrial pressure is relatively less, the valve will not open until later, since initially there is not enough pressure to snap it open. Thus, the timing of the opening snap is *inversely* proportional to the severity of mitral stenosis: the *more severe* the mitral stenosis, the *earlier* the opening snap.

Mitral Regurgitation. During systole, the ventricles contract, ejecting blood into their respective outflow tracts (Left Ventricle->Aorta, Right Ventricle->Pulmonary Artery). This contraction is quite forceful, and the job of the mitral and tricuspid valves is to shut tightly so as to prevent backflow and maximize forward flow. In mitral regurgitation, the mitral valve allows backflow into the left atrium during ventricular contraction.

Recall that if mitral regurgitation exists for a long time, the heart will compensate by dilating to accommodate the increased blood volume (which can cause systolic dysfunction, an S3, etc.). If cardiac dilatation exists for another reason (e.g., genetic, drugs, aortic regurgitation), this dilatation stretches the ring-like mitral valve, preventing it from closing optimally. So mitral regurgi-

tation can lead to left ventricular dilatation *or* it can be the result of ventricular dilatation. Aside from ventricular dilatation, mitral regurgitation can be caused by degeneration of the valve (mitral valve prolapse, also known as myxomatous degeneration), rheumatic fever, endocarditis, or ischemic heart disease.

Where is the regurgitated blood going in mitral regurgitation? Back into the left atrium. So chronic mitral regurgitation can lead to left atrial dilatation. Forward flow is diminished since what was supposed to be part of the cardiac output is sent *backward* into the atria. Since pressure increases *backward* through the left atrium to the lungs, this can cause shortness of breath. If mitral regurgitation develops over a long period of time, dilatation of the atrium can allow it to adapt to accommodate the backflow, preventing significant elevations in pulmonary pressure. Alternatively, if mitral regurgitation occurs *acutely* (e.g., papillary muscle rupture secondary to ischemia), there is no time for compensatory dilatation of the left atrium to occur. Without the compensation of a dilated atrium, the pressure in the lungs acutely elevates due to the sudden onset of backward flow. Pulmonary congestion is a prominent symptomatic feature in acute mitral regurgitation, whereas in more chronic mitral regurgitation, the fatigue/forward flow symptoms are more prominent. The acute problem is not well tolerated by the pulmonary system, and urgent surgical replacement of the valve is often necessary.

Fig. 1-9B. The murmur of mitral regurgitation. Is the murmur of mitral regurgitation systolic or diastolic? In mitral regurgitation, blood flows *backward* across the mitral valve. This occurs during systole when the ventricles contract, so this is another systolic murmur, occurring between S1 and S2. How can you distinguish it from the murmur of aortic stenosis, which is also systolic? A subtle difference is that mitral regurgitation lacks the crescendo-decrescendo pattern that is present in aortic stenosis. Since the regurgitant mitral valve flops back with the onset of systole, the murmur is usually relatively constant from S1 to S2 (*holosystolic* or *pansystolic murmur*).[2]

Other manifestations of mitral regurgitation. Associated findings can also help distinguish between aortic stenosis and mitral regurgitation as causes of a systolic murmur. Mitral regurgitation can be accompanied by an S3. Why? S3 can be thought of as blood splashing against blood already in the ventricle. In mitral regurgitation, all of the blood that got inappropriately ejected back into the atrium then returns to the ventricle during diastole: splash!

---

[2] Mitral valve *prolapse*, a specific type of mitral regurgitation, causes a mid-late systolic crescendo murmur, often initiated by a systolic click.

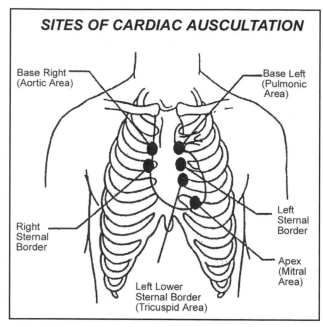

SITES OF CARDIAC AUSCULTATION

Figure 1-10. From Chizner: *Clinical Cardiology Made Ridiculously Simple*, MedMaster, 2006 (Courtesy of W. Proctor Harvey, M.D.)

Atrial dilatation from mitral regurgitation can lead to atrial fibrillation, as in mitral stenosis.

Fig. 1-10. Sites of cardiac auscultation. Another distinguishing factor on physical exam is *where* the murmur is heard best and where it radiates. Aortic stenosis is best heard over the aortic valve region in the *right*[3] upper sternal border, and it radiates straight up to the carotids. One classically hears the murmur of mitral regurgitation over the cardiac apex, and it radiates to the left axilla.

Finally, another way to distinguish between the systolic murmurs of aortic stenosis and mitral regurgitation is through physical exam maneuvers. While a full discussion of the cardiac physical exam maneuvers is beyond the scope of this text, a quick review of one maneuver will be helpful. If you ask the patient to clench his/her fists, what does this accomplish? This is one way to increase the systemic vascular resistance by clamping down on the arteries in the hand/arm. Why would a change in systemic vascular resistance affect a murmur? Given the choice of going through what is now a path with *greater resistance* (the body with clenched fists) and simply flowing back across the regurgitant mitral valve, the blood chooses the mitral valve (the path

[3] The pulmonary artery comes from the right heart and the aorta comes from the left heart, *but* because of the way the anatomy is situated, the aortic area is on the (patient's) right of the patient's sternum and the pulmonic area is on the (patient's) left of the patient's sternum.

of least resistance). Thus, this maneuver will *increase the intensity of the mitral regurgitation murmur*, while leaving the aortic stenosis murmur unchanged. Why would the aortic stenosis murmur remain unchanged? The main point of resistance responsible for the murmur in aortic stenosis is the valve itself, so changes in resistance distal to this point (i.e., clenched fists) will have little or no effect on the murmur of aortic stenosis.

Aside from aortic stenosis and mitral regurgitation, what other cardiac pathology could lead to a systolic murmur? Where else could the blood go during systole? If there is a ventricular septal defect, blood flow through this hole can also create a murmur, and this too would occur during systole.

Tricuspid Valve

Tricuspid Stenosis. The pathophysiology in tricuspid stenosis is essentially the same as in mitral stenosis, except that it occurs on the right side of the heart. The murmur is diastolic and best heard at the left lower sternal border. Just as mitral stenosis leads to left atrial dilatation, tricuspid stenosis results in right atrial dilatation/increased pressure. How can one see a barometer of this right-sided pressure? The jugular vein is connected to the superior vena cava, which is connected to the right atrium, and thus increased pressure in the right heart can lead to elevated jugular venous pressure (JVP).

Tricuspid Regurgitation. Tricuspid regurgitation also has a similar pathophysiology to its counterpart on the left, mitral regurgitation. Because of increased regurgitation of blood into the right atrium and elevated right atrial pressure, the JVP can be elevated, as in tricuspid stenosis. The systolic murmur of tricuspid regurgitation is best heard at the left lower sternal border and increases with inspiration.

Pulmonary Valve

Pulmonic Stenosis. Unlike aortic stenosis, which typically arises from calcification with age, pulmonic stenosis is almost always the result of a *congenital anomaly* of the valve. Since blood passes across this valve during systole, the murmur is systolic (as in aortic stenosis). The murmur of pulmonic stenosis can be heard more prominently over the patient's *left* upper sternal border.

Pulmonic Regurgitation. In pulmonary hypertension, the normally low-pressure system in the lungs develops high pressure. Due to the high pressure, the pulmonary artery may dilate, and this can lead to a separation of the leaflets of the pulmonic valve, resulting in pulmonic regurgitation. The murmur occurs during diastole, as with aortic regurgitation, though it occurs over the pulmonic valve region (on the patient's left). Pulmonic regurgitation lacks the changes in pulses and blood pressure seen with aortic regurgitation, since the right heart ejects into the lungs, and is thus not responsible for what is measured in the peripheral pulses.

Review of Valves I: Review by Pathology

Fig. 1-11. Summary of valvular pathology.

- There are four valves, any of which can be regurgitant or stenotic. (A stenotic valve can also be regurgitant. Stenotic valves are hard to open and can also be hard to shut. Thus, a stenotic valve can permit some regurgitation.)

- *Aortic stenosis* greatly increases the work of the left heart, which can cause hypertrophy (and thus diastolic dysfunction, associated with S4) and can lead to syncope, angina/infarction, and congestive heart failure. Since blood normally passes forward across the aortic valve during systole, aortic stenosis causes a systolic murmur.

- *Aortic regurgitation* allows blood to flow back into the heart after systole, thus decreasing systemic blood pressure during diastole, resulting in a widened pulse pressure. Increased volume demand on the heart can lead to left ventricular dilatation (and thus systolic dysfunction, associated with S3 and heart failure symptoms). Since the blood is flowing back after systole, aortic regurgitation causes a diastolic murmur.

- *Mitral stenosis* increases the pressure in the left atrium, causing it to enlarge. Since blood passes across the mitral valve into the left ventricle during diastole, mitral stenosis causes a diastolic murmur.

- *Mitral regurgitation* occurs when the mitral valve does not fully prevent backflow across the valve during systole. This leads to a systolic murmur.

- In **both** *mitral* pathologies, increased left atrial pressure leads to increased pulmonary pressure, which can cause dyspnea. Also, both mitral pathologies can lead to left atrial dilatation, which can cause atrial fibrillation.

- Though *tricuspid and pulmonic valve* pathologies do occur, they are rarer than left-sided valvular disease. Murmurs can mimic the counterparts on the left, but right heart failure signs/symptoms (elevated JVP, edema) would be predominant (if pathology is severe enough to cause signs/symptoms).

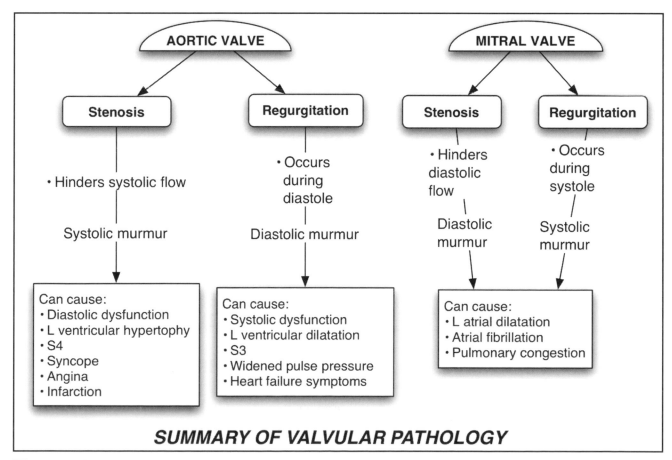

Figure 1-11

Review of Valves II: Review by Murmur

Fig. 1-12. Summary of murmurs.

Systolic Murmurs occur between S1 and S2. During systole, blood flows across the aortic and pulmonic valves, so *stenosis* of either of these valves can lead to a systolic murmur. The closed mitral (on the **left**) and tricuspid (on the **right**) valves prevent backflow during systole (their closure *is* S1). If they are incompetent, allowing for regurgitation, this too will create a systolic murmur. The only other direction blood could go during systole would be through a ventricular septal defect. Thus, causes of a systolic murmur include *aortic stenosis, pulmonic stenosis, mitral regurgitation, tricuspid regurgitation,* and *a ventricular septal defect.* Note that a systolic aortic flow murmur can also occur in normal individuals, in pregnant women, or in cases of pathologically increased flow (e.g., in a patient with anemia or a fever).

Diastolic Murmurs occur between S2 and S1. During diastole, blood flows across the mitral and tricuspid valves, so if either of these is stenotic, this would lead to a diastolic murmur. The closure of the aortic and pulmonic valves (S2) ends systole and begins diastole. If this closure is incomplete, blood will leak back during diastole, so aortic and pulmonic regurgitation can also lead to diastolic murmurs. Thus, causes of a diastolic murmur include *mitral stenosis, tricuspid stenosis, aortic regurgitation,* and *pulmonic regurgitation.*

Notice that stenotic valves produce murmurs when blood is flowing in the *forward/normal direction* across them, whereas regurgitant valves produce murmurs when blood is flowing *backward/the wrong way* across them.

Diseases of the Electrical System: Arrhythmias

The electrical system of the heart conducts impulses to the cardiac muscle, causing it to contract in an organized, rhythmic way. An *arrhythmia* is an abnormal heart rhythm: a rhythm that is too slow, too fast, and/or irregular. If the electrical activity of the heart is uncoordinated, then muscular contraction will be uncoordinated. A ventricular arrhythmia can thus lead to inefficient ventricular contraction, leading to an immediate drop in forward flow. This can cause hypotension, syncope, or, in some cases, sudden death.

Fig. 1-13. The cardiac conduction system. Each cardiac muscle cell (*myocyte*) spontaneously depolarizes at some intrinsic rate. Cells from different parts of the heart depolarize *at different rates.* The fastest cells are in the atria. As one moves down the heart, there is a *decreasing* rate of spontaneous depolarization (i.e., the slowest spontaneous firing rate occurs in ventricular cells). The cardiac myocytes are connected, so the heart beats at the rate of whichever cells are depolarizing the *fastest.* The cardiac myocytes that depolarize fastest are those that make up the *sinoatrial (SA) node.* Sinoatrial node impulses travel to the myocytes of the atria,

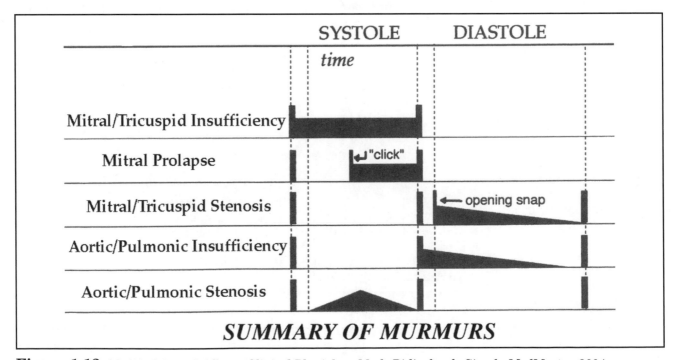

Figure 1-12. Modified from Goldberg: *Clinical Physiology Made Ridiculously Simple,* MedMaster, 2004

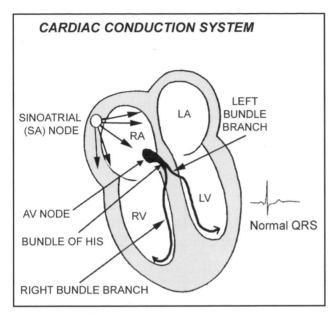

CARDIAC CONDUCTION SYSTEM

Figure 1-13

resulting in their synchronized depolarization and contraction. The electrical impulse then travels to the *atrioventricular (AV) node,* where it is held up by a built-in delay before proceeding to the bundle of His and bundle branches. Finally, the electrical signal spreads across the ventricles by way of the Purkinje fibers. This causes the ventricles to contract as a unit.

Fig. 1-14. Components of the EKG. The P wave represents the electrical depolarization that occurs just prior to *atrial contraction.* The flat interval until the next spike represents the time where the impulse is held up in the AV (atrioventricular) node before passing to the ventricles (this is called the *PR interval*). The QRS complex represents ventricular depolarization and the T wave represents ventricular repolarization.

The U wave can sometimes be seen in normal patients following the T wave, but it is not always visible. When seen, the U wave may represent further depolarization in the ventricle or repolarization of the Purkinje system. The U wave can become more prominent in bradycardia (slow heart rates) or electrolyte abnormalities (e.g., hypokalemia).

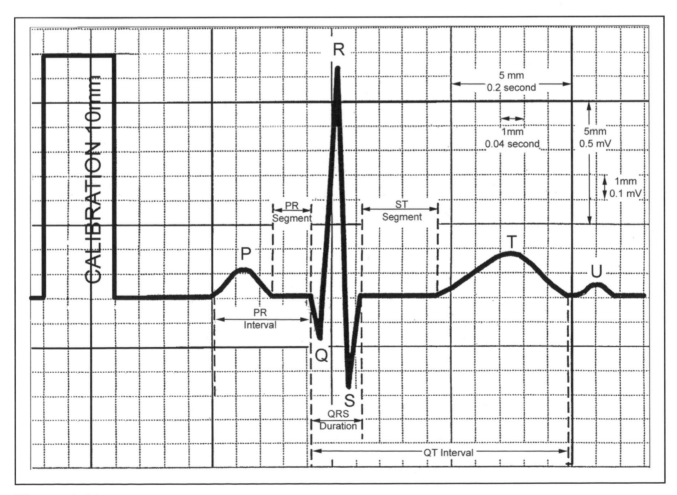

Figure 1-14

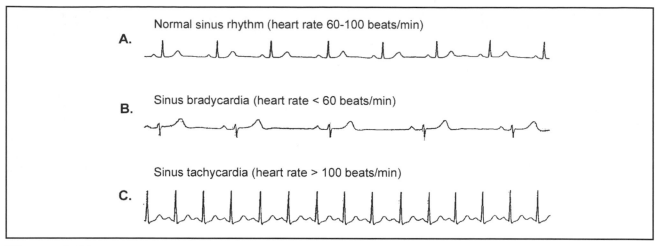

A. Normal sinus rhythm (heart rate 60-100 beats/min)

B. Sinus bradycardia (heart rate < 60 beats/min)

C. Sinus tachycardia (heart rate > 100 beats/min)

Figure 1-15

Fig. 1-15. Bradyarrhythmia (bradycardia) vs. tachyarrhythmia (tachycardia). Arrhythmias are first classified as either *too slow* (bradyarrhythmia or bradycardia) or *too fast* (tachyarrhythmia or tachycardia). The next level of classification is *where* the aberration is coming from in the conduction pathway (atria vs. ventricles).

The term arrhythmia can be confusing to musicians, because some of the arrhythmias are in fact perfectly rhythmic, just faster or slower than normal. A heart rate can be regular (i.e., a normal rhythm), regularly irregular (i.e., an abnormal rhythm which is repeated over and over), or irregularly irregular (i.e., a totally random pattern).

Bradyarrhythmia (Bradycardia)

Fig. 1-16. Causes of bradycardia. Bradyarrhythmia (bradycardia) is usually defined as a heart rate less than 60 beats per minute. For a slow heart rate to occur, there must either be a *problem with the SA node* (such that the impulses it is generating are at a slower rate) or there must be a *block* somewhere in the conduction system. Slower heart rates can also occur in normal people (e.g., trained athletes).

Slow SA Node. Why would the SA node fire more slowly than usual? A decrease in SA node firing rate can be a normal physiological response (e.g., during sleep) or the result of ischemia, certain drugs, or increased vagal tone. Increased vagal tone refers to increased activity of the vagus nerve (cranial nerve X), which provides the parasympathetic input to the heart. The parasympathetic nervous system slows heart rate ("rest and digest"), while the sympathetic nervous system increases heart rate ("fight or flight").

Fig. 1-15B. Sinus bradycardia rhythm strip. How would bradycardia secondary to a slow SA node look on EKG? The P wave should appear normal and the PR interval (which indicates the *conduction* of the impulse) should also appear normal. The difference in sinus bradycardia would be that the **rate** *would be slowed*: the number of P and QRS complexes per unit time will be decreased, but they will appear normal in configuration.

Abnormal Conduction (Heart Block). In heart block, the sinus node pulses away at its normal rate, but the conduction is blocked somewhere along the route to the ventricles. The block can occur in the AV node, in the bundle of His, or in the bundle branches (Fig. 1-13). There are four types of heart block: First-degree, Second-degree Mobitz type I (also known as Wenckebach), Second-degree Mobitz type II, and Third-degree (also known as complete heart block).

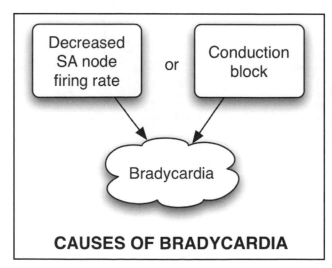

Figure 1-16

Each cell of the heart has its own intrinsic rate. If the pace generated by the SA node slows *below* the intrinsic rate of cells in the AV node, those cells can *escape* the pacemaker's rhythm and generate *junctional escape beats*. If there is heart block at the AV node or below, the ventricular cells can generate escape beats.

Fig. 1-17. Ventricular escape beats. On EKG, how would the QRS of a ventricular escape beat look? Normally the QRS is narrow since the electrical impulse is conducted rapidly to both ventricles via the Purkinje fibers, and depolarization of the muscle then proceeds uniformly. If some isolated ventricular cells produce an escape beat, the depolarization will spread in a less organized fashion, resulting in a *widened QRS*.

Fig. 1-18. Rhythm strips of first-, second-, and third-degree heart block. How would AV block manifest on EKG? The PR interval represents the time that the impulse travels through the AV node. *In first-degree heart block, the PR interval is lengthened* (criteria for diagnosis is > 0.2 seconds).

Second-degree heart block is further divided into two types of blocks. In Mobitz type I (also called Wenckebach), the PR interval progressively increases until finally an atrial impulse is not conducted at all. This

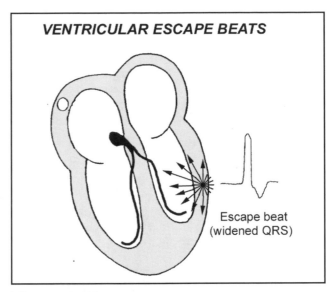

Figure 1-17. Modified from Chizner: *Clinical Cardiology Made Ridiculously Simple*, MedMaster, 2006

leads to a pause, followed by a normally conducted beat, and then the cycle repeats. In Mobitz type II, the AV node does not conduct some proportion of incoming atrial impulses to the ventricles. This causes ventricular beats to be intermittently dropped entirely.

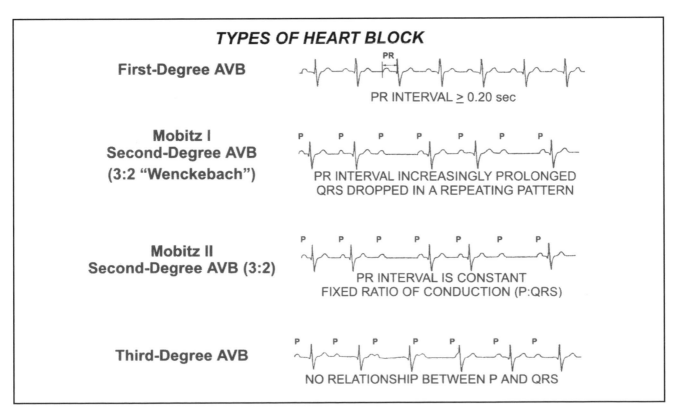

Figure 1-18. Modified from Chizner: *Clinical Cardiology Made Ridiculously Simple,* MedMaster, 2006

In *third-degree* heart block, there is *no conduction at all* from the atria to the ventricles. Since the SA node's signal does not reach the ventricles, the cells around the AV node start firing at their own intrinsic rate, which is around 30-50 beats per minute. Since the atria and ventricles then function totally independently of each other in third-degree heart block, this is a form of *AV dissociation.*

In summary, bradycardia can be caused by a slow SA node or *decreased conduction.*

Treatment of Bradycardia. To increase heart rate, treatment can either *increase rate directly* (beta agonists such as isoproterenol or implantation of a pacemaker) or *decrease inhibition* (anticholinergics such as atropine, which decrease parasympathetic stimu-lation of the heart). Implantation of a pacemaker is usually necessary for second-degree Mobitz type II or third-degree heart block.

Tachyarrhythmias

Tachyarrhythmias are classified by whether they originate above or within the ventricles. Arrhythmias originating in the atria or AV node are called *supraventricular* (i.e., above the ventricle) tachyarrhythmias.

Supraventricular Tachyarrhythmias

Fig. 1-19. Supraventricular Tachyarrhythmias.

Sinus tachycardia is simply an increase in the SA node firing rate above 100 (See Fig. 1-15C). This can happen as the sympathetic nervous system's response

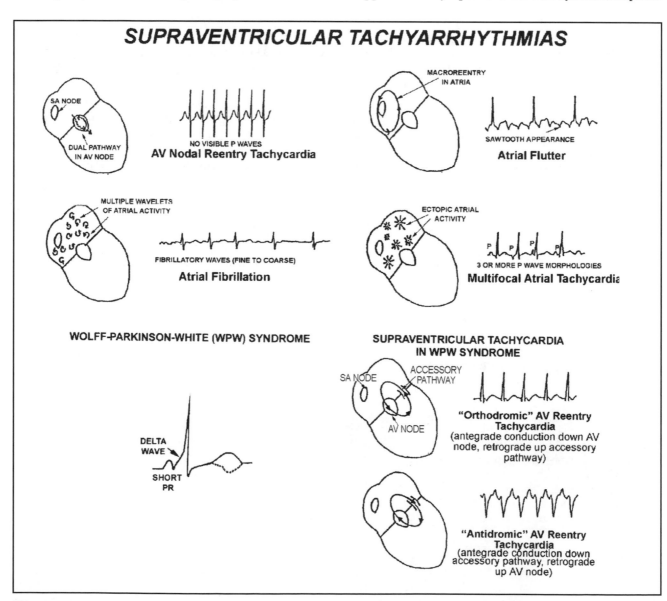

Figure 1-19. Modified from Chizner: *Clinical Cardiology Made Ridiculously Simple*, MedMaster, 2006

to either a physiologic state (e.g., exercise, fight/flight) or a pathophysiologic condition (e.g., fever, pulmonary embolus).

In *multifocal atrial tachycardia (MAT)*, multiple sites in the atria take on very fast rhythms. This can occur in patients with pulmonary disease. What would the EKG look like? If multiple sites in the atria fire, there will be *multiple P wave morphologies*: the P waves will have several different appearances and can occur at irregular intervals.

Atrial flutter and *atrial fibrillation* are common arrhythmias that have similar underlying pathophysiology, both involving *reentrant circuits*. Reentrant circuits are circular pathways in which electrical impulses can travel around the circle, reactivate the starting point, and create an endless loop.

In *atrial flutter*, a reentrant circuit in the atrium allows electrical impulses to spin around the loop at very high speed instead of following the normal conduction pattern. If you imagine this current looping around the atrium, you can also imagine the EKG: a *saw-tooth* appearance to the P waves. In atrial flutter, the atrial rate is typically between 200-400 beats per minute.

In *atrial fibrillation*, there are many reentrant circuits spinning around in the atria. The EKG appears as a wavy, chaotic, disorganized baseline without recognizable P waves. Rates in the atria can be over 400 beats per minutes, but due to the refractory period of the AV node, the ventricular rhythm cannot reach this speed. Usually the ventricle gets no faster than 100-150 beats per minute unless there is an accessory pathway (discussed below). Since the beats that *do* make it through are essentially random, the ventricular rhythm is *irregularly irregular*. Causes of atrial fibrillation include a variety of heart diseases (e.g., coronary disease, valvular disease, cardiomyopathy, heart failure), pulmonary disease, pulmonary embolism, hyperthyroidism, and hypertension. Atrial fibrillation can also occur idiopathically.

Because fibrillating atria quiver instead of contracting, blood flow within them is quite turbulent. This leads to an increased risk of clot formation in the atria. If a clot forms in the left atrium, it can pass to the left ventricle and then out the aorta. This could lead to stroke (if it goes up the carotids), mesenteric ischemia (if it lodges in the GI vascular bed), renal ischemia (if it lodges in the renal artery), etc. Patients with atrial fibrillation are thus often given *anticoagulants* to prevent clot formation in the atria.

The next two tachyarrhythmias also have reentrant circuits. AV nodal reentrant tachycardia (AVNRT) has a reentrant circuit involving the AV node itself. Atrioventricular reciprocating tachycardia (AVRT) has a reentrant circuit that involves the atrium, AV node, ventricle, and an accessory pathway.

AVNRT develops when the refractory period becomes altered in pathways through the AV node. There are normally two pathways through the AV node, one of which is slower than the other. In AVNRT, a change in the refractory period of the slower pathway allows the electrical impulse to inappropriately come back up to the atrium after its normal path down the AV node. Thus, the EKG can manifest a P wave *after* the QRS complex, and this P wave may be inverted since the impulse comes backward up through the atria.

In *AVRT* (e.g., Wolff-Parkinson-White syndrome), there is an *accessory pathway* that allows impulses to flow to the ventricles directly from the atria and vice versa. If the accessory pathway functions in the *retrograde* direction (*orthodromic*), a reentrant loop occurs (from atria to AV node to ventricles *back* to the atria via the accessory pathway). This cycling of the impulse causes the tachycardia. In orthodromic Wolff-Parkinson-White, the impulse travels first normally down the AV node to the ventricles, so the QRS will be normal. If the accessory pathway functions in the *anterograde* direction (*antidromic*), the atrial impulses bypass the AV node, go directly to the ventricles, and then return to the atria retrogradely via the AV node. What would the antidromic EKG look like? First, there would be *a shortened PR interval* because the impulse bypasses the built-in delay of the AV node. Second, since part of the ventricle is activated early through the accessory pathway, the QRS can appear abnormal. The upstroke of the QRS reflects this in what is known as a *delta wave*. A delta wave is a more gradual beginning to the QRS, as opposed to the normal sharp upstroke that occurs with normally conducted electrical activity. If a patient with an accessory pathway were to develop atrial fibrillation, this rapid rate can be conducted to the ventricles via the accessory pathway, which has none of the built-in delays of the normal system. This can lead to extremely rapid ventricular rates, which can be deadly.

Summary of the supraventricular tachyarrhythmias. Either the sinus node itself can take on a faster rate (sinus tachycardia); multiple sites in the atria can take on the role of firing (multifocal atrial tachycardia); a large atrial reentrant loop can form in the atria, leading to atrial flutter; or multiple reentrant loops in the atria can lead to atrial fibrillation. Reentrant circuits can also involve the AV node itself (AVNRT) and/or an accessory pathway (AVRT, Wolff-Parkinson-White).

Ventricular Tachyarrhythmias. In *ventricular tachyarrhythmias*, the fast rate originates in the ventricle. If the ventricles depolarize in any way other than by the normal conduction system, this depolarization will spread in a disorganized fashion, resulting in a *widened* QRS.

Aside from loss of the atrial kick at the end of diastole, the overall ability of the heart to do its job should *not* be greatly impaired by *atrial* arrhythmias (assuming otherwise normal ventricular function). In marked contrast, *sustained ventricular arrhythmias lead to uncoordinated muscular activity in the ventricle, which can suddenly decrease forward flow*. Thus, sustained ventricular arrhythmias are often emergencies in need of defibrillation.

Fig. 1-20. Ventricular arrhythmias. *Ventricular tachycardia* can result from a *reentrant circuit in the ventricle* or from a *group of ventricular cells firing at an increased rate*. For example, a myocardial infarction can lead to an area of dead tissue. This area can have abnormal electrical conduction properties, thus creating a reentrant circuit, which can result in extremely high ventricular rates.

Ventricular fibrillation results from multiple reentrant circuits in the ventricles, just like atrial fibrillation results from multiple reentrant circuits in the atria. The electrical (and thus muscular) activity in ventricular fibrillation is even more uncoordinated than that of ventricular tachycardia because of the multiple circuits, and cardiac output can thus be even more severely impaired. Without immediate intervention, this can even lead to sudden death. Ventricular fibrillation may result from ischemia or infarcted areas of ventricular tissue, similar to the mechanism described above for ventricular tachycardia. Ventricular fibrillation may also result from ventricular tachycardia.

Torsades de Pointes is French for twisting of the points, and describes a specific type of ventricular tachycardia. The name refers to the EKG appearance of this ventricular arrhythmia, since it appears to turn around the horizontal. Causes include anything that can prolong the QT interval, such as certain anti-arrhythmics (e.g., quinidine, sotalol) and other drugs, hypocalcemia and other electrolyte abnormalities (see endocrine chapter), cardiac ischemia, and congenital long QT syndrome. Torsades can lead to syncope and/or ventricular fibrillation.

Treatment of Tachyarrhythmia. Tachyarryhthmias are treated with drugs that decrease cardiac myocytes' rate of firing. This can be accomplished either by *decreasing sympathetic stimulation of the heart* or by acting at ion channels to *alter portions of the cardiac action potential,* e.g., decreasing upstroke, increasing threshold, prolonging repolarization. Drugs that decrease sympathetic stimulation of the heart include beta-blockers, called Class II antiarrhythmics. Drugs that alter the cardiac action potential include: Class I antiarrhythmics (sodium channel blockers, e.g., quinidine, lidocaine), Class III antiarrhythmics (which act at various ion channels and as beta blockers, e.g., amiodarone, sotalol), and Class IV antiarrhythmics (calcium channel blockers, e.g., verapamil).

If an arrhythmia does not respond to pharmacologic therapy, or in an emergency, electrical defibrillation may be necessary. Additionally, regions of tissue responsible for generating the arrhythmia can be ablated surgically or via catheter techniques.

Review of Arrhythmias

In summary, arrhythmias are abnormal heart rhythms that can be too slow, too fast, and/or irregular. If the rate is too slow, either the SA node (the pacemaker) is firing too slowly (*sinus bradycardia*),

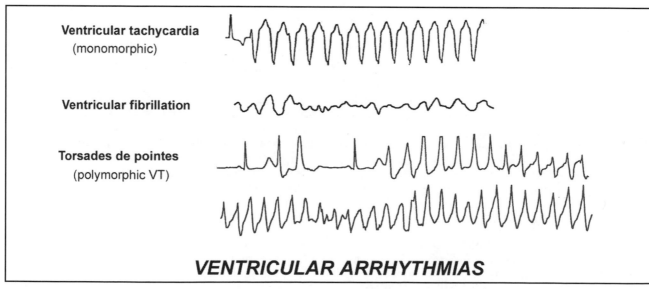

Figure 1-20. Modified from Chizner: *Clinical Cardiology Made Ridiculously Simple*, MedMaster, 2006

or the SA node is working fine, but there is a block of the signal somewhere along the conduction pathway (*heart block*). Tachyarrhythmias are heart rates that are too fast, and are generally divided into those which originate in the atria and/or AV node (i.e., supraventricular: sinus tachycardia, MAT, atrial flutter, atrial fibrillation, AVNRT, AVRT, Wolff-Parkinson-White) and those that originate in the ventricles (ventricular tachycardia, ventricular fibrillation, torsades de pointes). Atrial tachycardias can be dangerous for two reasons: 1) they can lead to turbulent flow in the atria, which can lead to thrombus formation and embolization (e.g., to the cerebral vasculature leading to stroke) and 2) they can transmit to the ventricle via the AV node (with some holdup) or via accessory pathways (directly), causing very fast ventricular rates. Ventricular tachyarrhythmias are dangerous because ventricular function can be so severely compromised as to cause an immediate decrease in forward flow. This can result in sudden death in some cases if immediate intervention does not occur.

Diseases of the Heart's Vasculature: Angina and Myocardial Infarction

The *coronary arteries* provide the heart's blood supply. If this blood supply is compromised, oxygen supply to the heart can be insufficient, decreasing cardiac function.

Diabetes, smoking, high blood pressure, high cholesterol, and many other factors can lead to blood vessel injury and inflammation, which can result in *atherosclerotic plaque* formation in blood vessels. This narrows the vessel lumen, hardens the blood vessel, and can predispose to clot formation in the vessel. In the coronary vasculature, this can cause *angina* and/or *myocardial infarction* (heart attack).

Angina and Myocardial Infarction

During exertion, the heart beats both harder and faster to supply oxygen to the muscles. Vasodilation of the coronary vasculature increases blood flow to the cardiac muscle to meet its increased demand for oxygen. The situation is one of economics in that cardiac function is determined by how the supply (in this case of oxygenated blood) meets the demand (the cardiac muscular demand for oxygen).

Now imagine a heart with bad atherosclerotic disease of the coronary vessels. The vessel lumens are narrowed and thus blood supply to the heart is diminished. In milder cases, the heart may still be fine at rest. However, increasing exertion can get the heart into trouble because diseased vessels are not only narrow, but they also cannot adequately vasodilate. In economic terms, the vessels cannot supply sufficient

oxygen for the heart's demand, and this can manifest as chest pain/tightness and/or shortness of breath. This situation is known as *stable angina*. The heart is stable at rest, but with exertion, supply of blood through the narrowed vessels cannot keep up with demand. The classic story is that a patient has progressively increased limitations on how much they can exert themselves before they have problems. For example, a patient might say "I was previously able to walk four blocks, then I would have to catch my breath...now I can only walk two..." or "I used to have to rest once halfway up the steps in my house, now I have to rest three or four times..."

With increasing occlusion of the coronary vessel(s), even the demands of the resting heart may be too great for what the diseased vessel(s) can supply. When the patient experiences angina even *without* exertion, or when the level of exertion necessary to cause anginal symptoms decreases, this is *unstable angina*. Unstable angina is a precipitous state; it means that one or more coronary vessels is nearly totally occluded. If an atherosclerotic plaque ruptures, coronary thrombosis can ensue, causing the occlusion to proceed to 100%. If collateral flow is inadequate, the tissue supplied becomes ischemic. Without oxygen, a portion of the muscle can die, and this is known as *myocardial infarction* (or heart attack). Myocardial infarction can present as chest pain unrelieved by rest (sometimes radiating down the left arm or into the jaw or neck), dyspnea, nausea/vomiting, sweating, fever and/or other signs of distress. Myocardial infarction can also be entirely asymptomatic or cause minor symptoms that the patient disregards (*silent myocardial infarction*).

Variant, or *Prinzmetal's angina* occurs secondary to intermittent *vasospasm*, as opposed to vascular occlusion. It can thus occur at any time and is not related to the person's activity.

Complications of Myocardial Infarction

Depending on which vessel occludes, different regions of the heart can be affected, causing a variety of consequences. Ischemia of the conduction system can cause arrhythmias. If a large enough area of muscle infarcts and becomes nonfunctional, heart failure symptoms can occur (*ischemic cardiomyopathy*). In ischemic cardiomyopathy, there is less effective pumping because part of the muscular wall has a damaged area that does not move as well as the rest. If the ischemic area is in the left ventricle (e.g., occlusion of the left anterior descending artery), this could lead to left heart failure with pulmonary congestion (backup) and decreased forward flow. If the right coronary artery is the site of occlusion, this can affect the right ventricle, leading to right heart failure signs (e.g., JVD). Infarction of the papillary muscle can cause it to rupture, leading to acute mitral regurgitation. Infarction of the ventricular wall itself can result in its rupture, either at the septum or in the free wall. A septal rupture will lead to a ventricular septal defect and a new *systolic* murmur. As for ventricular free wall rupture, remember that the heart sits in the pericardial sac. If the ventricle ruptures and the heart bleeds into this sac, the blood can quickly surround the heart, preventing it from adequately filling. This is known as *tamponade* and can be quickly fatal.

Treatment of Angina and Myocardial Infarction

Treatment of Angina. Dietary and lifestyle modifications are necessary to prevent further progression of atherosclerotic diseases (e.g., reduction in fat intake, quitting smoking, weight loss). In patients with elevated cholesterol, cholesterol-lowering drugs may also be initiated (Fig. 1-21). Aspirin or other platelet inhibitors can be used to inhibit thrombosis formation. In angina, myocardial demand for oxygen exceeds the ability of the coronary vasculature to supply it. Two treatment angles for remedying this mismatch are possible: *decrease the heart's demand for oxygen* and *increase the vasodilation of the coronary vessels.* Decreasing the heart's demand for oxygen can be accomplished by beta-blockers and calcium channel blockers (both of which decrease both heart rate and contractile force). Increased vasodilation is accomplished with nitrates, which dilate the coronary vasculature, and can thus also be used as quick relief for anginal symptoms. Nitrates also dilate veins, decreasing the heart's work by decreasing preload. Calcium channel blockers also increase coronary vasodilatation and decrease coronary vasospasm. For the latter reason, they are also used in the treatment of variant (Prinzmetal's) angina. If coronary occlusion is very advanced, angioplasty, stenting, or bypass surgery can be performed. The former two procedures seek to open existing vessels, while the latter uses vein grafts (usually the saphenous vein from the leg), artery grafts (usually from the radial artery), or connection of the blocked coronary artery to the internal mammary artery to create an alternate pathway for blood flow, bypassing areas of occlusion.

Treatment of Myocardial Infarction. If an area of the heart is ischemic due to vascular occlusion, the goal is to reperfuse the heart. Thrombolytic drugs such as streptokinase and tissue plasminogen activator (t-PA) or procedures such as angioplasty with coronary stenting can accomplish this goal. In addition to the treatments discussed above for angina (lifestyle modifications, nitrates, cholesterol-lowering agents, beta blockers, calcium channel blockers, aspirin), ACE inhibitors and anticoagulants (e.g., heparin) are components of treatment for myocardial infarction as well as prevention of a subsequent myocardial infarction.

VASCULAR DISEASE OUTSIDE THE HEART: PERIPHERAL ARTERIES AND AORTA

Emboli

An embolus can be a clot (*thrombus*), cholesterol plaque, fat, tumor fragment, amniotic fluid, or an air bubble that travels from *somewhere to somewhere else.* For example, a clot (thrombus) that forms in a fibrillating atrium and travels through the arterial system (as an embolus) can affect the cerebral vasculature (causing stroke), the vascular supply of the gut (causing mesenteric ischemia), or the renal vasculature (causing renal ischemia). These are examples of *arterial* emboli.

A common site for *venous* clot formation is in a deep vein, known as deep venous thrombosis (DVT). This most commonly occurs in deep leg veins. One cause of pulmonary embolus can be deep venous thrombosis (DVT) in the leg. Thrombus from the DVT can travel to the right heart and then to the pulmonary artery. Venous thrombosis can occur in any *hypercoagulable state* (see hematology Chapter 6).

Consider the case of a young patient who has a stroke but is *not* in atrial fibrillation and has *no* atherosclerotic disease. One possible cause would be a hypercoagulable state. What if the patient is found to have recurrent DVTs and strokes? Hopefully you are saying, "Wait! The patient has *venous* thrombosis and is ending up with strokes?! How can that be if the venous return is to the right heart? Shouldn't the patient have pulmonary emboli instead of strokes?" What could account for this? If the patient has an atrial or ventricular septal defect, a clot from the venous side can cross through this defect from right atrium to left atrium and lead to a stroke (*paradoxical embolus*). One cause of paradoxical embolus is a *patent foramen ovale,* a congenital defect leaving a hole that connects the atria.

Peripheral Vascular Disease

Atherosclerosis can occur in any artery, which can cause symptoms and signs related to the ischemia of the affected organ, such as mesenteric ischemia, stroke, renal ischemia, retinal ischemia, etc. The same risk factors and pathophysiological circumstances that lead to coronary arterial atherosclerosis can also cause atherosclerosis of peripheral arteries with similar consequences.

Atherosclerotic lesions of peripheral vasculature can cause *claudication,* which is analogous to angina in the heart: exertion involving the muscles supplied by the compromised vessels leads to pain and weakness, which is relieved by rest. Further occlusion of the arteries can lead to symptoms even at rest (*rest pain*), analogous to unstable angina in the heart. The symptoms and signs of peripheral vascular disease are often referred to as "the 6 Ps": pallor, pulselessness, pain, paresthesias (uncomfortable sensory disturbances), paralysis, and poikilothermia (cold temperature). Changes in hair, nail, and skin can also occur in the affected region(s). Commonly affected sites include the buttocks/thighs (caused by disease of the distal aorta and/or iliac arteries; ischemia here can also cause impotence in men) and the calves (caused by disease of the popliteal and femoral arteries). Less commonly, the arms (supplied by the subclavian arteries) may be affected.

Diagnosis can be confirmed by Doppler ultrasound, angiography, and/or ankle-brachial index of blood pressure (ABI). The ABI compares the blood pressure at the ankle with that in the arm. Normally, these should be equivalent, yielding a ratio of 1. A lesser ratio demonstrates decreased blood pressure at the ankle as compared to the upper extremity and indicates peripheral vascular disease of the lower extremity.

Like treatment of atherosclerotic heart disease, treatment of peripheral vascular disease involves dietary and lifestyle modifications (exercise, cholesterol reduction, smoking cessation, etc.) as well as angioplasty and/or surgical bypass.

Atherosclerosis of the Aorta

Aortic Aneurysm

Atherosclerosis is one cause of aortic aneurysm (dilatation of the aorta). Atherosclerosis-induced aortic aneurysm occurs more commonly in the abdominal portion of the aorta. Other causes of aortic aneurysm in either the thoracic or abdominal portions include connective tissue diseases (such as Marfan Syndrome and Ehler's-Danlos Syndrome), infections (e.g., syphilis), and vasculitis. Aortic aneurysms may be asymptomatic or may cause symptoms related to pressure on nearby structures, especially in the case of thoracic aortic aneurysms (e.g., compression of esophagus or trachea leading to dysphagia or cough). An abdominal aortic aneurysm may be palpable as a pulsating mass on abdominal exam. Depending on size and rate of expansion, surgical repair is often necessary to prevent rupture.

Aortic Dissection

Aortic aneurysm/rupture is distinct from *aortic dissection*. Aortic dissection is a tear in the intima of the aorta into which blood can flow, furthering the tear. Trauma, hypertension, syphilis, and connective tissue diseases such as Marfan Syndrome and Ehler's-Danlos Syndrome can predispose to aortic dissection. Dissection presents as "tearing/ripping" chest and/or back pain. On physical exam, loss of pulses and different blood pressures between the two arms may be present. Other consequences of dissection can include stroke (leading to neurological deficits), myocardial infarction, aortic regurgitation (leading to a diastolic murmur), and/or tamponade (leading to hypotension, muffled heart sounds, and elevated JVP). Chest X-ray may demonstrate a widened mediastinum. Emergency surgical repair is often necessary, and beta-blockers can be used to reduce blood pressure while awaiting surgery.

Lipids and Lipid-Lowering Drugs

Since elevated lipids are a risk factor for developing atherosclerosis, maintaining low serum lipids is one goal of prevention of atherosclerotic disease.

Fig. 1-21. Lipid processing pathways and lipid-lowering drugs. Lipids are processed in the body via two pathways: the *exogenous pathway*, which absorbs fats from the digestive tract into the circulation, and the *endogenous pathway*, which transports fats synthesized in the liver between the liver and the peripheral tissues. LDL (low density lipoprotein) is often referred to as "bad cholesterol" and HDL (high density lipoprotein) as "good cholesterol," because LDL largely transports cholesterol to the periphery (where it may be incorporated into atherosclerotic lesions), and HDL mostly transports cholesterol back to the liver from the periphery.

Aside from dietary modification to decrease lipid intake, what sites of pharmacologic intervention are possible?

Treatments affecting the exogenous pathway:

- *Lipid absorption can be inhibited* (e.g., ezetimibe).

- *Bile acids can be sequestered in the GI tract*, promoting their loss and hence increasing conversion of hepatic cholesterol to bile acids for secretion (bile acid sequestrants, also known as resins, e.g., cholestyramine).

Treatments affecting the endogenous pathway:

- *HDL can be increased* by nicotinic acid or fibrates (e.g., gemfibrozil).

- *Hepatic cholesterol production can be decreased* by the following mechanisms:
  - *Inhibiting the enzyme HMG Co-A reductase,* a rate-limiting step in cholesterol synthesis (e.g., statins)
  - *LDL can be decreased* (nicotinic acid decreases hepatic production of VLDL; it also raises HDL by mechanisms less well understood).

Fibrates and nicotinic acid also *lower triglycerides.*

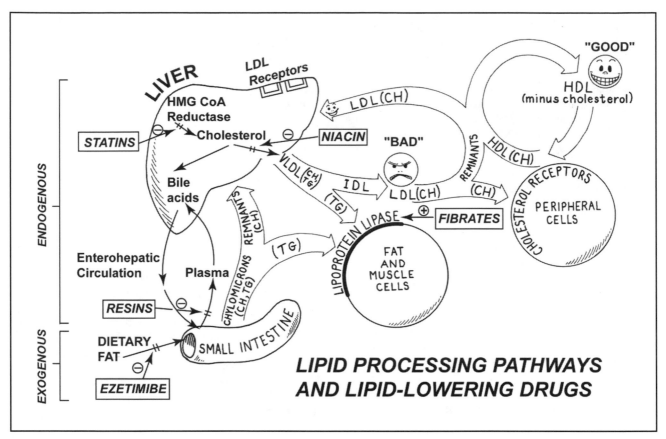

Figure 1-21. Modified from Goldberg: *Clinical Biochemistry Made Ridiculously Simple,* MedMaster, 2004

Vasculitis

Vasculitis is an inflammation of blood vessels that can be caused by *infection* (Hepatitis B or C, Epstein Barr virus, cytomegalovirus), *drugs* (penicillin, sulfonamides, quinolones), *autoimmune disease* (systemic lupus erythematosis, rheumatoid arthritis), or independent *vasculitic syndromes.*

Fig. 1-22. Vasculitis syndromes. The vasculitic syndromes are classified by the size of vessels that they affect (small vs. medium vs. large).

Symptoms/signs of any vasculitis can include constitutional symptoms (weight loss, fatigue, fever) as well as consequences of ischemia including skin rashes/ulcers, renal dysfunction, neuropathy, and/or bowel infarction. Other features are specific to specific vasculitis syndromes. Lab features used in diagnosis are included in the table. Infectious causes, drugs, and underlying systemic diseases must be ruled out before diagnosis of a vasculitic syndrome can be made. Arterial biopsy and/or angiogram is necessary for definitive diagnosis, and treatment involves immunosuppressive drugs, most commonly steroids.

Hypertension

Most cases of hypertension have no identifiable cause (*essential hypertension*). Before making the diagnosis of essential hypertension, causes of secondary hypertension must be ruled out. Secondary hypertension can be caused by any process that increases arterial resistance, blood volume, and/or cardiac output. Thus, potential culprits are the *kidneys, hormonal changes, changes in the blood vessels themselves,* or *drugs.*

Renal disease can cause failure to adequately excrete sodium and water, increasing intravascular volume. Additionally, stenosis of one or both renal arteries can lead to hypertension. This stenosis decreases blood flow to the kidney(s), causing increased renin secretion. This activates the renin-angiotensin-aldosterone axis, leading to increased blood volume (secondary to aldosterone increase) and increased arterial resistance (secondary to angiotensin increase). See Fig. 1-6. Renal artery stenosis can be caused by atherosclerosis or fibromuscular dysplasia of one or both renal arteries.

Figure 1-22 Vasculitis Syndromes

DISEASE	AFFECTED VESSELS	CLASSIC SYMPTOMS/ SIGNS (in addition to fever, malaise, weight loss, arthralgias/myalgias, rash)	DIAGNOSIS (ESR, CRP, WBC may be elevated in all)	TREATMENT	OTHER
Large Vessel					
Giant cell (Temporal) arteritis	Aortic arch and branches, especially temporal arteries and extracranial vertebral arteries	Typically > age 50. Headache, temple tenderness (pain when brushing hair), absent temporal pulses, visual loss, jaw claudication (pain when chewing)	ESR, CRP, biopsy of temporal artery	Steroids	Can co-occur with polymyalgia rheumatica (though either can occur separately). Polymyalgia rheumatica: Typically > age 50, pain/stiffness in neck, pelvis, shoulders
Takayasu's arteritis	Aorta and branches	More common in Asians; patients < 40; claudication in extremities; neurologic, cardiac, pulmonary, dermatologic findings; changes in pulses; bruits, hypertension, retinal changes	Angiography	Steroids +/– other immuno-suppressives	
Medium Vessel					
Polyarteritis nodosa (PAN)	(medium-sized arteries)	Mononeuritis multiplex, skin findings, abdominal angina, renal involvement, testicular infarction	No specific test	Steroids +/– cytotoxic agents	Possible association with Hepatitis B
Kawasaki's disease	(medium-sized arteries)	Disease of young children, more common in Asians. Fever, rash, conjunctivitis, myocarditis/heart failure, coronary aneurysms; any system: CNS, pulmonary, GI, renal	No specific test. Coronary aneurysms can be visualized with echo	Aspirin, IV Ig	
Small Vessel					
Wegener's granulomatosis	(small arteries)	Nasal/sinus, upper airway problems, pulmonary, glomerulonephritis	C-ANCA*	Cyclophos-phamide, Steroids	
Churg-Strauss vasculitis	(small arteries)	Asthma, allergic rhinitis most common but any system can be affected	Eosinophilia, P-ANCA*	Steroids	
Microscopic polyangiitis	(small arteries)	Skin findings, renal and pulmonary dysfunction (any organ system can be affected)	ANCA (more commonly P-ANCA*)	Cyclophos-phamide, Steroids	
Thrombangiitis obliterans (Buerger disease)	(small arteries)	Associated w/smoking, more common in young men (20s–40s); higher incidence in Ashkenazi Jews and Asians; claudication; Raynaud's in feet, legs, hands, and arms	Rule out scleroderma	Smoking cessation greatly improves prognosis	
Henoch-Schonlein purpura	(small arteries)	Most common in children; Purpuric rash, arthritis, abdominal pain, renal involvement; Commonly preceded by upper Resp. or GI infection	IgA in lesions on biopsy	Self-limited, steroids may help during symptoms	

*ANCA = antineutrophil cytoplasmic antibodies. ANCA may be involved in the pathogenesis of some vasculitis. C (cytoplasmic) and P (perinuclear) refer to patterns of histologic staining of these antibodies in different diseases. C-ANCA is more commonly associated with Wegener's, P-ANCA with Churg-Strauss and microscopic polyangiitis.

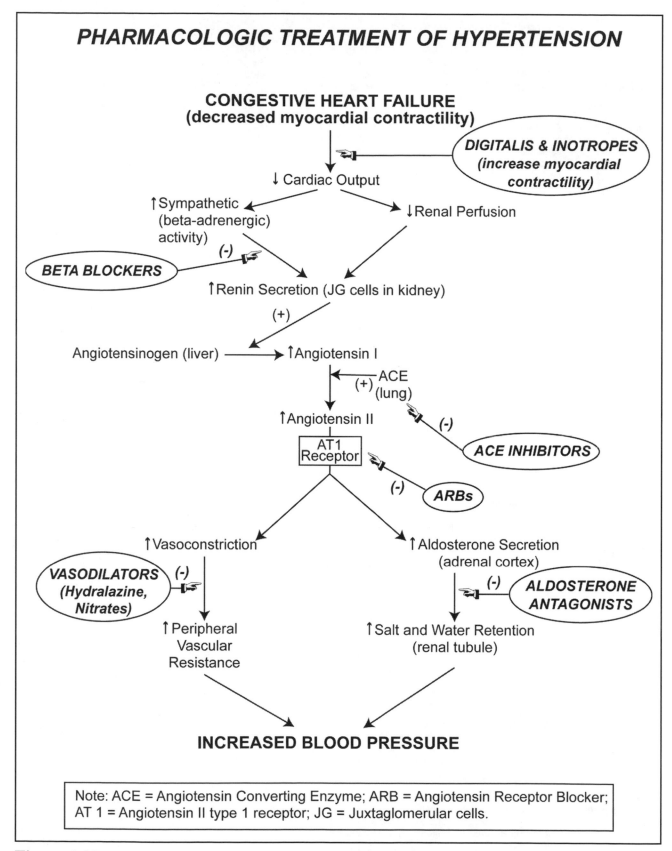

Figure 1-23. Modified from Chizner: *Clinical Cardiology Made Ridiculously Simple,* MedMaster, 2006

Hormonal changes that can cause hypertension include:

- Hyperaldosteronism (increased aldosterone → increased sodium reabsorption → increased blood volume)

- Increased cortisol, also known as Cushing's syndrome (when in excess, cortisol can stimulate aldosterone receptors)

- Hyperthyroidism (excess thyroid hormone increases cardiac output)

- Increased epinephrine/norepinephrine, e.g., secondary to pheochromocytoma (epinephrine/norepinephrine increase heart rate and arterial resistance.)

Changes in the arteries themselves that can lead to hypertension include aortic coarctation and vasculitis.

Consequences of Hypertension

Hypertension was discussed above as a cause of cardiac hypertrophy and myocardial infarction. Hypertension can also cause kidney damage (nephropathy), retinopathy, stroke, intracranial hemorrhage, aortic aneurysm, and aortic dissection.

Treatment of Hypertension

Lifestyle modifications such as exercise, weight loss, and dietary changes (such as sodium reduction) are an important component of managing hypertension.

Fig. 1-23. Pharmacologic treatment of hypertension. Pharmacologic treatment of hypertension aims to either *decrease blood volume* (diuretics) or *decrease arterial resistance*. Decreasing arterial resistance can be accomplished by direct vasodilation (e.g., hydralazine, nitrates) or inhibition of vasoconstriction. Inhibition of vasoconstriction can be accomplished by blocking the sympathetic system (alpha blockers), blocking calcium-activated smooth muscle contraction (calcium channel blockers), blocking aldosterone (aldosterone antagonists, e.g., spironolactone), and/or blocking the renin-angiotensin system (ACE-inhibitors, angiotensin receptor blockers (ARBs)).

CARDIAC INFECTION, INFLAMMATION, AND NEOPLASIA

Fig. 1-24. Sites of cardiac inflammation. Infection and inflammation of the heart can affect any of its three layers: endocardium, myocardium, pericardium.

Endocarditis

Endocarditis, inflammation of the endocardium, can result from noninfectious or infectious causes. Noninfectious causes of endocarditis include hypercoagula-

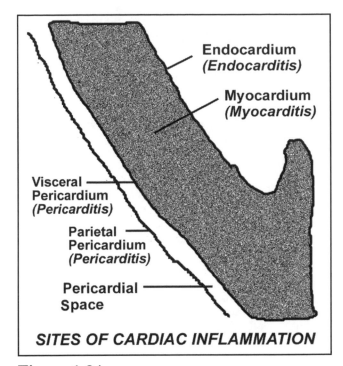

SITES OF CARDIAC INFLAMMATION

Figure 1-24

ble states (which can lead to thrombus formation on valves) and inflammatory conditions such as systemic lupus erythematosis. Lupus-induced endocarditis is called *Libman-Sacks endocarditis*.

Infection can occur on a native valve or a prosthetic valve. Any valvular disease can predispose to infectious endocarditis. Common bacterial causes of endocarditis include *Streptococcus viridans* and *Staphylococcus aureus*. The course of infective endocarditis can be acute or subacute, and symptoms generally include fever and a new heart murmur. Infectious emboli can form and lead to a pulmonary embolus (if the embolus comes from the right heart), or stroke, renal dysfunction, and/or peripheral vasculitic lesions (if the embolus comes from the left side). Blood cultures and echocardiography are used to confirm the diagnosis, demonstrating bacteremia and vegetations on the valve, respectively.

IV drug abuse is a common cause of endocarditis. On which valve would you expect an IV drug abuser to have endocarditis? Drugs injected into the venous system can cause infectious material to travel to the right heart, infecting the tricuspid (and/or more rarely the pulmonary) valve. *Staphylococcus aureus* is the most common cause of IV drug-related endocarditis.

Treatment of infective endocarditis involves extended IV antibiotic therapy. If the damage to the valve is enough to induce heart failure, surgical replacement of the valve may be necessary.

If a patient is known to have valvular pathology that could predispose to endocarditis (e.g., congenital lesion, rheumatic heart disease, prosthetic valve), antibiotic prophylaxis is given prior to any procedure that could induce transient bacteremia (e.g., dental work, surgery).

Rheumatic Fever and Rheumatic Heart Disease

Acute rheumatic fever is a complication of Group A streptococcus infection of the upper respiratory tract. Due to what is thought to be an autoimmune response triggered by the bacterium, an inflammatory response occurs that can affect the heart, central nervous system, skin, and joints. Acute rheumatic fever manifests as fever, joint pain, subcutaneous nodules, chorea (uncontrollable purposeless movements), and/or other motor disturbances occurring a few weeks after a sore throat. The long-term effects of the inflammation in the heart can include mitral stenosis and/or regurgitation as well as aortic stenosis and/or regurgitation (*rheumatic heart disease*).

Myocarditis

Myocarditis can be caused by *infection* (Coxsackie B virus is the most common viral cause, though various other viruses, bacteria, and parasites can cause myocarditis), *inflammatory disease* (e.g., lupus, dermatomyositis), or *toxins* (e.g., drugs, radiation). Depending on the severity, any symptom/sign of congestive heart failure may be present. Treatment is directed toward the underlying cause and alleviating heart failure symptoms/signs if present.

Pericarditis

The heart is contained within the pericardial sac. The visceral pericardium lines the outer surface of the heart and connects to the parietal pericardium, which forms the pericardial sac.

The pericardium can become inflamed (*pericarditis*) secondary to infectious or noninfectious causes. Infection can be caused by viruses (echovirus and Coxsackie B are the most common), tuberculosis, or bacteria (e.g., *Streptococcus*, *Staphylococcus*, gram negatives). Noninfectious causes of pericarditis include connective tissue diseases (e.g., lupus, rheumatoid arthritis), drugs, malignancy, renal failure, radiation, trauma to the heart, and myocardial infarction (*Dressler's syndrome* is the name given to postmyocardial infarction pericarditis). Pericarditis can also occur idiopathically. Chest pain in pericarditis is *pleuritic*, meaning that it gets worse with deep inspiration. The pain is often affected by position; it gets better when the patient leans forward and worse when the patient lies down. Patients with pericarditis

are often febrile. On auscultation, one may hear a *pericardial rub*, the sound of the inflamed pericardial layers rubbing against each other. Treatment depends upon the etiology: viral pericarditis is generally self-limited, while bacterial pericarditis requires antibiotics and, often, drainage of infection from the pericardial space. Treatment may also include anti-inflammatories such as aspirin.

Constrictive pericarditis can be a consequence of any of the above etiologies of pericarditis. In constrictive pericarditis, the pericardium becomes rigid and impairs filling of the chambers of the heart. This leads to backup of flow and impaired forward flow, resulting in signs and symptoms similar to those in left and right heart failure. A classic sign of constrictive pericarditis is *Kussmaul's sign*: a rise in the JVP during inspiration. During inspiration, the decrease in intrathoracic pressure brings blood into the heart. If constrictive pericarditis inhibits the right heart's ability to accept that blood, it will back up into the venous system, producing Kussmaul's sign. Often the pericardium must be surgically removed for definitive treatment of constrictive pericarditis.

Any cause of pericarditis can also result in a *pericardial effusion*, an accumulation of fluid in the pericardial sac. If this happens rapidly (i.e., cardiac injury leading to bleeding into the sac), it can cause *tamponade*, severe restriction of cardiac motion, which is often fatal. Signs include hypotension (from decreased forward flow), increased JVP (from increased backup), and distant heart sounds (since the fluid in the pericardium muffles the sounds' transmission to the stethoscope). To treat tamponade, fluid is removed from the pericardial space by needle aspiration (*pericardiocentesis*).

If pericardial effusion occurs over a more prolonged time course, gradual stretching of the pericardium can accommodate the effusion. If asymptomatic, the patient can be observed without intervention, but drainage of the fluid by pericardiocentesis or surgery (*pericardial window*) is necessary if hemodynamic compromise arises.

Cardiac Neoplasia

The most common neoplasias of the heart are metastases. Metastases can affect the heart itself or the pericardium.

Atrial Myxoma

Atrial myxoma is the most common primary cardiac tumor. It is most commonly benign and found in the left atrium. Because these tumors tend to be shaped like a ball on the end of a stalk, they can "bob" around, causing intermittent, position-dependent symptoms (e.g., syncope, dyspnea). Emboli from the tumor can cause vascular occlusion (which could lead to stroke, mesenteric ischemia, renal ischemia, retinal artery occlusion). Constitutional symptoms (e.g., fever, fatigue, weight loss) may also occur.

If the myxoma is in the atrium, what type of murmur would you expect it to cause? Atrial contraction occurs at the end of diastole, so an atrial tumor can cause a diastolic murmur. If the myxoma blocks the mitral valve, a diastolic rumble may be heard. The motion of the tumor on its pedicle can cause a "tumor plop" sound during diastole. The murmur caused by atrial myxoma can be position-dependent.

Atrial myxomas are treated by surgical removal.

CONGENITAL HEART DISEASE

The embryological development of the heart is complex, and many errors can occur along the way: 8/1000 births have some type of congenital heart defect.

Fetal Circulation

Fig. 1-25. The fetal circulation. The fetal lungs are nonfunctional and mostly collapsed. After all, the fetus is bathed in fluid, so it would not do much good to have the lungs breathe. So how does the fetus get oxygenated blood? From the mother via the umbilical vein. It is called the umbilical *vein* because it is coming *towards* the baby's heart (remember *artery* = *a*way from heart), but do not be fooled: the umbilical vein is carrying oxygenated blood to the baby.[4] The umbilical vein connects to the fetal venous system, which eventually returns blood to the fetal right atrium via the inferior vena cava (IVC). If this blood enters the fetal *venous* system, it will be mixed with deoxygenated blood that is on its way back to the heart. However, this inferior vena cava blood + oxygenated blood from the umbilical vein is still more oxygenated than blood coming from the superior vena cava (SVC).

Notice that both the relatively more oxygenated blood from the IVC and the less oxygenated blood from the SVC both mix in the right heart. However, the IVC enters at an angle such that the blood is directed towards the *foramen ovale*, a passageway in the intra-atrial septum that allows communication between the atria. Thus, the more oxygenated blood

---

[4] What are the only other veins that carry oxygenated blood? The pulmonary veins (from the lungs to the left atrium).

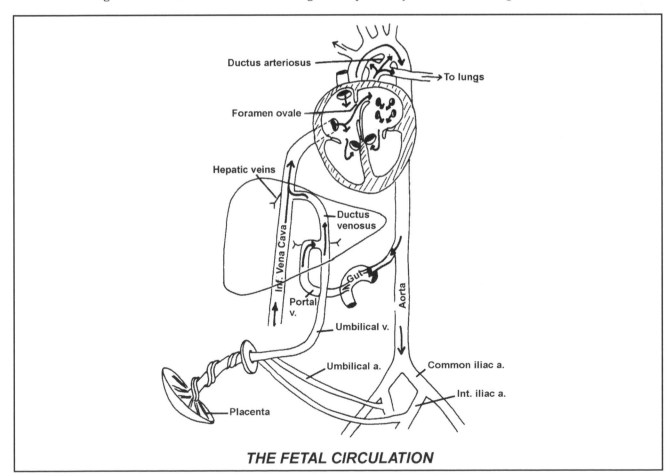

THE FETAL CIRCULATION

Figure 1-25. Modified from Goldberg: *Clinical Anatomy Made Ridiculously Simple,* MedMaster 2004

from the IVC makes it across to the left heart (which can then pump it to the body). What about the remaining blood from the SVC and IVC that returns to the right atrium and passes to the right ventricle? It would not be of much use to have it travel through the lungs since they cannot yet oxygenate blood (in fact, the developing lungs use oxygen from the very little blood they do get for their own development). Most of the blood from the right heart ejected through the pulmonary artery passes through a shunt called the *ductus arteriosus,* which connects the pulmonary artery to the aorta. Thus, the lungs are almost entirely bypassed either by direct passage from the IVC to the right atrium through the foramen ovale to the left atrium or from the right ventricle through the pulmonary artery through the ductus arteriosus to the aorta.

When the baby takes its first breath after birth, the newly expanded lungs offer far less resistance than they did while they were collapsed. This favors flow from the right heart/pulmonary artery to the lungs, as opposed to the ductus arteriosus. The decrease in flow through the ductus arteriosus along with a decrease in prostaglandin levels causes the ductus arteriosus to close.[5] The changes in pressure also result in closure of the foramen ovale. These shunt closures lead to the establishment of the adult circulation as described in Fig. 1-1.

Classification of Congenital Heart Disease

Congenital heart disease is divided into pathologies that cause *cyanosis* ("blue babies") and those that do *not* cause cyanosis. For cyanosis to occur, deoxygenated blood must somehow bypass the lungs and make it into the systemic circulation. What would allow deoxygenated blood to get from the venous system/right heart to the left side of the body? Though your first guess might be some kind of intracardiac shunt (e.g., atrial septal defect (ASD), or ventricular septal defect (VSD)), realize that due to relatively higher pressure in the left heart vs. the right, ASD/VSD should *not* normally lead to cyanosis. The only situation in which a septal defect could lead to cyanosis would be if there is a VSD *and* right heart pressures are abnormally elevated so as to overcome left heart pressures. Tetralogy of Fallot is an example of this. Normally, however, any communication between the 2 circulations should *not* lead to cyanosis.

---

[5] Prostaglandin levels are high during gestation, which also helps keep the ductus open. One can take advantage of this fact in the treatment of some congenital heart disease by keeping the ductus open after birth by prostaglandin administration, or by closing it with anti-inflammatories (e.g., indomethacin) if it remains open.

Cyanotic Heart Disease

Tetralogy of Fallot

Fig. 1-26. Tetralogy of Fallot. *Tetra* means four, and there are four components of the pathology here: a *VSD,* an *overriding aorta* (i.e., one which spans the middle portions of both ventricles), and *right ventricular hypertrophy* (leading to a boot-shaped heart on a chest X-ray) secondary to *pulmonic stenosis.* The stenotic pulmonary artery causes the deoxygenated blood from the right ventricle to flow through the VSD instead of the pulmonary artery. This blood then flows from the left ventricle into the aorta. This mixes the venous and oxygenated blood supplying the systemic circulation, which causes cyanosis. If a baby feeds or exerts her/himself, s/he will need increased blood flow to various parts of the systemic circulation. The arteries in these areas will dilate, thus decreasing the resistance in the systemic circulation, which *encourages* blood to go from right to left (by making the path of least resistance even less resistant). This leads to increasing cyanosis, and these episodes are known as "Tet spells" ("tet" is short for tetralogy). If the decrease in systemic resistance increases right-to-left flow, how do you think a patient could try to relieve these symptoms? If there were a way to *increase* systemic resistance, this would raise left-sided pressure. Increased left-sided pressure will shunt a little more blood back to the right so it can go through the pulmonary system and get oxygenated. Children do this by squatting, which increases resistance in the arterial system, and thus decreases right-to-left shunting. Treatment is surgical: patching shut the VSD and widening the pulmonary outflow tract.

Transposition of the Great Arteries

Fig. 1-27. Transposition of the great arteries. In this condition, the aorta and pulmonary artery connect to

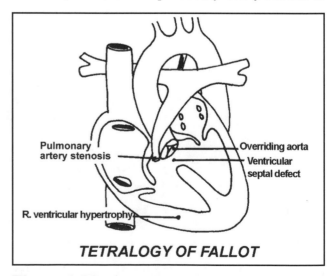

Figure 1-26. From Goldberg: *Clinical Anatomy Made Ridiculously Simple,* MedMaster 2004

the wrong ventricles: the pulmonary artery to the *left* ventricle and the aorta to the *right* ventricle. Thus, de-oxygenated venous blood returns to the right heart and then is ejected into the aorta to the systemic circulation, which then returns to the right heart, etc. The left heart receives blood from the lungs and then ejects into the lungs, and then the blood comes back to the left heart and then is returned to the lungs, etc. The result is two parallel loops instead of a continuous progression. In utero, the communications between the two circulations via the foramen ovale and ductus arteriosus allow for enough mixing to maintain oxygenation of tissues. However, when these close at birth, there is no way of getting oxygenated blood to the tissues, which can be deadly. If diagnosed in utero, efforts are made to keep the ductus arteriosus open after birth (by administering prostaglandins) until surgery can be performed to attach the great vessels to their appropriate ventricles.

Other Causes of Cyanotic Heart Disease

There are other less common cardiac anomalies that can lead to cyanosis, such as a single ventricle, hypoplastic left heart, totally anomalous pulmonary venous return, and many others. The main point to keep in mind is that for a cardiac lesion to cause cyanosis, there must either be a right-to-left shunt (e.g., tetralogy of Fallot) *or* the blood must somehow be bypassing the lungs (e.g., transposition of the great arteries). *Non*-cardiac causes of cyanosis in the newborn are discussed in case #3 in Chapter 10.

Noncyanotic Congenital Heart Disease
Atrial Septal Defect (ASD) and Ventricular Septal Defect (VSD)

Since left heart pressure normally exceeds right heart pressure (with a few exceptions e.g., tetralogy of Fal-

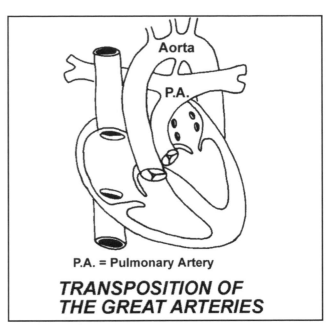

P.A. = Pulmonary Artery

TRANSPOSITION OF THE GREAT ARTERIES

Figure 1-27. From Goldberg: *Clinical Anatomy Made Ridiculously Simple*, MedMaster 2004

lot), blood flows through ASDs and VSDs from *left to right*. This results in an increased amount of blood handled by the right heart.

Fig. 1-28. Catheterization findings in ASD and VSD. Although these defects can be detected by murmur on physical exam and then visualized by echocardiography, sometimes catheterization is performed. Catheterization will demonstrate increased oxygenation of the blood in the right side of the heart compared to normal patients. If there is an ASD or VSD, blood in the right heart will be a mixture of venous return from

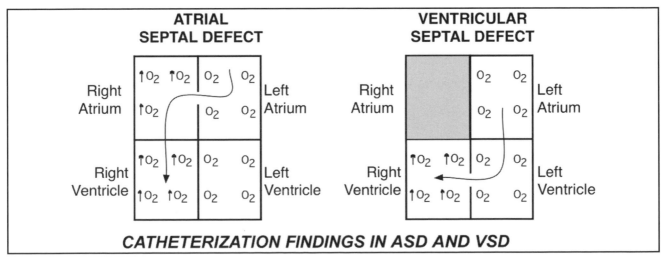

CATHETERIZATION FINDINGS IN ASD AND VSD

Figure 1-28

the right side of the body (deoxygenated) *and* oxygenated blood that has traversed the defect from the left heart. If there is only a VSD, *only* the right ventricle will have this elevated O_2. Since the leak is from the left ventricle to the right ventricle, the blood in the right atrium should still be purely venous deoxygenated blood. This is in contrast to *ASD* where both the right atrium *and* the right ventricle have increased O_2 (since oxygenated blood passes from the left atrium to the right atrium via the ASD and then from the right atrium to the right ventricle).

Atrial Septal Defect (ASD). A small ASD can be asymptomatic, but a large ASD can lead to significant overload of the right ventricle, which can result in its enlargement. In such cases, surgical repair of the ASD is necessary. Since there is not really a substantial amount of pressure across the ASD, the blood flow across the ASD itself does not create a murmur. However, due to the *volume overload of the right heart,* increased flow across both tricuspid and pulmonic valves can produce murmurs during diastole and systole, respectively. Additionally since the amount of blood ejected by the right heart becomes greater than that ejected by the left, pulmonic valve closure occurs *later* than aortic valve closure. This causes a fixed split of S2. Diagnosis is made by echocardiography or MRI.

Ventricular Septal Defect (VSD). The murmur of VSD occurs when the ventricle contracts, i.e., a holosystolic murmur. A VSD causes increased flow to the lungs, which can eventually cause such severe pulmonary hypertension that the pressure in the right heart overcomes the pressure in the left heart, reversing the shunt. This is Eisenmenger syndrome (Fig. 1-29).

Fig. 1-29. Eisenmenger syndrome. The left ventricle normally has a harder job than the right ventricle, ejecting to the entire systemic vasculature instead of the low-pressure pulmonary system. Thus, the left ventricle is stronger than the right ventricle. So when the heart squeezes, if there is a hole, the stronger left ventricle wins and pushes blood over to the right side. Now the flow through the lungs is increased since the right heart is pumping extra blood (i.e., it is pumping both the venous return from the body and the oxygenated blood from the left ventricle that passes through the defect). This causes the pressure to be so high in the lungs that the right-sided system eventually starts to be under higher pressure than the left. At that point, the right side starts to win, pushing blood through the VSD to the left side. The blood in the right heart has not yet been oxygenated by the lungs, and so when it passes to the left side, the body gets some blood without oxygen, leading to cyanosis. This is *Eisenmenger syndrome*: a left-to-right shunt causing pulmonary and right heart pressures to increase so that the shunt *reverses,* resulting in blood flow from right to left through the defect, causing cyanosis.

Patent Ductus Arteriosus (PDA)

The ductus arteriosus serves as an in utero connection between the pulmonary artery and the aorta. In the fetal circulation, this allows blood ejected by the right heart (which contains oxygenated blood from the mother) to pass from the pulmonary artery to the aorta, bypassing the lungs since they would not be oxygenating this blood anyway. At birth, the ductus arteriosus closes. What would happen if the ductus arteriosus did *not* close at birth? As with all other shunts we have described, the *left-sided pressure is*

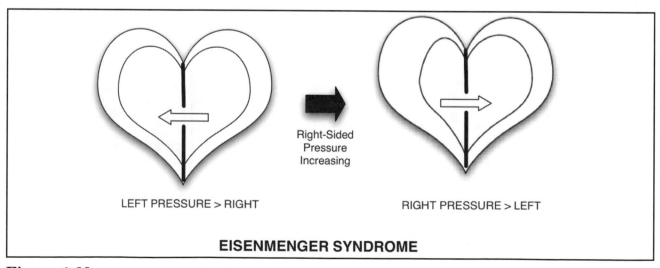

EISENMENGER SYNDROME

Figure 1-29

higher than right-sided pressure, so flow across the PDA will be *from aorta to pulmonary artery*, the *opposite* of in utero. The result is that oxygenated blood from the aorta passes to the pulmonary artery, and then goes for another trip to the lungs and back to the left heart and round and round again. This increases the work of the left heart since it is now responsible for the normal pulmonary venous return *and* the extra blood that comes through the shunt. This extra work can lead to heart failure. Also, as with other left-to-right shunts, pulmonary blood flow increases, which can lead to elevated pulmonary arterial pressure. This elevated pulmonary arterial pressure can subsequently result in right heart failure and/or sufficiently elevated pulmonary artery pressure so as to reverse flow through the PDA (analogous to Eisenmenger syndrome). This would allow deoxygenated blood from the pulmonary artery to pass to the aorta, causing cyanosis.

If there is a patent ductus arteriosus, blood flows through it *constantly* throughout the cardiac cycle, resulting in a *continuous machine-like murmur*.

Since prostaglandins keep the ductus open, anti-inflammatories (i.e., indomethacin) can be used to close the ductus. If this treatment fails, surgical ligation can be performed.

Pulmonic Stenosis

Pulmonic stenosis can occur in adults, but it occurs more commonly as a congenital lesion. Similar to the effect of aortic stenosis on the left ventricle, pulmonic stenosis causes the right ventricle to hypertrophy. If severe, this can cause right heart failure. The murmur is systolic. Pulmonic stenosis can occur as part of tetralogy of Fallot or independently.

Congenital Aortic Stenosis

Congenital aortic stenosis is similar in pathophysiology to adult aortic stenosis: a congenitally stenotic valve increases the workload on the left ventricle, leading to hypertrophy. Hypertrophy can result in fatigue, dyspnea, syncope, and eventual congestive heart failure, depending on the severity. What kind of murmur occurs in aortic stenosis? Systolic ejection murmur.

Coarctation of the Aorta

Coarctation of the aorta is a congenital narrowing of the aorta that can occur anywhere along its length. Most commonly it occurs near the ductus arteriosus. A severe coarctation increases the resistance facing the left ventricle, and can thus lead to congestive heart failure.

Clinical manifestations of coarctation of the aorta. How does the heart respond to increased resistance in adult aortic stenosis? Hypertrophy. Left ventricular hypertrophy is also one potential consequence of aortic coarctation. Additionally, in a neonate, the body will take advantage of collateral vessels along the undersurface of the ribs to supply the lower portion of the body. One manifestation of this is the radiologic finding of *rib notching*: the enlarged collateral vessels under the ribs actually wear away at the rib surface over time due to their increased blood flow, and these notches can be seen on chest X-ray.

What type of murmur would coarctation of the aorta cause? When is blood passing through the murmur-producing area? Blood flows through the aorta during systolic ejection, and thus aortic coarctation produces a *systolic ejection murmur*.

Coarctation of the aorta can also result in higher blood pressure in the upper extremities than in the lower extremities. Why? If the coarctation occurs distal to the brachiocephalic, common carotid, and left subclavian arteries, these vessels will all get *normal* flow, while the circulation distal to the coarct will get diminished flow. If the coarct occurs *distal to the brachiocephalic* take-off but *proximal to the left subclavian take-off*, there will be higher blood pressure in the right arm than in the left.

Fig. 1-30. Aortic coarctation. Depending on whether the coarctation occurs *proximal* or *distal* to the ductus arteriosus, different manifestations can occur. The ductus arteriosus is distal to the brachiocephalic artery (which gives rise to the right common carotid artery and right subclavian artery), the left common carotid artery, and the left subclavian artery. If the narrowing occurs *proximal* to the ductus (preductal coarctation), but still distal to the three vessels mentioned above, what happens in utero? The three vessels of the arch are *proximal* to the obstruction, and so blood from the left ventricle easily goes through these to the head and upper extremities. While the ductus is open in utero, blood from the pulmonary artery flows through the ductus arteriosus to the aorta distal to the obstruction to supply the lower body, and all is well.

What happens when the ductus closes at birth? The head and upper extremities receive normal blood flow since they occur proximal to the obstruction. The lower half of the body, however, has reduced blood flow, due to the narrowing of the aorta and the loss of the "detour" via the ductus arteriosus. What would be the consequence of this? Blood pressure would be much higher in the upper extremities than the lower extremities. What if the ductus failed to close in preductal coarctation? Again, the upper body will be normally supplied by the left ventricle, but the lower body will be supplied by the pulmonary artery through the ductus arteriosus to the aorta. This results in the delivery of a mixture of deoxygenated and oxygenated blood to the

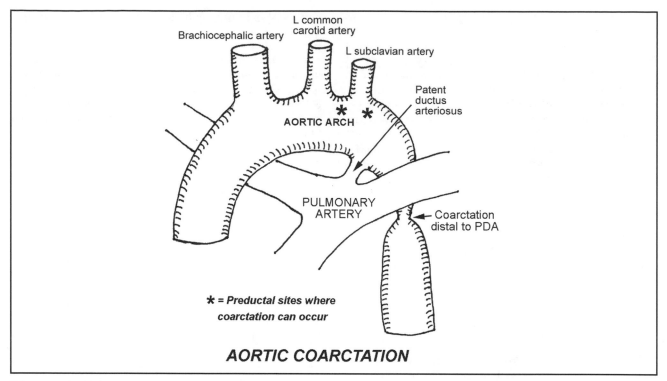

Figure 1-30. From Goldberg: *Clinical Anatomy Made Ridiculously Simple,* MedMaster 2004

lower half of the body. This can lead to *differential cyanosis,* in which the upper half of the body appears normal while the lower part of the body is cyanotic.

In *post-ductal* coarctation, the clinical consequences depend on the severity. As mentioned above, a very severe coarctation can lead to heart failure.

Review of Congenital Heart Disease

Congenital heart disease can be divided into diseases that cause cyanosis and those that do not. In heart diseases that cause cyanosis, blood must have some way of bypassing the lungs. This can occur either via trans-position of the great arteries, or a shunt (but *only* if the right ventricle pressures are higher than the left ventricle pressures through the shunt, e.g., tetralogy of Fallot). Aortic coarctation can cause differential cyanosis if it is preductal *and* the ductus fails to close. The other pathologies are either "things left open" (ASD, VSD, PDA), or "things not fully opened" (aortic and pulmonic stenosis). "Things left open" can lead to increased left-to-right flow, which can result in pulmonary hypertension and right heart failure. "Things not fully opened" can lead to increased work of the chamber ejecting through the stenosed valve and subsequent heart failure.

CHAPTER 2. THE PULMONARY SYSTEM

COMPONENTS OF THE PULMONARY SYSTEM

The lungs oxygenate the blood and eliminate carbon dioxide from it. The lungs contain two basic components: the *tracheo-broncho-alveolar system* (i.e., the airways and air sacs) and *blood vessels*.

Fig. 2-1A. Schematic of lung components. The functional unit of the lungs is the alveolus and its capillary.

The alveolus is basically a *sac* that fills with air when one breathes in and allows that air to pass across a *membrane* into a *blood vessel* (an alveolar capillary). Then the alveolus contracts back down like a deflating balloon to let carbon dioxide out and begin the cycle anew. The alveoli are the final branches of the airways (trachea → bronchi → bronchioles → alveoli). What could cause this system to fail? A problem with the sac (alveolus), the airways (trachea/ bronchi/ bronchioles), their membranes, or the blood vessels.

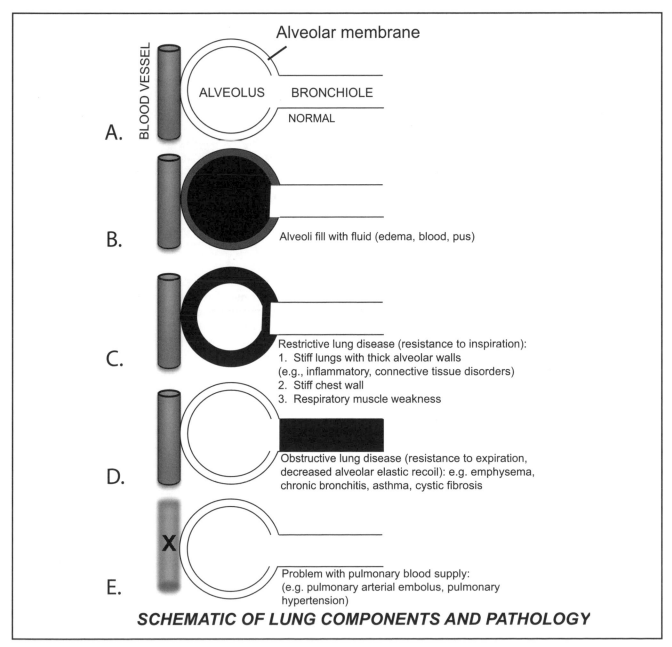

SCHEMATIC OF LUNG COMPONENTS AND PATHOLOGY

Figure 2-1

Alveolar Sac/Airway

All the sac has to do is fill up with oxygen, and all the airways have to do is serve as a conduit for inspired/expired gases. What problems could affect the alveolar sac and/or airways?

- The sac is already filled with something other than air (Fig. 2-1B).

- The sac does not open adequately (Fig. 2-1C).

- The sac is unable to expire adequately due to either obstruction of the airways or decreased elastic recoil of the sac itself (Fig. 2-1D).

Fig. 2-1B. *The sac is already filled with something other than air.* What could fill the sac? Pus (pneumonia) or fluid (edema or blood). Any process that clogs the alveoli diminishes their ability to hold oxygen (and thus decreases their ability to oxygenate the blood in their capillaries). One cause of filled alveoli is cardiogenic pulmonary edema: when the heart fails and blood backs up into the lungs, the elevated pressure causes transudation of fluid into the alveolar sacs, preventing adequate filling with oxygen. A non-cardiogenic cause of pulmonary edema is acute respiratory distress syndrome (ARDS), which can occur in septic shock, trauma, etc. In ARDS, inflammation causes the pulmonary capillaries to be leaky, resulting in pulmonary edema. Aside from pus and edema fluid, blood can fill an alveolus if there is pulmonary hemorrhage. This can occur in Goodpasture's syndrome or secondary to lung cancer, for example.

Fig 2-1C. *The sac does not open adequately.* The sac cannot open adequately if it faces some *restriction* to doing so *(restrictive lung disease)* or if the brain does not tell it to do so *(central sleep apnea)*. *Restrictive lung disease* can be due to stiff lungs, a stiff chest wall, or respiratory muscle weakness. Any of these causes of restriction create a situation where the airway *cannot open all the way and is difficult to keep open, so it collapses quickly.* Restrictive lung disease is discussed later in this chapter.

If you were to blow out all the air in your lungs and then hold your breath for a really long time, eventually you would either gasp for air or pass out. This is because the brain detects decreased oxygen *(hypoxia)* and increased carbon dioxide *(hypercarbia)* and demands a breath. So one reason that the sac would not open is if the brain is not doing its job. In *central sleep apnea,* there is thought to be diminished sensitivity of central receptors in the brain for this hypoxia/hypercarbia as well as a diminished response to these stimuli. The centers in the brainstem that "tell the lungs to breathe" stop working on occasion such that while asleep, these patients actually stop breathing. This is different from *obstructive sleep apnea,* where the upper airway collapses due to structural abnormalities. In both types of

sleep apnea, the result is daytime drowsiness because of frequent awakening at night caused by apnea.

Fig. 2-1D. *The sac is unable to expire adequately.* Suppose the sac opens, takes in its oxygen, and passes the oxygen across the membrane to the blood without problem. But then, suppose that when it was going to blow off the waste and breathe in again, it was somehow unable to do so. How could this happen? Either *obstruction of the airway* or *inadequate elastic recoil of the alveoli.* The alveoli are the final branching of a tree that begins with the trachea. The trachea bifurcates into the bronchi, which branch into bronchioles, which branch into alveoli. An *obstruction* anywhere would prevent the alveolus from returning to its deflated state and thus lead to retention of carbon dioxide and inability to initiate a new cycle. How could the airway become obstructed? A foreign body (like an aspirated peanut in a child), a tumor, or chronic mucus plugging *(chronic bronchitis* or *cystic fibrosis)* could all produce a mechanical obstruction. Additionally, airway obstruction can occur if the airways are *hyper-reactive* (causing them to constrict in response to cold and/or exercise and/or allergens as in *asthma)* or if *damage to lung parenchyma causes increased collapsibility of the airways (emphysema).* In emphysema, the damaged lung architecture also causes a *decrease in the elastic recoil of alveoli,* decreasing the force of expiration. Each of these disease processes will be discussed in greater detail below under *obstructive lung disease.*

Membrane

The alveolar membrane allows O_2 across to the blood and CO_2 out from the blood. Any disease that causes destruction or thickening of this membrane can reduce the diffusion of oxygen across it. Destruction of portions of the membrane can occur in emphysema, leading to a decrease in surface area available for gas exchange. Thickening of the alveolar membrane occurs in diseases that cause *fibrosis* of the lungs (e.g., connective tissue disease; hypersensitivity; exposure diseases such as silicosis, beryliosis, asbestosis, etc.). These diseases also cause *restrictive pulmonary disease,* because fibrotic thickening restricts proper expansion of the lung. Unless there is extremely severe thickening of the membrane, oxygen diffusion is usually adequate for the body's needs at rest, but can become inadequate for the needs of the body with activity. This can lead to exertional dyspnea. What else can lead to exertional dyspnea? Angina from decreased heart perfusion due to atherosclerosis in the coronary arteries. So when you think about exertional dyspnea, the lung and the heart are both potential pathophysiological culprits.

Blood Vessels

Fig. 2-1E. The goal of the pulmonary vasculature is to bring blood to the lungs to pick up oxygen and release carbon dioxide. An obstructed blood vessel (i.e., from a *pulmonary embolus*) could prevent transport of blood to the lungs for gas exchange. Another disease of the pulmonary blood vessels is *pulmonary hypertension*, elevated pressure in the pulmonary vascular system.

What if there were a change in the blood itself? For example, if the oxygen-carrying capacity of the blood decreases, it does not matter how good the lungs are at oxygenating the blood since the blood cannot adequately receive the oxygen. Thus, *anemia* can decrease the body's ability to provide oxygen to the tissues. If the oxygen-carrying capacity of the blood decreases, how will the body compensate? It will try to obtain more oxygen by breathing more deeply and faster and by circulating the existing blood volume faster to get the most mileage out of it. This can cause shortness of breath and tachycardia. So causes of shortness of breath include not only cardiac and pulmonary problems, but also hematologic ones.

OBSTRUCTIVE AND RESTRICTIVE LUNG DISEASE

An important concept in pulmonary pathophysiology is the distinction between obstructive and restrictive lung disease. If there is obstruction anywhere in the airways this will make it difficult for *air to get out*. Causes of obstruction include:

1. *Mechanical obstruction of the airways* (e.g., foreign body, tumor, chronic mucus plugging in chronic bronchitis)

2. *Increased resistance in the airways* (e.g., airway thickening from inflammation in chronic bronchitis)

3. *Increased tendency for airway closure* (a component of asthma and emphysema)

Restrictive lung disease makes it difficult to get the air *in*. Restrictive lung disease can be caused by:

1. Stiff lungs (e.g., interstitial lung disease)

2. A stiff chest wall (e.g., kyphoscoliosis, ankylosing spondylitis, obesity)

3. Respiratory muscle weakness (neurological or neuromuscular disease)

Mnemonic: *o*bstruction makes it hard to get the air *o*ut, restri*c*tion makes it hard to get the air *i*n,

Obstructive Lung Diseases

Emphysema

Under the microscope, the lungs look like honeycombs: empty air spaces surrounded by alveolar membranes. When you breathe in, those membranes are flexible, and they stretch, allowing air in, and then they relax, pushing air back out.

If we take this honeycomb-like lung architecture and start tearing out some of the alveolar membrane, we are left with *bigger, floppier* alveoli and bronchioles (as opposed to a lot of little tight ones in the normal lungs). There are two consequences of this floppiness: the *alveoli have decreased elastic recoil,* and the *bronchioles are more likely to collapse*. Because of the decreased elastic recoil in these floppy alveoli, they are weaker in expelling air than normal "tighter" ones (imagine an old used balloon as opposed to a brand-new stiff difficult-to-blow-up one). This decreased elastic recoil, combined with the increased collapse of bronchioles, leads to *difficulty getting air out*. If the lungs have trouble expiring, this leads to *hyperinflation* and *air trapping*. In addition, destruction of alveolar membranes decreases the surface area available for gas exchange. This is *emphysema*, one type of chronic obstructive pulmonary disease (COPD). In emphysema, the alveolar walls are progressively destroyed (e.g., by smoking or alpha-1 antitrypsin deficiency), leading to dilatation of distal air spaces. The resulting baggy, flabby alveoli do not exhale well, and the bronchioles collapse too easily, causing *obstruction* of the airways.

Symptoms and Signs of Emphysema. Patients with emphysema may take a deep breath in and then have a *prolonged expiratory phase* because of the obstruction to expiration. Their lungs may get so bad at exhaling that they recruit *accessory muscles* (e.g., intercostals, abdominal muscles) to help exhale. What will you hear as the air tries to leave through obstructed airways? If you just blow through your wide-open mouth, it sounds like rushing air. To whistle, you must make a very small hole with your lips for the air to come out of. So a small hole with air rushing through it gives high-pitched noise. Similarly, obstructed airways lead to *wheezing* on exam.

If you were to take a very big deep breath, hold it, and then try to keep breathing in but with your chest still expanded, that would give you the sense of what it is like to have a COPD or asthma flare. During a flare, patients breathe at high lung volumes, which can be fatiguing to the point that respiratory failure can ensue. Breathing at high lung volumes can also cause hyper-expansion on chest X-ray: the lungs appear too big (mostly in the superior-inferior axis) and flatten the diaphragm. An emphysema patient may also have a barrel-shaped chest.

Pulmonary Function Testing

The pulmonary function test (PFT) used to distinguish obstructive from restrictive disease is the *FEV1/FVC ratio* (forced expiratory volume in one second divided by forced vital capacity). FVC is the amount of air that can be forcefully expired after a maximal inspiration. FEV1 is how much air one gets out in the first second during this task. If a *normal* person tries to force all of the air out of the lungs, a little remains, known as the *residual volume*; one just cannot get it all out no matter how hard one tries. This is because at a certain point in expiration, the intrathoracic pressure exceeds the pressure in the airways, and the airways collapse. This airway collapse normally causes some residual volume to be left in the lungs.

Pulmonary Function Tests in Emphysema

Fig. 2-2. FEV1/FVC ratio in obstructive lung disease. With floppy emphysematous lungs, one cannot exhale as much in the first second as a normal healthy person can. So FEV1 goes down. Although there is *increased residual volume* in obstructive disease because of difficulty getting rid of air, most of the air can eventually be expired, just very slooooowwwwllllly. So if the top number goes down and the bottom one essentially stays the same, the FEV1/FVC ratio will *decrease. In emphysema the FEV1 is decreased and the FVC is the same or decreased (though less so than FEV1), leading to a **decrease** in FEV1/FVC ratio.* A decreased FEV1/FVC ratio is the hallmark PFT finding in obstructive lung disease.

The destruction of alveolar walls in emphysema leads to reduced surface area for oxygen uptake. A test called the *diffusion capacity of the lungs for carbon monoxide* (DLCO) measures diffusion of carbon monoxide across the alveolar membrane, assessing overall diffusion capacity of the lungs. DLCO *decreases* in emphysema. Note that in other obstructive lung diseases where there is *no* alveolar destruction (e.g., asthma), DLCO will *not* decrease. Only the decreased FEV1/FVC ratio is present in *all* obstructive lung diseases.

Smoking is the most common cause of emphysema. A rarer genetic cause, *alpha-1 antitrypsin deficiency*, should be considered in a non-smoker who develops emphysema. Liver disease (cirrhosis) can also develop in alpha-1 antitrypsin deficiency. Here is a logical way of remembering the different pathologic findings between alpha1-antitrypsin emphysema and smoking-induced emphysema: if a gene is missing *in every cell in the lungs* as is the case in alpha-1 antitrypsin

deficiency, do you expect the lungs to be destroyed focally or all over? All over. This is known as *panlobular (panacinar)* emphysema, which is seen in alpha-1 antitrypsin deficiency-induced emphysema. Emphysema from smoking mostly destroys the lungs *nearer where the smoke enters* (i.e., adjacent to the airways that bring the smoke in), thus *centrilobular emphysema* is the characteristic pathologic finding of smoking-related emphysema.

Chronic Bronchitis

In chronic bronchitis, the airways clog with mucus, causing resistance to airflow. Imagine blowing through a toilet paper tube: easy. Now imagine filling it with wads of wet paper towels until the lumen is practically obliterated: difficult. This is what is going on in the lungs in chronic bronchitis. Airways are filled with mucus plugs that *obstruct* expiration. Since the main pathophysiologic process here is *obstruction*, the FEV1 will be decreased and so the FEV1/ FVC ratio will go *down,* just like in emphysema. Emphysema and chronic bronchitis are both called COPD: their underlying pathophysiology is obstructive, and this is reflected in their similar PFT findings.

Smoking is the main cause of chronic bronchitis. Some patients have features of both chronic bronchitis and emphysema. These patients usually have some degree of shortness of breath on exertion, since pulmonary function is impaired. However, respiratory infection can lead to a COPD *flare* in which the patient gets acutely worse. This is due to an increase in obstruction, which results in increased breathing difficulty.

Asthma

In asthma, another type of obstructive lung disease, the airways are *hyper-reactive*. Possible triggers of this hyper-reactive response include allergens, cold air, and exercise. Hyper-reactivity refers to the fact that the airways are more likely to constrict in response to these stimuli. Just as with other causes of obstruction, these patients can have hyper-expansion, wheezing, prolonged expiratory phase, accessory muscle recruitment, and reduced FEV1. *The difference between asthma and COPD is that asthma is **reversible** bronchoconstriction*: the patient and PFTs improve after the exacerbation ends (usually

$$\text{OBSTRUCTIVE LUNG DISEASE} \longrightarrow \frac{FEV_1 \Downarrow}{FVC \longleftrightarrow} = FEV_1 / FVC \text{ ratio} \downarrow$$

THE FEV1/FVC RATIO IN OBSTRUCTIVE LUNG DISEASE

Figure 2-2

with treatment), and the patient can breathe normally again. With the other obstructive diseases (i.e., chronic bronchitis and emphysema), there is a *chronic* decrease in lung function, which worsens further in acute exacerbations. As in emphysema, patients having an asthma exacerbation breathe at high lung volumes due to the obstruction, and can thus fatigue the respiratory muscles to the point of respiratory failure, sometimes requiring intubation and mechanical ventilation.

When examining a patient having an asthma flare, *pulsus paradoxus* may be noted. During the flare, increased lung volumes lead to very high negative pressures in the chest, causing more venous return to get "sucked in." This increased venous return can be dramatic enough to distend the right ventricle to the point of compressing the left ventricle, thus affecting left ventricular outflow. Left ventricular outflow is the source of the peripheral circulation (and hence the pulse). So when feeling the pulse of a patient having an asthma attack, one can feel decreased peripheral pulses during inspiration (*pulsus paradoxus*). Pulsus paradoxus can also occur in cardiac tamponade.

Treatment of Asthma and COPD Flare. How would you help a patient with COPD (or asthma) during a flare? There are two processes that you can correct: *closed airways* and *inflammation*. To open the airways, you must affect the pulmonary sympathetic and/or parasympathetic nervous systems.

The sympathetic nervous system is for fight or flight, the parasympathetic nervous system is for rest and digest. If you were about to fight (or flee from) a tiger, you would want your heart to beat fast to pump blood to your muscles for the strength to fight (or run away), your airways to be wide open so you could get enough oxygen, your eyes to open wide (pupillary dilation) to see the tiger, and your bowels and bladder to pause for a moment (i.e., no pit stops while you're running away).

The parasympathetic nervous system does the opposite: slows the heart, constricts the airways, constricts the pupils, and stimulates digestion, bowel movements, and urination. Though it does not exactly fit into this logical framework, the parasympathetic system mediates penile erection, and the sympathetic system mediates ejaculation.

Fig. 2-3. Bronchodilation. Back to the airways: The *sympathetic system opens* the airways and the *parasympathetic system constricts them*. So in an asthma or COPD flare where we want to *open* the airways, we need to *stimulate the sympathetic* system and/or *inhibit the parasympathetic* system. *Sympathetic* stimulation in the lungs works through beta-2 receptors, so you would want *agonists* of these receptors, e.g., albuterol. The *parasympathetic* system in the lungs works through acetylcholine, so you would want to *inhibit* this with anticholinergics, such as ipratropium.

When would you *not* want to use a beta agonist to open the airways? Recall that beta *blockers* are used in certain arrhythmias and also to slow the heart so as to decrease its energy needs when a patient has angina. Giving a beta-agonist to a patient who needs beta-blockers is obviously quite a bad idea, because

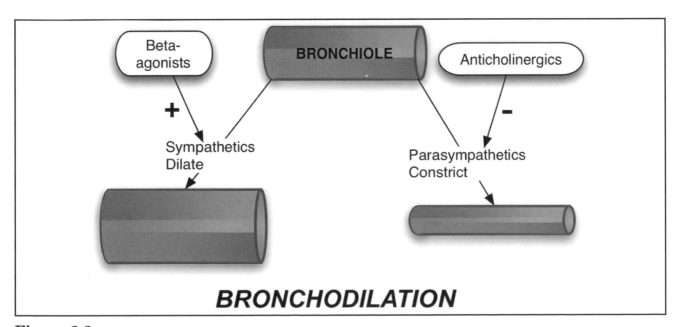

Figure 2-3

these beta agonists can increase heart rate, thus worsening angina.

As for treating the inflammation, steroids such as prednisone can decrease this component of the flare. Since infection is thought to contribute to flares in COPD patients, antibiotics are sometimes used in the treatment of an acute COPD flare.

Cystic Fibrosis

Cystic fibrosis is another cause of obstructive lung disease. Cystic fibrosis is caused by a mutation in the CFTR (cystic fibrosis transmembrane conductance regulator) protein, an epithelial cell chloride transporter found in exocrine glands. The defective gene is inherited in an autosomal recessive pattern. The problem with chloride transport leads to water flow abnormalities, causing secretions to become more viscous. These viscous secretions in the lungs can cause obstruction, which predisposes to pulmonary infection. Repeated infection and consequent inflammation lead to COPD. Viscous mucus in cystic fibrosis can also cause pancreatic insufficiency (resulting in malabsorption and, in some cases, diabetes), biliary obstruction, and intestinal obstruction.

Symptoms/signs can include: delayed passage of meconium (the first stool in infancy), floating foul-smelling stools (from the malabsorption of fats), failure to thrive, cough, recurrent pulmonary infections, and dyspnea.

Diagnosis is confirmed by a chloride sweat test, which will show an elevated level of chloride in the sweat. Treatment involves drugs that break down the thick mucus (DNAse enzyme, called *dornase* or *Pulmozyme*), bronchodilators, regular percussion of the back and chest to help clear secretions, antibiotic treatment of infection, replacement of pancreatic enzymes, and dietary supplements to remedy malabsorption. If the lungs are severely damaged, lung transplant may be necessary.

Bronchiectasis

Bronchiectasis, abnormal dilatation of a bronchus, can occur congenitally or secondary to any infection that leads to inflammation and destruction of the airway. The recurrent infections of cystic fibrosis are a common cause of bronchiectasis. The dilated airways are easily collapsible, and thus bronchiectasis can be considered a chronic obstructive pulmonary disease. Patients with bronchiectasis may be asymptomatic, or may have intermittent symptoms related to infections, including cough, production of purulent, foul-smelling sputum, and/or hemoptysis (coughing up blood). Antibiotics are used to treat infections, and surgical resection of the affected lung lobe may be necessary in certain cases if antibiotic treatment fails or if there is excessive hemoptysis.

Restrictive Lung Disease

Restrictive lung disease can occur if the lungs are stiff (fibrotic disease), if the chest wall is stiff, or if the respiratory muscles are weak. Any of these can prevent adequate lung expansion. The causes of restrictive lung disease include:

1. **Stiff lungs**, i.e., interstitial lung disease secondary to:
   - pneumoconiosis, e.g., to asbestos, beryllium, silicon, etc.
   - hypersensitivity pneumonitis ("farmer's lung," "bird breeder's lung," chemical exposure)
   - connective tissue disorder: scleroderma, rheumatoid arthritis, lupus, myositis
   - drug toxicity: amiodarone, bleomycin, methotrexate, radiation
   - other: idiopathic pulmonary fibrosis, sarcoid, bronchiolitis obliterans organizing pneumonia (BOOP), eosinophilic granuloma

2. **Stiff chest wall**: kyphoscoliosis, ankylosing spondylitis, obesity

3. **Respiratory muscle weakness**: Guillain-Barré, amyotrophic lateral sclerosis (ALS), multiple sclerosis, muscular dystrophies, myasthenia gravis, spinal cord injury

In restrictive lung disease due to stiff lungs, the alveolar walls become thick and inflexible (in contrast to becoming weak and flimsy as occurs in emphysema). What would this do to airflow? (1) The stiff alveoli contract more quickly and more forcefully, and (2) stiff airways are less likely to collapse. So lungs with restrictive disease are "too good" at getting rid of their air because they are stiff, and snap back to their original shape instead of relaxing back to it. In contrast to increased residual volume seen in COPD patients, patients with restrictive disease generally have *decreased* residual volume.[1] At first this may not seem so bad, but if the lungs get too stiff, it is hard to take a good deep breath (or even a good normal breath).

Pulmonary Function Tests in Restrictive Lung Disease

Fig. 2-4. FEV1/FVC ratio in restrictive lung disease. Restriction of the lungs decreases total lung capacity (TLC), so both FEV1 and FVC are reduced in restrictive lung disease. If both FEV1 and FVC decrease proportionally, the FEV1/FVC ratio remains normal. However, in some instances of restrictive lung disease, FEV1 can decrease *less* than FVC because the in-

---

[1] There is an exception to this: in restrictive disease caused by respiratory muscle weakness, expiratory muscles can be affected. If *expiratory* muscles are weak, full exhalation cannot take place, and residual volume increases.

$$\text{RESTRICTIVE LUNG DISEASE} \longrightarrow \frac{FEV_1 \downarrow}{FVC \downarrow(\downarrow)} = FEV_1 / FVC \text{ ratio} \longleftrightarrow \text{ or } \uparrow$$

(Total lung capacity decreases)

FEV1/FVC RATIO IN RESTRICTIVE LUNG DISEASE

Figure 2-4

creased elastic recoil of stiff lungs or a stiff chest wall can preserve some of the force of the FEV1. If the FEV1 decreases less than the FVC, the FEV1/FVC ratio can be *greater* than normal. Thus, the FEV1/FVC *ratio* in restrictive disease either *increases* or *remains normal.*

If restrictive disease occurs secondary to pulmonary fibrosis (see causes above), this leads to a thick alveolar membrane, resulting in a *diffusion defect*. At rest this might not be a problem, but the patient can have severe drops in blood oxygenation with exercise or even with mild activity, depending on the severity of disease. Pulmonary fibrosis leads to a marked *decrease* in diffusion. A decreased DLCO is a hallmark of pulmonary fibrotic disease.

Symptoms and Signs of Restrictive Lung Disease

Patients with restrictive disease can become very short of breath because of the increased work necessary to open the lungs. Accessory muscles may be recruited to help inhale (e.g., sternocleidomastoid) during inspiration. What might you hear on auscultation of a patient with restrictive lung disease? *Crackles* are the sounds of the stiff alveoli popping open. They sound like velcro under the stethoscope.

Treatment of Restrictive Lung Disease

Treatment of restrictive lung disease is directed toward the underlying etiology. In fibrosis secondary to inflammatory lung disease, steroids are generally used to reduce inflammation.

Review of Obstructive and Restrictive Lung Disease

Starting from the simple anatomical understanding that the lungs contain airways that end in alveoli, alveolar membranes, and blood vessels, we can develop a framework for thinking about pathologies of the lung by considering how these different components are affected. The role of the alveoli is to fill with O_2 (which passes across the alveolar membrane) and release CO_2. If the alveoli clog with pus, blood, or fluid, these functions decrease.

If the airways are obstructed, the alveoli cannot contract as well, making it hard to get air *out*. This leaves the lung hyper-expanded with retained CO_2. Obstruction can occur from a foreign body, asthma (in which case the obstruction is reversible), chronic mucus plugging (chronic bronchitis, cystic fibrosis), or destruction of the alveolar membrane leading to floppy collapsible airways (emphysema). Chronic bronchitis and emphysema are known as COPD and can occur either separately or together, often in smokers. Emphysema can also occur in alpha-1 antitrypsin deficiency. (The pathology in alpha-1 antitrypsin deficiency is panlobular, as opposed to centrilobular in smoking-induced emphysema). In COPD, the PFTs show a *decreased FEV1* (the amount of air that can be blown out in 1 second — think of those floppy alveoli slowly contracting against high resistance/collapsed airways), but with *normal or decreased FVC*. This leads to a *decreased FEV1/FVC ratio* in obstructive lung disease. These patients breathe at high lung volumes, can end up retaining CO_2, and can demonstrate wheezing, prolonged expiratory phase, and/or accessory muscle use on physical exam, and hyper-expansion on chest X-ray. Pulmonary obstruction also occurs in asthma, leading to similar symptoms, signs, and PFTs. In asthma, however, the changes in pulmonary function are *reversible*.

In restrictive lung disease, it is hard to get air *in*. The causes include intrinsic lung disease, any cause of a stiff chest wall, or respiratory muscle weakness. Restrictive lung disease leads to a decrease in total lung capacity, but FEV1 can decrease less than FVC, resulting in an *increased or normal FEV1/FVC ratio*. If the cause is pulmonary fibrosis, a diffusion defect can also occur, due to thickening of the alveolar membrane. This manifests as a decrease in DLCO and can cause insufficient blood oxygenation with exercise or even mild activity, depending on the extent of disease. The opening of stiff air sacs sounds like crackles on auscultation.

PULMONARY HYPERTENSION

Pulmonary hypertension is an increase of pressure in the pulmonary vasculature.

Causes of Pulmonary Hypertension

Fig. 2-5. Causes of pulmonary hypertension. Pulmonary hypertension can arise from problems in the left heart, right heart, or the pulmonary vasculature itself. The *left heart could have decreased forward flow*, causing a backup into the pulmonary system, e.g., heart failure, valvular dysfunction, cardiomyopathy, arrhythmia. For the right heart to be responsible for increased pulmonary pressure, there would have to be an *increase in flow from the right heart,* e.g., ventricular septal defect (see Chapter 1) or any other significant left-to-right shunt. Problems with the *pulmonary vasculature* itself (e.g., vasculitis, primary pulmonary hypertension) or problems that affect the lung architecture such that vessels are secondarily compressed (e.g., interstitial lung diseases) can also lead to pulmonary hypertension.

Additionally, *hypoxic vasoconstriction* can cause pulmonary hypertension. If there is an area of the lung that is not receiving much oxygen (e.g., one filled with pus from pneumonia), it is in the lung's best interest to shunt blood *away* from this area to a region of lung where it is more likely to be oxygenated. Hypoxic vasoconstriction accomplishes this: In areas of the lung where oxygen tension is low, the blood vessels constrict so blood will go elsewhere. When there is one area of isolated hypoxia, you can see how this mechanism would be helpful. But if the *whole* lung suffers from hypoxia (e.g., high altitude, COPD, hypoventilation from restrictive diseases of the lungs/chest wall/muscles), then all of the blood vessels of the pulmonary vasculature perceive hypoxia, and they will *all* constrict. This is obviously maladaptive, and can result in pulmonary hypertension.

So the origin of pulmonary hypertension is either *pulmonary* (i.e., disease in the vessels themselves or pulmonary disease that secondarily affect the vessels) or *cardiac*. Cardiac causes of pulmonary hypertension are *backup from the left heart* or *increased flow from the right heart*.

Pulmonary hypertension creates extra resistance for the right heart, since the right heart pumps into the pulmonary vascular system. If uncorrected, this can lead to right-sided hypertrophy and failure (*cor pulmonale*).

RESPIRATORY INFECTIONS

Smoking causes inflammation and decreased mucociliary function in the respiratory tract. It predisposes to any of the infections listed below, and smoking cessation contributes to speedier recovery from these infections.

Fig. 2-6. Sites of respiratory infections.

Rhinitis

Rhinitis, inflammation of the nasal mucosa, can be *allergic* ("hay fever," in response to pollen, dust, animals) or *infectious* ("the common cold" usually adenovirus, rhinovirus). The symptoms/signs include stuffed nose, rhinorrhea ("runny nose"), sneezing, cough, sore throat, etc. Since infectious rhinitis is self-limited, treatment is generally geared towards relieving symptoms (e.g., antihistamines, pseudoephedrine, nasal steroids). Allergic rhinitis is also treated symptomatically, along with reduction of exposure to allergen. In severe cases of allergic rhinitis, desensitization via immunotherapy ("allergy shots") may be considered.

Sinusitis

Sinusitis is inflammation of the sinuses. If mucus outflow from the sinuses becomes impaired, the mucus trapped in the sinuses can create an environment that facilitates bacterial growth, leading to sinusitis. Most commonly, mucus outflow becomes impaired by inflammation, and

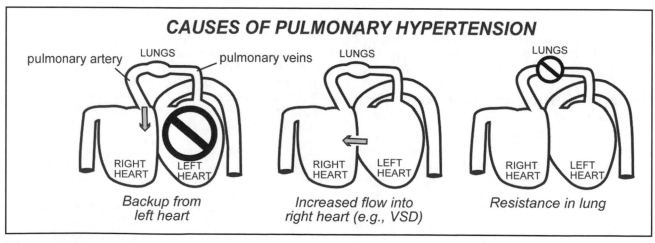

CAUSES OF PULMONARY HYPERTENSION

pulmonary artery — LUNGS — pulmonary veins — LUNGS — LUNGS

RIGHT HEART LEFT HEART — *Backup from left heart*

RIGHT HEART LEFT HEART — *Increased flow into right heart (e.g., VSD)*

RIGHT HEART LEFT HEART — *Resistance in lung*

Figure 2-5

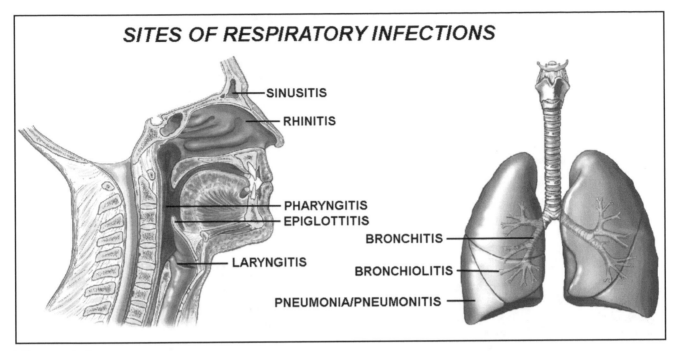

Figure 2-6

swelling resulting from an upper respiratory infection. However, predisposition to sinusitis can occur with any cause of sinus inflammation (e.g., allergic rhinitis) and/or obstruction (e.g., nasogastric/nasotracheal tubes, nasal polyps, anatomical abnormality such as a deviated septum). The most common causes of sinusitis are *Streptococcus pneumoniae, Hemophilus influenzae,* and *Branhamella (Moraxella) catarrhalis*. Symptoms include rhinitis symptoms (which may have gone away and returned), foul-smelling mucus, pain/pressure around the eyes and cheeks (especially when leaning forward, which increases pressure on the sinuses), and headache. Treatment is aimed at relieving obstruction with nasal spray decongestants (e.g., oxymetazoline or phenylephrine), treating the infection with antibiotics, and treating allergies, if present. In chronic sinusitis (greater than 3 months), surgical relief of obstruction may be necessary if other treatments are unsuccessful.

Pharyngitis

Pharyngitis, inflammation of the pharynx, can be caused by viruses (adenovirus, rhinovirus, parainfluenza virus, and many others) or bacteria (Group A beta-hemolytic streptococci, *N. gonorrhoeae, C. diphtheriae, H. influenzae, Moraxella catarrhalis*). Symptoms include sore throat, fever, and other signs of infection (malaise, chills, etc.). Signs may include cervical adenopathy, enlarged tonsils with or without exudates, and pharyngeal erythema. Although tonsillar exudates (white patches on the throat) are popularly thought to

distinguish viral from bacterial pharyngitis, they can be present with either etiology. The causative organism is determined by throat culture, and appropriate antibiotic treatment for this organism is initiated. Untreated group A beta hemolytic streptococcus pharyngitis can lead to rheumatic fever (see Chapter 1).

Laryngitis

Laryngitis, inflammation of the larynx, can be caused by vocal strain, GERD (gastroesophageal reflux disease), or viral infection (rhinovirus, adenovirus, influenza, and many more). Symptoms include hoarseness and any upper respiratory infection (URI) symptoms. Viral cases are self-limited, vocal strain requires vocal rest, and GERD-induced pharyngitis requires treatment of GERD. Prolonged hoarseness by itself requires a search for an underlying cause such as a neurological/neuromuscular disorder or neoplasia compressing the recurrent laryngeal nerve (e.g., head/neck cancer or vocal cord polyp).

Epiglottitis

Epiglottitis is inflammation of the epiglottis. Most commonly caused by *Hemophilus influenza* B, epiglottitis is rarely seen in the U.S. today because of vaccination against this organism. It is most commonly seen in young children. An inflamed epiglottis can lead to drooling (failure to clear secretions), respiratory distress, stridor (a high-pitched inspiratory sound), a muffled voice, and a classic posture: sitting forward with neck extended to ease breathing ("tripoding"). Pharyngeal exam should be avoided in patients with suspected epiglottitis because it can precipitate spasm, resulting in sudden airway closure. Antibiotics are used to treat the infection. Patients must be monitored closely; tracheal intubation may be necessary if respiratory failure appears imminent.

Bronchitis

Bronchitis is inflammation of the bronchi. *Chronic* bronchitis, a type of COPD, is discussed above. *Acute* bronchitis is typically viral (rhinovirus, respiratory syncytial virus, adenovirus, influenza virus, parainfluenza virus). Cough and other upper respiratory symptoms are typically present. Although viral bronchitis typically resolves spontaneously, the cough itself can be palliated by anti-tussives (e.g., Robitussin) and/or bronchodilators.

Bronchiolitis

Bronchiolitis is inflammation of the bronchioles. This typically occurs in infants and is most commonly caused by respiratory syncytial virus (RSV). It can also be caused by adenovirus, influenza virus, and parainfluenza virus. Symptoms can range from typical upper respiratory symptoms to symptoms of respiratory distress (wheezing, nasal flaring, tachypnea, tachycardia, etc.). Treatment is supportive and depends on severity (oxygen, fluids, and/or mechanical ventilation if necessary). Treatment with the antiviral ribavirin is controversial.

Pneumonitis

Pneumonitis refers to *inflammation* of the lungs rather than infection. Such inflammation can be due to radiation, chemical inhalation (e.g., in factories, or from chlorine, pesticides, etc.), or hypersensitivity to an environmental antigen (e.g., "farmer's lung" from moldy hay, "bird breeder's lung," etc.). Acute hypersensitivity pneumonitis can present as cough, dyspnea, malaise, and/or fever 4-6 hours after exposure. Chronic and/or recurrent exposure to toxins can lead to pulmonary fibrosis, causing restrictive lung disease.

Pneumonia

Pneumonia is an infection of the lung parenchyma, and can be viral, bacterial, or fungal. Pathogens can reach the lungs from inhalation/aspiration or from hematogenous spread from other sites of infection in the body. Aspiration pneumonia occurs when vomit or food particles are inhaled, for example during alcohol/drug intoxication, trauma, seizure, stroke, or other loss of consciousness. Aspiration can also lead to the subacute formation of a pulmonary abscess (area of necrosis in lung) or empyema (pus in the pleural space).

Streptococcus pneumoniae is the most common cause of pneumonia, though many other bacteria (including *Staphylococcus aureus, Hemophilus influenzae, Chlamydia pneumoniae, Moraxella catarrhalis, Legionella pneumophila, Klebsiella pneumoniae, Mycoplasma pneumoniae, Coxiella burnetii*) and viruses (including RSV, parainfluenza, and influenza) can also cause pneumonia. Fungal pneumonia (e.g., *Pneumocystis carinii, Cryptococcus neoformans, Aspergillus fumigatus*) can occur in immunocompromised patients (e.g., patients with HIV, patients undergoing chemotherapy).

Symptoms/signs of pneumonia include fever, cough (usually productive of sputum), chest and/or abdominal pain, and, if there is an area of consolidation (which most commonly occurs in bacterial pneumonia), dullness to percussion, egophony, and decreased breath sounds.

Chest X-ray findings in pneumonia. Bacterial pneumonias tend to affect one lobe of the lung, appearing as a region of consolidation on X-ray, while viral and fungal pneumonias tend to produce more diffuse interstitial patterns.

Treatment of pneumonia involves antibiotics for the offending organism and respiratory support if necessary.

Tuberculosis (TB)

Mycobacterium tuberculosis can affect any organ system, causing pneumonia, tuberculous osteomyelitis, meningitis, pericarditis, adrenal tuberculosis, and/or renal tuberculosis. *Miliary* TB refers to widespread TB infection. Exposure to TB is generally through inhalation. Inhaled droplets can cause a primary infection presenting as pneumonia, for example, in children, elderly, and immunocompromised patients (e.g., HIV/AIDS). More often, initial infection remains asymptomatic; tuberculosis bacteria are contained in granulomas in the lung (tubercles), which can calcify (*Ghon focus*). A *Ghon complex* is the presence of a Ghon focus plus calcified granulomas(s) in perihilar lymph nodes. These may be seen on X-ray. Aside from the radiologic signs, latent asymptomatic TB infection may be identified by PPD (purified protein derivative) testing. A PPD is the injection of protein antigens from killed TB. If an individual has been exposed to TB, an immune response will occur, causing an area of induration at the site of injection. Once exposed, patients may remain asymptomatic for long periods, with about a 5% chance per year of progressing to reactivation or secondary TB (the risk in immunocompromised patients is about 10%/year). Symptoms of reactivation TB can include cough, hemoptysis, and constitutional symptoms such as fever, weight loss, and/or night sweats. Additionally, any of the organ systems mentioned above may be affected. Treatment includes isoniazid, rifampin, ethambutol, and pyrazinamide.

LUNG CANCER

Lung cancer is commonly caused by smoking, though radiation and other environmental exposures (e.g., asbestos) can also increase risk of developing lung cancer. Pathologically, lung cancer is divided into *small cell lung cancer* and *non-small cell lung cancer* (large cell carcinoma, squamous cell carcinoma, and adenocarcinoma). Small cell lung cancer is its own category because it is generally more aggressive, yet also more amenable to chemotherapy, and it is also associated with certain *paraneoplastic syndromes*. A paraneoplastic syndrome occurs when a tumor causes signs/symptoms unrelated to direct effects of the tumor itself or metastases.

Lung cancer can cause pulmonary symptoms (cough, dyspnea, hemoptysis), constitutional symptoms (fever, weight loss, fatigue, night sweats), symptoms related to compression of nearby structures such as the esophagus (dysphagia), recurrent laryngeal nerve (hoarseness), superior cervical ganglion (Horner's syndrome: ptosis, miosis, anhidrosis), superior vena cava (superior vena cava syndrome: facial/arm swelling, headache orthopnea, jugular venous distension), and symptoms related to paraneoplastic syndromes. Paraneoplastic syndromes most commonly associated with small cell lung cancer include syndrome of inappropriate anti-diuretic hormone secretion (SIADH) (discussed in Chapter 3), ectopic adrenocorticotrophic hormone (ACTH) production (discussed in Chapter 5), and Lambert-Eaton Syndrome, a myasthenia gravis-like syndrome (discussed in Chapter 7). Squamous cell carcinomas of the lung can release parathyroid hormone-related protein (PTHrP), causing hypercalcemia. Other squamous cell carcinomas of the head and neck can also release PTHrP. PTHrP is discussed in Chapter 5.

Treatment of lung cancer involves surgery, chemotherapy, and radiation, and depends upon the stage of the disease as determined by tumor size, local extent, lymph node involvement, and distant metastasis.

DISEASES OF THE PLEURA AND PLEURAL SPACE

The lungs are covered by a thin membrane, the pleura, which has two layers: one lines the lungs; the other lines the chest wall, with a space between them called the pleural cavity. Pathologically, the pleura can become inflamed (*pleuritis / pleurisy*) and an effusion can occur in the pleural cavity (*pleural effusion*).

Pleuritis (Pleurisy)

Pleuritis (also called pleurisy) is inflammation of the pleura. Pleuritis can be caused by pulmonary infection, hematogenous spread of infection to the pleura, penetrating chest trauma, esophageal rupture, asbestos, neoplastic cells, or inflammatory disease.

Pleuritic pain is a sharp, stabbing chest pain that is made worse by breathing in or coughing. It is caused by the inflamed portions of the pleura rubbing against each other. Although it is characteristic of pleural inflammation, it can also be caused by other pulmonary pathology such as pulmonary embolus, pneumonia, or lung cancer. A *pleural friction rub*, though only rarely heard on auscultation, is diagnostic of pleuritis. Pleural friction rub is a grating sound that persists through the entire respiratory cycle.

Although aspirin can relieve the pain of pleuritis, treatment of the underlying cause is necessary.

Inflammation of the pleura usually leads to a *pleural effusion*, fluid in the pleural space.

Pleural Effusion

Pleural effusions are classified as either *transudates* or *exudates*. *Trans*udates (hydrothorax) are accumulations of fluid arising from fluid excess alone with no change in vascular permeability, while *ex*udates are caused by inflammatory conditions that increase vascular permeability. Thus, exudates tend to have a higher content of protein, cells, and/or solid materials than transudates. A transudate can be caused by congestive heart failure, cirrhosis, nephrotic syndrome, or hypoalbuminemia. Exudates can be caused by any of the causes of pleuritis (e.g., infection, neoplasia, inflammatory disease, asbestosis) as well as uremia or pancreatitis. *Light's criteria* state that the fluid is exudative if any of the following are met: pleural fluid protein/serum protein ratio > .5, pleural fluid LDH/serum LDH > .6, or pleural fluid LDH level > 2/3 upper limit for serum LDH. The first criterion demonstrates the inflammatory nature of exudates, since the increased vascular permeability leads to a higher concentration of protein in the pleural fluid than would be caused by a transudate. LDH is an indicator of inflammation, and is thus more highly elevated in exudates.

Empyema, pus in the pleural space, can be a complication of pneumonia, or it can be caused by penetrating chest trauma or esophageal rupture.

A pleural effusion can cause dyspnea, pleuritic chest pain, and/or a pleural friction rub. The accumulation of fluid between the lung and the chest wall leads to dullness on percussion and decreased/absent breath sounds. Chest radiograph will reveal an opacity that may hide the angle of the diaphragm (*blunting of the costophrenic angle*).

Thoracentesis to remove the fluid is necessary for diagnosis and as a therapeutic measure. The fluid can be analyzed for infectious organisms, malignant cells, inflammatory cells, and other clues to an underlying etiology.

Chylothorax, Hemothorax, and Pneumothorax

Lymph in the pleural space (*chylothorax*) can be caused by trauma to or obstruction of the thoracic duct. Blood in the pleural space (*hemothorax*) can occur from trauma or ruptured aortic aneurysm.

Pneumothorax is air in the pleural space, and can be spontaneous, iatrogenic, or traumatic. Spontaneous pneumothorax occurs from rupture of an alveolus. This can occur secondary to any underlying pulmonary disease or idiopathically. Idiopathic spontaneous pneumothorax occurs more commonly in tall young people. Iatrogenic pneumothorax refers to introduction of air into the pleural space during mechanical ventilation, or from procedures such as thoracentesis, central line placement, or lung biopsy, where the lung may be punctured. Traumatic pneumothorax can occur from a penetrating chest wound or rib fracture puncturing the lung. Pneumothorax can cause chest pain and/or dyspnea, or it can be asymptomatic, if small. Physical exam may reveal decreased breath sounds and increased resonance to percussion. On chest X-ray, pneumothorax appears as a line or pocket of radiolucency (darkness) between the lung and the chest wall. Smaller pneumothoraces may resolve spontaneously, whereas larger ones may require removal of the air by syringe aspiration or chest tube placement.

A *tension pneumothorax* occurs when air enters the pleural space but cannot exit, for example from a penetrating chest wound. A tension pneumothorax can collapse the lung on the affected side and cause compression of mediastinal structures, which can be fatal. Symptoms and signs are similar to those discussed above for pneumothorax, and can also include absent breath sounds on the affected side, hypotension, and jugular venous distension. Quick removal of air with a large bore needle is usually curative.

PULMONARY PHYSICAL EXAM

Percussion

Tap a drum and you get a nice hollow, resonant sound. Tap a brick and you get a dull thud. By analogy, if you tap a lung filled with air (as it should be), you hear a nice hollow, resonant sound. If you tap a lung filled with fluid or pus, you hear a dull thud. What would make the lung sound hyper-resonant (more resonant than usual) to percussion? Hyper-resonance to percussion must mean that there is more air than usual. This can occur in asthma or COPD from hyper-expansion/air trapping. Hyper-resonance can also occur with a pneumothorax, since the thorax is filled with air surrounding the lung.

Fremitus, Egophony, and Pectoriloquy

Solids and liquids conduct sound better than air. Fremitus, egophony, and whisper pectoriloquy take advantage of this phenomenon. Tactile fremitus is when one feels the vibrations on a patient's back as the patient speaks. To assess egophony, one asks the patient to say "e" (as in eat) and listens through the stethoscope to hear whether it sounds like "a" (as in say or bay). Whisper pectoriloquy is when one asks the patient to whisper a phrase and listens to the patient's back through a stethoscope. What do these have in common? All of them test how well the lungs and thorax conduct sound. Since a normal lung is filled with air, and since air does not conduct sound so well, whispering and speaking should be faintly audible and faintly vibratory to the touch, respectively, and saying "e" should sound like "e." If there is edema fluid or consolidation (e.g., pus in pneumonia), that area of the lung will be more solid than air-filled lung, and so it will conduct sound better. *If the lung is filled with something other than air, it will be dull to percussion, have increased vibration felt on tactile fremitus, have increased audibility of whisper pectoriloquy, and have conversion of "e" to "a" (egophony).*

Clubbing

Clubbing is the swelling of the fingertips, leading to reduction in the angle between the nail and the nail bed. Clubbing can be caused by many pulmonary diseases. It is not known exactly why this occurs. Other causes can include cyanotic heart disease, malignancy, inflammatory bowel disease and genetic primary clubbing disorders (e.g., pachydermoperiostosis, familial clubbing).

CHAPTER 3. THE RENAL SYSTEM

OVERVIEW OF KIDNEY FUNCTION

Roles of the kidneys:

- *Filtration of the blood*
  - *— to remove wastes*
  - *— to maintain appropriate concentrations of electrolytes*
  - *— to maintain acid / base balance*

- *Regulation of blood volume and blood pressure*

- *Activation of vitamin D* (to 1,25-dihydroxy-vitamin D3; the hydroxy in the 25 position comes from the liver and the hydroxy in the 1 position from the kidneys)

- *Production of erythropoietin*

If the kidneys fail, there can be an increase of wastes in the circulation, disequilibrium of fluids and electrolytes, decreased activation of vitamin D (which can result in decreased calcium absorption and subsequent hypocalcemia), and/or decreased erythropoietin (which can lead to anemia).

ACUTE RENAL FAILURE

Fig. 3-1. Classification of acute renal failure. The kidneys get blood from the renal arteries, filter the blood, reabsorb some substances back into the blood, and excrete wastes as urine. Urine travels through the collecting system into the ureters then to the bladder, where it is stored until it passes through the urethra to the outside world.

If the cause of renal failure is a decrease in *blood supply* to the kidneys (renal perfusion), this is called *prerenal failure.*

If the cause of renal failure is a problem *within the kidneys,* this is *intrinsic renal failure.*

Postrenal failure is due to a problem in the *collecting system* (ureters/bladder/urethra), e.g., obstruction by stones or tumor.

Prerenal Failure

In prerenal failure, the kidneys do not get an adequate blood supply, and thus cannot adequately filter the blood. Any circumstance that can cause decreased blood volume (*hypovolemia*) can lead to deceased renal flow (e.g., hemorrhage, dehydration). Atherosclerotic disease of the renal arteries can also decrease flow to one or both kidneys.

Another cause of prerenal failure is *effective volume depletion.* This is when the kidneys are not adequately perfused despite the fact that the blood volume is *not*

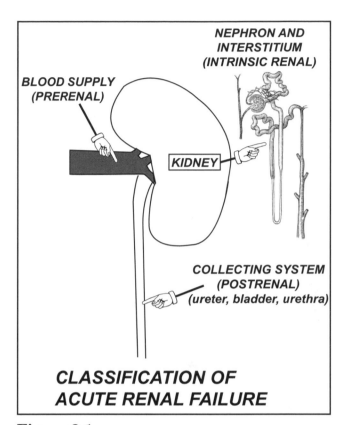

Figure 3-1

actually depleted (in fact it is increased in some instances). Two examples of effective volume depletion are congestive heart failure and cirrhosis. In congestive heart failure, the heart does not pump adequately, leading to *decreased renal perfusion.* Cirrhosis is scarring of the liver that can impede blood flow through the hepatic portal system, causing portal hypertension. Due to this blockage in the venous return, blood pools in the gut's venous system. Again, the *effective* blood volume that reaches the kidneys decreases, because a large volume of the body's blood supply stagnates in the mesenteric veins. This decreased renal perfusion can result in prerenal failure (*hepato-renal syndrome*).

So prerenal failure can occur from an actual decrease in the amount of blood reaching the kidneys (hypovolemia) or effective volume depletion (e.g., congestive heart failure or cirrhosis). An important point about prerenal failure is that the *kidneys themselves are, in principle, healthy;* if the blood supply is restored in a timely fashion, they will work again. The only problem is that the *kidneys do not receive the usual amount of blood to filter,* so they cannot do an adequate job filtering. How would the kidneys (or an individual kidney) react to low blood volume? *The kidney(s) will try to reabsorb sodium and water in an attempt to replenish intravascular volume.* This point will become important when we discuss the lab findings that are used to distinguish prerenal failure from intrinsic renal failure, namely BUN/creatinine ratio and fractional excretion of sodium (FENa). With *real* hypovolemia (e.g., hemorrhage, dehydration), increased sodium and water reabsorption is crucial for attempting to maintain blood pressure. In effective volume depletion, increased sodium and water reabsorption by the kidneys can be detrimental (see Fig. 1-6).

Intrinsic Renal Failure

The functional unit of the kidneys is the *nephron.* Each nephron contains a *glomerulus* (tuft of capillaries and filtration surface for filtering the blood), a *tubule* (for reabsorption and secretion of various ions and molecules; parts include proximal tubule, loop of Henle, distal convoluted tubule), and a *collecting duct* (further reabsorption/secretion and delivery of urine to the ureters for delivery to the bladder). The one million or so nephrons of each kidney are surrounded by an *interstitium* containing blood vessels and connective tissue.

The causes of intrinsic renal failure include diseases of the glomeruli (*glomerulopathies*) and tubules (*tubulointerstitial diseases*), both discussed in more detail below. Some causes of intrinsic renal failure have a more chronic time course (e.g., some of the glomerulopathies), while some are more acute phenomena (e.g., some of the glomerulopathies, ischemia or drug/toxin-induced damage to one or both kidneys causing *acute tubular necrosis*). In contrast to prerenal failure, in intrinsic renal failure, *one or both kidneys have been damaged and do **not** work properly.* This is important to keep in mind when using laboratory findings to diagnose the etiology of acute renal failure. In both hypovolemia (prerenal) and drug/toxin-induced renal failure (intrinsic renal), the onset of renal failure can be acute. Thus, when clinical assessment cannot distinguish between acute prerenal and acute intrinsic renal failure, laboratory tests may be helpful.

Laboratory Distinction Between Prerenal and Intrinsic Renal Failure

One of the functions of the kidneys is to filter, and the rate at which the kidneys do so is known as the *glomerular filtration rate* (GFR). Since *creatinine* is freely filtered and only small amounts are secreted, it can serve as a measure of how well the renal filtering mechanism is working. Additionally, creatinine concentration is easily measurable in the serum. If the serum creatinine level rises, this indicates that the glomerular filtration rate of this compound is inadequate, and that renal function is impaired.

Serum BUN/Creatinine Ratio. One laboratory finding that distinguishes acute prerenal from acute intrinsic renal failure is the *blood urea nitrogen (BUN) to creatinine ratio* in the *blood,* (i.e., *not* in the urine). As one or both kidneys fail (whether it is pre-, post-, or intrinsic renal failure), the ability to filter creatinine diminishes and the plasma creatinine rises. Thus, an elevated serum creatinine signifies renal failure of some sort. In prerenal failure, one or both the kidneys *"knows"* that it is not getting enough fluid, and so the kidneys reabsorb sodium and water in an attempt to increase intravascular volume to correct the perceived hypovolemia. One can imagine that *BUN is one of those other things that is also reabsorbed as part of this process[1]* and the *ratio of BUN to creatinine will be > 20:1.* In other words, in *any* type of renal failure, creatinine rises. In *prerenal* renal failure, since the kidneys fail due to either volume depletion or effective volume depletion, the kidneys go on a reabsorbing spree in an attempt to restore intravascular volume. This spree is reflected in a rise in BUN out of proportion to the rise in creatinine. Sodium reabsorption is also part of the spree, which will become important in a moment.

In *intrinsic renal* failure, the creatinine rises, but since there is *no* hypovolemia, the kidney *does not* respond by reabsorbing. Thus, the *BUN/creatinine ratio will be < 20:1.* Another way to remember this is that if the kidney is failing due to internal pathology, it cannot change what it reabsorbs anyway because it is not working properly, so it will *not* cause a disproportionate rise in BUN. This is in contrast to prerenal failure, where decreased renal perfusion causes the kidney(s) to increase reabsorption. This results in a disproportionate rise in BUN in prerenal failure. *Thus, prerenal failure: BUN/Cr > 20:1, intrinsic renal failure: BUN/Cr < 20:1.*

Urine Sodium. In prerenal failure one or both kidneys are not adequately perfused. In actual hypovolemia the kidneys observe that the volume status is low; in effective volume depletion, the kidneys "think" that volume status is low. The end result is the same: the kidneys try to increase intravascular volume by reabsorbing sodium and water. What would this do to the *urine?* If sodium and water are being reabsorbed from the tubular fluid, the urine will be *very concentrated,* but have a *low concentration of sodium* (typically less than 20 meq/L). In contrast, in a kidney failing due to internal pathology, there is *no* hypovolemia, so the kidney is not trying to hold onto anything. Also, its ability to reabsorb is diminished, and so it *wastes both water and sodium.* This leads to a *dilute* urine but an *increased excretion of sodium* in intrinsic renal failure (typically greater than 40 meq/L).

---

[1] This is not exactly what happens but it is a useful way of remembering the lab findings. Because prerenal failure increases water reabsorption in the nephron, this increases the concentration of urea left behind in the nephron. Since this increases the concentration gradient of urea from nephron to blood, urea diffuses down this concentration gradient, and serum BUN rises.

CHAPTER 3. THE RENAL SYSTEM

Fractional Excretion of Sodium (FENa). You might ask, "If the kidneys in prerenal failure hold onto sodium and water, this should make the urine quite concentrated. Wouldn't this cause the urine concentration of sodium to actually end up being *high* (due to the extremely concentrated urine) in prerenal failure? And then in intrinsic renal failure, due to the very dilute nature of the urine, shouldn't urine sodium concentration actually be *low* because the urine is so dilute?" Initially, when aldosterone is the main hormone counteracting perceived volume depletion in prerenal failure, sodium is mainly what is reabsorbed, resulting in the pattern of urine sodium concentrations discussed in the previous paragraph. Dehydration will also cause ADH (antidiuretic hormone) to be secreted from the posterior pituitary, and ADH increases *water* reabsorption. As the ADH system kicks in, the kidneys begin to actively pull *water* out of the tubular fluid. This makes the urine sodium *concentration* less reliable in determining whether the failure is prerenal or intrinsic renal because *both* urine sodium *and* water concentrations are changing. A more accurate clinical measurement is the *FENa (fractional excretion of sodium).* This measures the percent of filtered sodium that gets *excreted.*

$$FENa = \frac{\text{amount of sodium excreted}}{\text{amount of sodium filtered}} \times 100$$

$$[= (UNa \times PCr) / (PNa \times UCr) \times 100)]$$

(U = urine, P = plasma, Na = sodium, Cr = Creatinine)

In prerenal failure, the kidneys perceive a low volume state (real or effective), and thus actively reabsorb sodium to try to increase intravascular volume. Thus, of the sodium filtered, *relatively little sodium is excreted*, and so FENa in prerenal failure is quite *low* (typically less than 1%). In intrinsic renal failure, there is no volume depletion and the damaged kidney is less able to reabsorb sodium. This leads to *relatively more sodium being excreted* than in prerenal failure, which results in a higher FENa (typically higher than 2%) in intrinsic renal failure.

Fig. 3-2. Lab tests to distinguish prerenal from intrinsic renal failure. In summary, in any type of renal failure the creatinine will be elevated. If intravascular volume decreases (or in effective volume depletion), i.e., prerenal failure, the kidney tries to increase volume by

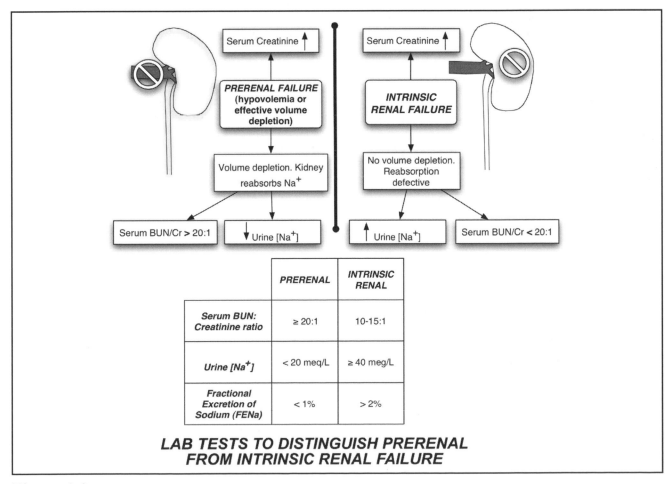

	PRERENAL	INTRINSIC RENAL
Serum BUN: Creatinine ratio	≥ 20:1	10-15:1
Urine [Na⁺]	< 20 meq/L	≥ 40 meg/L
Fractional Excretion of Sodium (FENa)	< 1%	> 2%

LAB TESTS TO DISTINGUISH PRERENAL FROM INTRINSIC RENAL FAILURE

Figure 3-2

49

holding onto salt and water, leading to a *concentrated urine* (because the body is conserving water) but a *low urine sodium concentration*. This is because part of the body's attempt to restore intravascular volume is to hold onto sodium (which water follows), and thus the urine sodium is low. As part of its reabsorption spree, imagine that the kidney holds onto BUN disproportionately more than creatinine's accumulation.

Imagine the normal kidneys as a very selective sieve, keeping certain substances and excreting others. If the kidneys fail due to an internal problem (intrinsic renal failure, e.g., acute tubular necrosis), imagine that the sieve's holes are damaged so that they are not as selective as before. Water and sodium pour through and *urine sodium concentration is high* but *the urine is dilute*. One could imagine that BUN is also spilling through the broken sieve as a way of remembering the lower BUN/Cr ratio in intrinsic renal failure.

Postrenal Failure

Postrenal refers to the ureters, bladder, and urethra. Blockage here can occur from passage of renal *stones* into the ureters, or a *tumor* in the genitourinary system (e.g., bladder, prostate) or adjacent systems (e.g., bowel, ovary). This blockage can cause renal failure. Ultrasound, CT, MRI or intravenous pyelogram can demonstrate obstruction. Any time there is obstruction of a tube, the portion of the tube proximal to the obstruction will dilate; in ureteral obstruction, ultrasound can demonstrate dilation of the ureter proximal to the site of obstruction (*hydroureter*) with dilatation of the renal pelvis (*hydronephrosis*). In acute renal failure it is prudent to rule out obstruction.

Causes of Intrinsic Renal Pathology: Diseases of Tubules and Glomeruli

Tubulointerstitial disease can be caused by drugs (e.g., antibiotics, chemotherapy agents), endogenous toxins (e.g., light chains in multiple myeloma), ischemia, immune processes (e.g., autoimmune diseases or transplant reaction), and/or infection (pyelonephritis).

The *glomerulopathies* can be divided into those causing *nephrotic* syndrome and those causing *nephritic* syndrome.

Nephrotic Syndrome

Signs of nephrotic syndrome include *edema, proteinuria* (which causes foamy urine), *hypoproteinemia*, and *hyperlipidemia*. In the glomerulopathies that cause nephrotic syndrome, there is damage to the filtering mechanism of the glomerulus, leading to protein wasting in the urine (proteinuria). This protein wasting decreases serum protein (hypoproteinemia, usually manifesting as hypoalbuminemia). The decreased serum

protein causes the intravascular fluid to be hypotonic to its surroundings (i.e., its concentration of *water* is greater than that of its surroundings). Water flows **out** of a hyp**o**tonic solution. So water will flow out of the hypotonic serum creating edema. The liver tries to increase the production of serum proteins (since they are being lost in the urine), and in so doing it also increases production of lipids, causing hyperlipidemia.

Mnemonics for the pathological findings in some of the more common causes of nephrotic syndrome:

- *Minimal change disease* has *no change* on light microscopy.[2]

- *Focal segmental glomerular sclerosis (FSGS)* has *focal segments* of glomerular pathology on light microscopy.

- *Membranous nephropathy* has thickening of capillary walls and subepithelial spikes. Mnemonic to remember this: make one word, "membranousssSpikes," and keep repeating it to yourself (membranousssSpikes membranousssSpikes membranousssSpikes).[3]

- The hallmark pathologic finding in *diabetic nephropathy* is Kimmelsteil Wilson nodules.

Nephritic Syndrome

The signs of nephritic syndrome include *hypertension, hematuria,* and *proteinuria*. Nephritic has *–iti(s)* in it, meaning inflammation. This inflammation is either due to systemic inflammatory/immune complex disease (e.g., vasculitis, lupus) or infection. Inflammation in the glomerulus leads to bleeding into the urine (*hematuria*) as well as renal vascular changes that produce hypertension.

Mnemonics for the pathological findings of some of the more common causes of nephritic syndrome:

- *Post-infectious glomerulonephritis* (usually post str**ep**: sub**ep**ithelial humps)

- *Ig A nephropathy* (**A** for mes**a**ngial deposits)

- *Membranoproliferative glomerulonephritis*: subendothelial deposits and mesangial deposits with a "tram track" appearance. Compare with membra-

---

[2] In minimal change disease, there are pathological changes seen with electron microscopy, namely effacement of the foot processes of podocytes. Podocytes are glomerular cells that normally have foot processes with spaces between them. These spaces form part of the filtration system of the glomerulus. Effacement in minimal change disease refers to the fact that the podocytes lose their foot processes, pathologically forming a continuous layer. This causes the filtration spaces between the podocytes to disappear.

[3] Do not confuse membranous nephropathy with membranoproliferative glomerulonephritis (discussed in the next section), which has different pathological findings. Remember membranoussssspikes.

nous: Membranoussssssspikes vs. Membr**ano**proliferative: sub**endo**thelial deposits.

A more complete discussion of the pathology of these entities can be found in any pathology text. This is just a quick way to remember the salient histopathological features of each disease.

Various systemic diseases can also affect the kidneys, including systemic lupus erythematosus (SLE) amyloid, Wegener's granulomatosis, scleroderma, hemolytic uremic syndrome (HUS), hypertension, and multiple myeloma.

CHRONIC RENAL FAILURE

Causes of chronic renal failure include diseases that affect either the kidneys or their blood supply, e.g., the glomerulopathies, hypertension, diabetes, SLE.

Fig. 3-3. Changes in serum chemicals in chronic renal failure. In advanced chronic renal failure, *sodium, potassium, hydrogen ion, magnesium, ammonia, and phosphate concentrations in the blood all* **increase**, *and* **calcium concentration decreases**. Sodium and water retention elevate intravascular volume, which can cause hypertension.

Why doesn't calcium accumulate like all of the other ions? Normally, the kidneys activate vitamin D (by adding the 1-OH to make 1,25-dihydroxy-vitamin D). In renal failure, vitamin D activation decreases. Without vitamin D, calcium cannot be absorbed from the diet, and the amount of calcium in the serum decreases. Thus, *calcium concentration decreases* in chronic renal failure.

Fig. 3-4. Parathyroid hormone (PTH) in chronic renal failure. Because of decreased calcium concentration in chronic renal failure, the parathyroid glands secrete parathyroid hormone in an attempt to increase blood calcium level. Increased parathyroid hormone in renal failure is called *secondary hyperparathyroidism*, since the parathyroids are hyperactive *secondary* to renal failure (see hyperparathyroidism in Chapter 5). So add parathyroid hormone to the list of things that go up in renal failure. One way that parathyroid hormone increases blood calcium is to release it from bone.

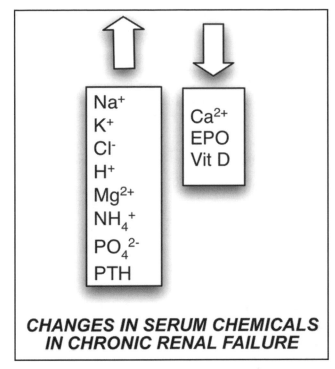

**CHANGES IN SERUM CHEMICALS
IN CHRONIC RENAL FAILURE**

Figure 3-3

Thus, bone is constantly being broken down, leading to *renal osteodystrophy*. Although this bone resorption can be asymptomatic, it can also cause weakness, bone pain, and a predisposition to fractures and tendon ruptures. In growing children with renal failure, renal osteodystrophy can result in skeletal deformities or growth retardation.

The kidneys produce erythropoietin. In renal failure, erythropoietin production decreases, which can result in decreased red blood cell (RBC) count (anemia).

If the kidneys fail, they cannot adequately excrete wastes (e.g., urea excretion to remove nitrogenous wastes from protein catabolism). Urea is one of the uremic toxins frequently examined by laboratory tests, but it is only one of the many toxins that build up. These toxins can lead to anything from fatigue,

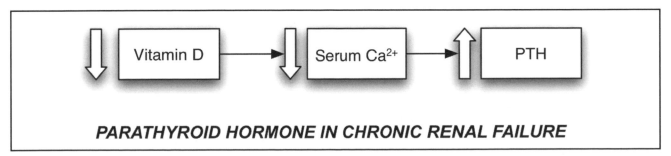

PARATHYROID HORMONE IN CHRONIC RENAL FAILURE

Figure 3-4

nausea, and mental status change to severe neurological dysfunction and coma.

URINARY TRACT INFECTION (UTI) AND URINALYSIS

Fig. 3-5. Urinary tract infection (UTI). UTI can occur anywhere in the genitourinary tract, leading to inflammation of the urethra (*urethritis*), the bladder (*cystitis*), and/or the kidneys (*pyelonephritis*). Though infectious agents can spread hematogenously to the urinary tract, most infections enter at the urethra and ascend. Ascent past the bladder to the kidneys is more likely if there is reflux of urine from the bladder back into the ureters(s) (*vesicoureteral reflux*), which can occur congenitally or due to neurologic dysfunction in the bladder (e.g., secondary to spinal cord injury or diabetic neuropathy). Other predisposing factors to UTI include catheterization, congenital anomalies of the genitourinary system, or any cause of obstruction (stones, tumor, pregnancy, enlarged prostate). Women are more prone to UTI than men, presumably because of a shorter urethra and/or urethral irritation during sexual intercourse.

Urethritis

Urethritis is commonly caused by sexual transmission of *N. gonorrhoeae* or *Chlamydia trachomatis*. Symptoms/signs include pain during urination (*dysuria*) and/or purulent urethral discharge.

Cystitis

Cystitis is typically caused by gram negative organisms (e.g., *E. coli, Proteus, Klebsiella, Enterobacter*) and less commonly by *Staphylococcus* (*aureus* and *saprophyticus*). It is more common in women. Symptoms can include increased urinary frequency, urgency (sudden necessity to urinate), dysuria, and suprapubic pain.

Pyelonephritis

Pyelonephritis is caused by the same organisms that cause cystitis. Symptoms include flank pain, fever, malaise, and any of the urinary symptoms listed under cystitis.

Urinalysis

Diagnosis of all of these disorders is confirmed by urinalysis/urine culture, which can demonstrate the presence of white cells (indicating inflammation) and infectious agents.

An important distinction must be made between *cells* and *casts* in urinalysis. If there are actual red blood *cells* or white blood *cells* in the urine with *normal* morphology, they must have entered it *after* the kidneys (i.e., in the ureters, bladder, or urethra). Had the cells entered in the kidneys, they would have been squashed and damaged in the glomeruli and/or tubules, and will appear deformed on microscopic urinalysis. So *cells* in the urine may signify lower urinary tract disease is their morphology is relatively normal, or renal disease if their morphology is abnormal. Red *cells* from the kidneys can occur in glomerulonephritis; red *cells* from the lower urinary tract can occur with urinary tract infection, nephrolithiasis (stones), hemorrhagic cystitis, or bladder cancer. White *cells* from the kidneys can occur in acute interstitial nephritis; white *cells* from the lower urinary tract can occur from infection, e.g., cystitis and urethritis.

Casts are conglomerates of protein and cells and *always* signify glomerular or tubular disease. More specifically, red cell *casts* occur in glomerular disease (remember the glomerulus is a tuft of blood vessels), while white and epithelial *casts* occur in acute tubular necrosis and pyelonephritis.

Leukocyte esterase (*LE*) and *nitrate* tests on the urine can be performed rapidly to screen for the white cells (LE) and bacteria (nitrate) in the urine, either of which can indicate UTI.

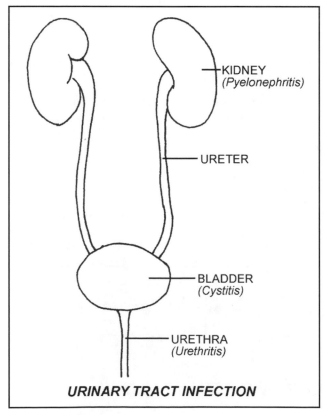

KIDNEY
(Pyelonephritis)

URETER

BLADDER
(Cystitis)

URETHRA
(Urethritis)

URINARY TRACT INFECTION

Figure 3-5

TUMORS OF THE URINARY TRACT

Smoking and occupational exposure to toxic chemicals can predispose to malignancy of the bladder and kidneys. Some hereditary syndromes (e.g., *von Hippel-Landau*) can predispose to renal cell carcinoma. Bladder cancer often presents as hematuria, but can also cause symptoms of urgency and frequency. Renal cell carcinoma also causes hematuria but may also present with flank pain and/or a palpable mass. Renal cell carcinoma can also cause a variety of *paraneoplastic syndromes*. A paraneoplastic syndrome occurs when a tumor causes signs/symptoms unrelated to direct effects of the tumor itself or metastases. Renal cell carcinoma can secrete erythropoietin (leading to polycythemia), parathyroid hormone-related protein (PTHrP, resulting in hypercalcemia), and/or renin (causing hypertension).

Wilms' tumor is a pediatric kidney tumor that often presents as an abdominal mass. Other symptoms/signs can include abdominal pain, hematuria, hypertension, and/or fever.

FLUIDS AND ELECTROLYTES

This section discusses the physiology and pathophysiology of water, sodium, potassium, and H^+/HCO_3^- (i.e., acid/base). Calcium metabolism and its disorders are discussed in Chapter 5.

Basic Concepts

Fig. 3-6. Hypertonicity, hypotonicity, and concentration gradients. Consider two solutions separated by a semipermeable membrane such that *only water* can diffuse between them. Substances flow from areas of higher concentration to areas of lower concentration in order to achieve equilibrium (*diffusion*). In Figure 3-6 on the left, *solution B is hypertonic to solution A* since is it has more sodium per solvent than solution A. *Solution A is hypotonic to B* since it has less sodium per solvent than solution B. You might first guess that because there is more solute in B, this solute will flow to A to achieve equilibrium. However, in this system, the membrane that separates the solutions *only allows passage of water*. Which way will water flow then? The goal is equilibrium, so water will flow from A to B, giving both solutions equal concentrations. Another way to think about it is that if B has more solute than A, then A has *more water* than B, and water will thus flow down *its* concentration gradient to the B side. Mnemonic: Water flows **o**ut of a hyp**o**tonic solution. *Osmotic pressure* is the name of the force that *pulls* water from A to B.

The simple system in Figure 3-6 is analogous to the separation of the extracellular space (i.e., interstitial and intravascular spaces) from the intracellular space by cellular membranes. Most substances cannot pass *freely* across cell membranes,[4] but water *can*, so we can make predictions about the effects of various disturbances in electrolytes on intravascular volume.

Sodium is the main extracellular cation. The body's goal is to maintain a constant **concentration** *of sodium* (i.e., amount of sodium per unit fluid volume). It does this in part by altering the amount of water present, either by excreting or retaining water via the kidneys, or by shifts of water from the cells to the

---

[4] Ions and solutes can pass across membranes via transporters and channels, but this is regulated and not free. The lipid bilayer of the cellular membrane allows free diffusion of water, gases, and nonpolar substances (e.g., steroid hormones). Ions, glucose, amino acids, etc. must pass by way of protein channels, transporters, etc.

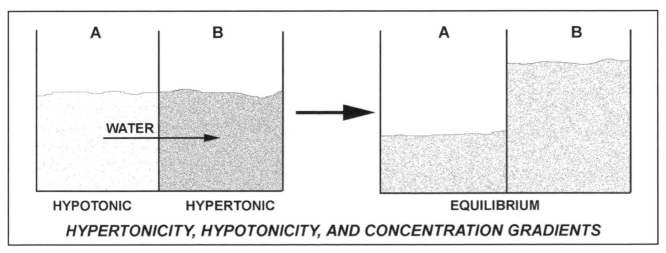

HYPERTONICITY, HYPOTONICITY, AND CONCENTRATION GRADIENTS

Figure 3-6

extracellular space (i.e., interstitial and intravascular spaces) and vice versa.

In pathological states such as hypernatremia, we are talking about the sodium *concentration*, *not* the absolute amount of sodium. In fact, if someone loses lots of water and salt, but more water than salt, sodium *concentration* increases (*hypernatremia*) despite a decreased total *amount* of sodium. If someone gains lots of water and salt but more water than salt, *concentration* of sodium decreases (*hyponatremia*) despite an increased *amount* of sodium. Thus, it is the *concentration* of sodium in which we are interested, not the absolute amount. This concentration depends upon the *volume of water* in which it is dissolved (i.e., plasma volume). Concentration will be referred to with brackets: as [Na⁺] or [sodium].

Fig. 3-7. Serum tonicity and intravenous (IV) solutions.

1. Hypertonic saline. This increases sodium concentration in the blood. Since sodium is a charged ion, it cannot pass *freely* through the cell membrane from the area of higher concentration to that of lower concentration; only water can do so. What will this increase in sodium concentration in the blood cause? Since water can diffuse, it will flow *from cells* to the intravascular space to dilute the increased sodium concentration. Thus, intravascular volume will increase in order to dilute the increased sodium load and prevent hypernatremia.

2. Hypotonic saline. This leads to a dilution of the intravascular fluid, which makes it hypotonic compared to the intracellular concentrations. Water flows *o*ut of a hyp*o*tonic solution, so this will cause water to flow from the intravascular space into the cells, causing some swelling of the cells (and preventing hyponatremia in the blood).

3. Isotonic saline. Since isotonic saline is at the *same* concentration as what is in the cells, no fluid shifts should occur. The intravascular *volume* will simply increase.

Based on the above physiology, one can determine what type of IV saline to use when replacing the intravascular volume of a hypovolemic patient (e.g.,

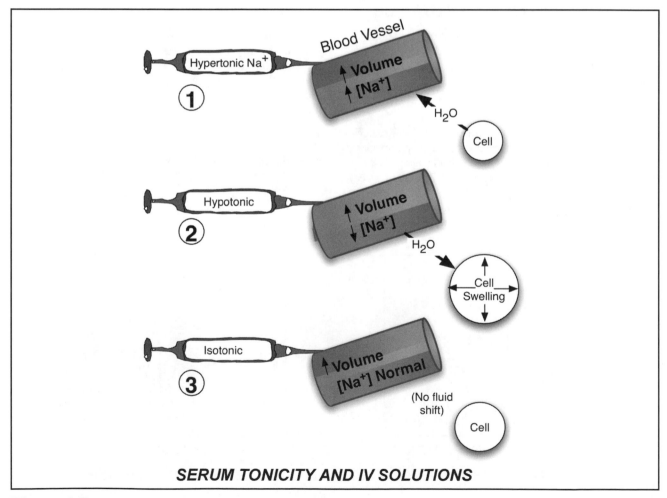

SERUM TONICITY AND IV SOLUTIONS

Figure 3-7

from blood loss, diarrhea, etc.). If a patient needs resuscitation or s/he cannot drink and needs maintenance fluids, one generally uses *isotonic* saline. Since it is isotonic to cellular fluid, an isotonic IV solution will increase intravascular volume without causing a shift of water into cells. In extreme cases of hypovolemia (e.g., shock), a *hypertonic* solution can be used. A hypertonic solution will stay in the intravascular space *and* pull more fluid into the intravascular space to try to dilute its hypertonicity (of course, it should not be so hypertonic so as to induce hypernatremia).

Electrolyte/fluid imbalances must be corrected slowly. Neurons depend upon appropriate electrolyte concentrations for electrophysiological function. Thus, in states of electrolyte imbalance, the brain will respond by transporting substances into the interstitium to compensate for this imbalance. If electrolyte/fluid imbalances are corrected too rapidly with IV fluids, the brain does not have time to re-equilibrate. This can cause *central pontine myelinolysis* (also known as *osmotic demyelination syndrome*) due to the dramatic fluid shifts that take place between the cells in the brain and the surrounding fluid.

Three additional key points to keep in mind:

- *AldosteRoNe causes Reabsorption of Na+ (sodium) and secretion of potassium.*

- *ADH (antidiuretic hormone) causes water reabsorption.*

- Sodium is the main *extra*cellular cation (higher concentration in the serum than in cells) and potassium is the main *intra*cellular cation (higher concentration in cells than in the serum).

Hypernatremia and Hyponatremia

Sodium (Na+) is the main extracellular cation: its concentration is much higher in the serum than inside cells.

Fig. 3-8. Hypernatremia and hyponatremia. Sodium concentration can increase *(hypernatremia)* or decrease *(hyponatremia)* and **in either case**, fluid volume can be increased *(hypervolemia)*, decreased *(hypovolemia)*, or remain relatively unchanged *(euvolemia)*.

The "-volemias" refer to *what is perceived on clinical exam* (i.e., edema in hypervolemia; dry mucous membranes and/or tenting[5] in hypovolemia). *Euvolemic* (normal volume status) states in both hyper- and hyponatremia *do* involve some fluid loss or gain, and are *not* truly euvolemic by a purist definition. The patients simply *appear* euvolemic on exam since the

aberration in volume status is not as extreme as in the other scenarios, and thus does not cause symptoms/signs of hypervolemia or hypovolemia. So the distinctions hyper-, hypo-, and eu- volemia refer to volume status as assessed *on clinical exam*.

Hypernatremia

Most generally, possible causes of increased serum sodium concentration (hypernatremia) include:

- Increase in serum sodium

- Increases in serum sodium and water/volume, but sodium increases *more* than water/volume

- Decrease in serum water/volume (which increases sodium *concentration*)

- Decreases in serum water/volume and sodium, but water/volume decreases *more* than sodium

Hypervolemic Hypernatremia. There must be an increase in volume *and* sodium to cause both hypervolemia and hypernatremia. Most commonly this is iatrogenic from the administration of sodium bicarbonate solutions or dialysis solutions. Primary hyperaldosteronism can also cause hypervolemic hypernatremia. In hyperaldosteronism, increased aldosterone increases sodium reabsorption, resulting in hypernatremia. Sodium reabsorption causes water to passively follow it, which is why hyperaldosteronism can cause hypervolemia.

Hypovolemic Hypernatremia. To become hypovolemic, there must be water loss, and to end up hypernatremic there must be *more water loss than sodium loss if one is losing both*. Such losses of water and/or sodium can be classified as *renal losses* or *extrarenal losses*.

Renal losses refer to *renal diseases* or *diuretics* that waste water and/or sodium. If the amount of water lost is greater than the amount of sodium lost, the result will be hypernatremia. If the amount of sodium lost is greater than the amount of water lost, this will result in hyponatremia.

Extrarenal losses of water and/or sodium can occur through sweat, stool, or fluid shifts from the intravascular space to the extravascular space, e.g., after major burns, surgery, etc.

If the clinical history and physical exam cannot distinguish between renal and extrarenal losses, *urine electrolytes* can. If the water/sodium losses occur extrarenally (i.e., sweating, diarrhea, fluid shifts from burns, etc.), the *kidneys will attempt to hold on to sodium, thus decreasing sodium concentration in the urine.* Thus, if the cause of hypovolemic hypernatremia is renal, there will be a higher concentration of sodium in the urine than if the losses are extrarenal.

---

[5] Tenting is when the patient's skin relaxes slowly when tugged upon, as opposed to falling right back into place. This is also called decreased *skin turgor*.

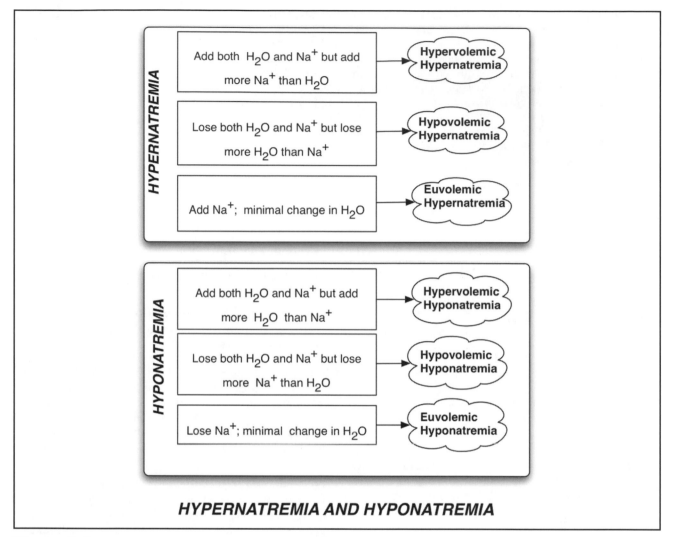

HYPERNATREMIA AND HYPONATREMIA

Figure 3-8

Typically these scenarios manifest as either urine [sodium] > 20 meq/L if the sodium losses are *renal* or urine [sodium] < 20 meq/L if the losses are *extra-renal*.

Euvolemic Hypernatremia. Although patients with euvolemic hypernatremia appear clinically euvolemic on physical exam, *they are in fact losing some water*. One cause of euvolemic hypernatremia is *hypodipsia*, or decreased water intake, usually caused by a hypothalamic lesion. Another cause of euvolemic hypernatremia is *diabetes insipidus*.[6] Diabetes insipidus is a loss of either antidiuretic hormone (ADH) *secretion* or a loss of ADH's *action*. ADH, secreted by the posterior pituitary, causes increased water reabsorption from the collecting ducts. *Increased ADH* increases water reabsorption, resulting in a more concentrated urine and a more dilute serum. *Decreased ADH* decreases water reabsorption, resulting in an increased and dilute urine output, and a more concentrated serum. Due to loss of ADH or its action in diabetes insipidus, urine output increases, leaving behind a more concentrated (hypernatremic) serum. Though there is some water loss (in the urine) in diabetes insipidus, the clinical picture is usually one of euvolemia.

There are two broad categories of diabetes insipidus. In *central* diabetes insipidus, posterior pituitary secretion of ADH decreases. In *nephrogenic* diabetes insipidus, the kidneys' *sensitivity* to ADH decreases. *Central diabetes insipidus* is usually secondary to some intracranial process (tumor, post-neurosurgery, head trauma, meningitis/encephalitis). *Nephrogenic diabetes insipidus* originates in the kidneys, either from a *congenital defect in the receptor* (X-linked

---

[6] Note: Diabetes insipidus differs from diabetes mellitus (which is also simply called "diabetes"). Diabetes *mellitus* is the disorder involving insulin, glucose, etc., discussed in Chapter 5.

hereditary nephrogenic diabetes insipidus) or from direct *toxicity* (e.g., from lithium, which is used in the treatment of bipolar disorder).

Diagnosis of diabetes insipidus. If diabetes insipidus is central, the posterior pituitary secretion of ADH will decrease, so serum ADH will be low. If the kidneys are not responding to ADH (nephrogenic diabetes insipidus), the posterior pituitary will increase ADH secretion in an attempt to stimulate the non-responding kidneys, so serum ADH will be high.

Fig. 3-9. Laboratory differentiation of central vs. nephrogenic diabetes insipidus. If you give IV ADH (also called ddAVP) to a patient and it works, you would know that the kidneys *are* able to respond to ADH, and thus, that the diabetes insipidus is *central*. If the IV ADH does *not* work, the kidneys must *not* be capable of responding to ADH, and thus the kidneys must be the problem (nephrogenic). How would you know if the IV ADH works? The urine will become more *concentrated* since ADH increases water reabsorption from the collecting system. If ADH does not work, the kidneys will continue to waste water and the urine will remain *dilute*. Thus, urine concentration in response to IV ADH can help evaluate whether diabetes insipidus is nephrogenic or central.

Fig. 3-10. Causes of hypernatremia.

Hyponatremia

Most generally, possible causes of decreased serum sodium concentration (hyponatremia) include:

- Decrease in serum sodium

- Decreases in serum sodium and water/volume, but sodium decreases *more* than water/volume

- Increase in serum water/volume (which decreases sodium *concentration*)

- Increases in serum water/volume and sodium, but water/volume increases *more* than sodium

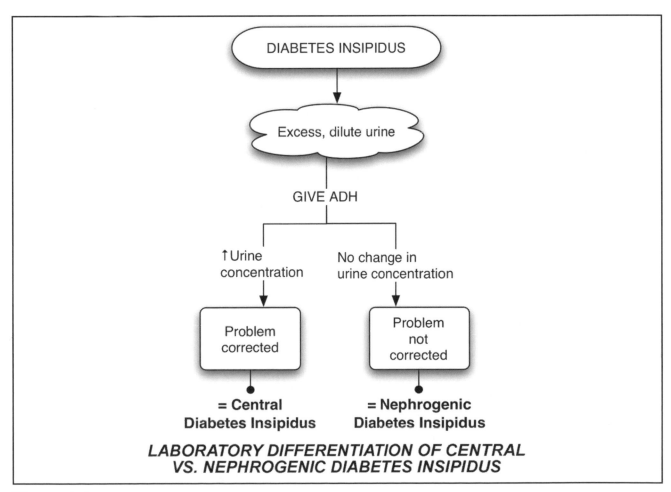

LABORATORY DIFFERENTIATION OF CENTRAL VS. NEPHROGENIC DIABETES INSIPIDUS

Figure 3-9

CAUSES OF HYPERNATREMIA

Hypervolemic hypernatremia
- **Iatrogenic (hypertonic saline)**
- **Hyperaldosteronism**

Hypovolemic hypernatremia
- **Renal losses (e.g., diuretics, renal disease)**
- **Extrarenal losses (e.g., sweating, diarrhea, fluid shifts [e.g., burns])**

Euvolemic hypernatremia
- **Diabetes insipidus**
- **Hypodipsia**

Figure 3-10

Hypervolemic Hyponatremia. To be hyponatremic with an increased intravascular volume, water is either being added or retained, such that the amount of sodium in the serum is diluted. Two situations where the body inappropriately increases the intravascular volume are heart failure and cirrhosis. In heart failure, due to decreased forward flow by the failing heart, the kidneys sense decreased perfusion and try to increase what it perceives as diminished intravascular volume (decreased effective circulating volume) via the renin-angiotensin-aldosterone system (Fig. 1-6). Additionally, perceived low volume activates ADH secretion further increasing water retention. Cirrhosis of the liver can lead to effective volume depletion secondary to pooling of blood in the mesenteric veins. This also decreases the amount of blood seen by the kidneys, resulting in subsequent reabsorption in an effort to increase what is perceived as a low intravascular volume. Thus, *urine* sodium concentration _____[7] in these situations, because the kidneys are attempting to retain sodium along with water. The amount of water retention exceeds that of sodium retention, resulting in the hypervolemic hyponatremia.

Hypovolemic Hyponatremia. To be hypovolemic *and* hyponatremic, there must be both water and sodium loss, but relatively more sodium loss than water loss. The *renal* and *extrarenal* causes of volume loss were discussed in hypovolemic hypernatremia. These are the basic ways that the body can lose fluid, and it is the *relative concentration of sodium in that fluid* that will determine whether the result is hyponatremia or hypernatremia. So any cause of volume loss can lead to hyper- or hyponatremia,

depending upon the concentration of sodium in the lost fluid. In hypovolemic hyponatremia, as with hypovolemic hypernatremia, we can examine the urine electrolytes for diagnosis: if the urine sodium concentration is greater than 20 meq/L, the kidneys must be losing the sodium. If urine sodium concentration is less than 20 meq/L, the sodium must be getting lost in some other way such as sweat, stool, or edema. In the scenarios of fluid loss secondary to excess sweating, diarrhea, or edema, the kidneys are appropriately holding onto sodium in an attempt to rectify the situation.

Euvolemic Hyponatremia can be caused by adrenal insufficiency, hypothyroidism, primary polydypsia, and syndrome of inappropriate antidiuretic diuretic hormone secretion (SIADH).

Excess water consumption (*primary polydipsia*) can be seen in patients with hypothalamic lesions, and *psychogenic polydipsia* can occur in psychiatric patients who drink excessively, either because of mental confusion or drug side effects. If the kidneys are working normally, these patients will also urinate large amounts (*polyuria*), thus usually maintaining clinical euvolemia.

Fig. 3-11. Distinguishing primary polydypsia from diabetes insipidus. Given that they both cause large urine output, how would you distinguish between diabetes insipidus and primary polydipsia? In diabetes insipidus, ADH is either not present or does not work, so lots of water is being lost in the urine. In contrast, in polydipsia, lots of water is being *added* to the plasma volume. *In diabetes insipidus, the diuresis leads to **decreased** intravascular volume (and thus **increased** serum sodium concentration). In polydipsia, the increase in plasma volume leads to hyponatremia.* Therefore, ***serum sodium concentration*** is a good way to distinguish between these two causes of polyuria: low serum sodium concentration in polydipsia, high serum sodium concentration in diabetes insipidus.

Fig. 3-12. Syndrome of inappropriate antidiuretic hormone secretion (SIADH). ADH secretion normally increases water reabsorption, thus increasing intravascular volume and diluting serum sodium. If ADH secretion occurs to the point of creating hyponatremia, it is clearly being inappropriately over-secreted. Hence the name for the syndrome: SIADH (Syndrome of Inappropriate Antidiuretic Diuretic Hormone). SIADH can result from intracranial pathology, a paraneoplastic syndrome,[8] pulmonary disease such as pneumonia or tuberculosis, or from drug toxicity, e.g., cyclophosphamide (used as a chemotherapy agent and

---

[7] decreases

[8] Paraneoplastic SIADH occurs when a tumor secretes ADH. Small cell lung cancer is a common culprit, though other tumors can secrete ADH as well.

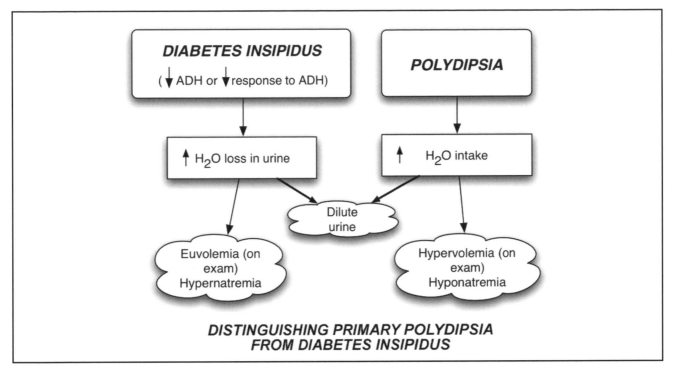

Figure 3-11

in some autoimmune diseases) and SSRIs (selective serotonin reuptake inhibitors, which are used to treat depression). What would you expect to find on urinalysis in SIADH? If ADH is over-secreted, the urine will be quite concentrated, since ADH causes water to be pulled out of the filtrate in the collecting duct. Thus, urine sodium concentration is typically elevated in SIADH.

Again, remember that the designation of euvolemic refers to what is seen on clinical exam most commonly, not necessarily the actual pathophysiology: in SIADH, there is some increase in volume, but this change in volume is usually not substantial enough to produce clinical signs of hypervolemia. Thus, SIADH generally causes *eu*volemic hyponatremia.

Fig. 3-13. Causes of hyponatremia.

Hyperosmolar Hyponatremia (Pseudohyponatremia). Osmolality refers to the amount of solute dissolved per kilogram solvent. Serum osmolality = $2 \times [Na^+] + [glucose]/18 + [urea]/2.8$

The normal value is around 290 mosm/kg.

Fig. 3-14. Hyperosmolar hyponatremia (pseudohyponatremia). An increase in glucose, lipids, proteins, or urea could raise serum osmolality, pulling water into the intravascular space to re-equilibrate things. This would lead to an increased water to sodium ratio and thus hyponatremia. Although the absolute *amount* of

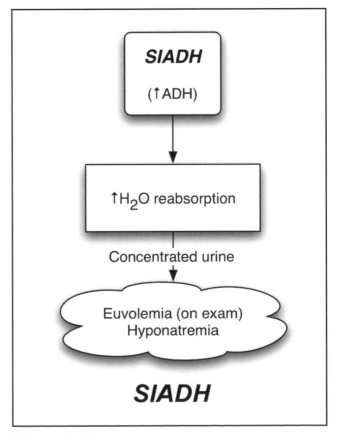

Figure 3-12

59

CAUSES OF HYPONATREMIA

Hypervolemic hyponatremia
- Cirrhosis
- Heart failure
- Nephrotic syndrome

Hypovolemic hyponatremia
- Renal loss
- Extrarenal loss

Euvolemic hyponatremia
- SIADH
- Polydipsia
- Adrenal insufficiency
- Hypothyroidism

Pseudohyponatremia
- ↑glucose
- ↑lipids
- ↑proteins
- ↑urea

Figure 3-13

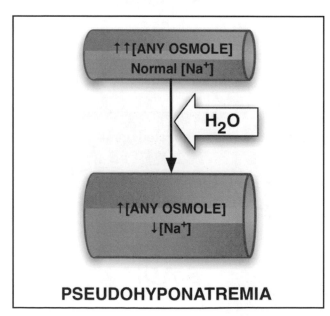

PSEUDOHYPONATREMIA

Figure 3-14

sodium is actually unchanged, the *concentration* of sodium is decreased by the water influx. In uncontrolled diabetes mellitus, the glucose concentration can raise the serum glucose levels to the point where lots of water is drawn into the intravascular space in an attempt to maintain fluid balance. This can result in hyponatremia and even hyperosmolar coma.

Fig. 3-15. Summary.

- The *hypervolemic* states are secondary to fluid overload:
  - An IV solution-generated hypernatremic one; hyperaldosteronism
  - An internally-generated hyponatremic one (e.g., CHF, cirrhosis, nephritic syndrome)

- The *euvolemic* states in both hyper- and hyponatremia include *aberrancies in ADH* or changes in water consumption:
  - Hypernatremia: diabetes insipidus, central (↓ADH secretion) or nephrogenic (↓ renal response to ADH); hypodipsia
  - Hyponatremia: increased ADH secretion (SIADH); polydipsia

- The *hypovolemic* states are secondary to fluid losses, either renal (e.g., diuretics) or extra-renal (diarrhea, sweating, blood loss, fluid shifts). Renal causes can be distinguished from extra-renal causes by urine [sodium]. Urine [sodium] is typically greater than 20 meq/L in renal losses and less than 20 meq/L in extra-renal losses.

When in doubt, remember the basics: in *hypernatremia* there is either net gain of salt or net loss of water. In *hyponatremia*, there is either net loss of salt or net gain of water.

Hyperkalemia and Hypokalemia

Potassium (K^+) is the main intracellular cation: its concentration is significantly higher inside cells than in the serum.

Hyperkalemia

Serum potassium concentration can increase secondary to three basic mechanisms:

- *Increased intake*

- *Decreased urinary excretion*

- *Increased movement of K^+ from the cells into the bloodstream*

Fig. 3-16. Causes of hyperkalemia

	HYPERNATREMIA	HYPONATREMIA
HYPERVOLEMIA	• Iatrogenic • Primary hyperaldosteronism	• Cirrhosis • Heart failure • Nephrotic syndrome
EUVOLEMIA	• Diabetes Insipidus (ADH↓) • Hypodipsia	• SIADH (ADH↑) • Polydipsia • Adrenal insufficiency • Hypothyroidism
HYPOVOLEMIA	• Renal vs. extrarenal losses	• Renal vs. extrarenal losses

Figure 3-15

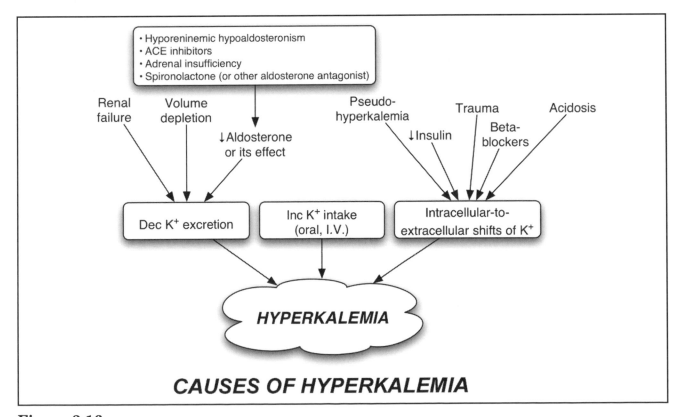

CAUSES OF HYPERKALEMIA

Figure 3-16

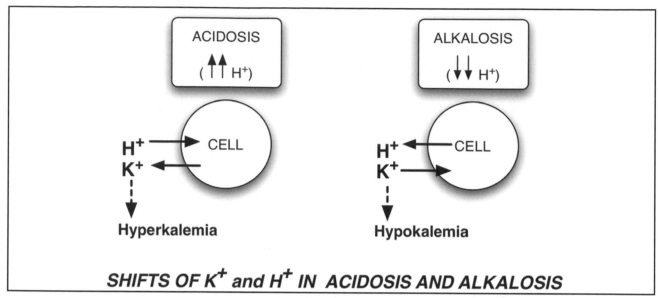

SHIFTS OF K⁺ and H⁺ IN ACIDOSIS AND ALKALOSIS

Figure 3-17

• *Increased intake*. Because of the body's mechanisms for regulating K⁺ (discussed below), it would be quite difficult to induce hyperkalemia by ingesting too much potassium *unless* there was a problem with the kidneys' excretion of potassium. A more likely cause of hyperkalemia due to increased intake would be an iatrogenic infusion of potassium at an inappropriately high dose.

• *Decreased excretion*: renal failure, volume depletion, and hypoaldosteronism.

 – In *renal failure*, the kidneys have difficulty filtering/excreting, resulting in increases in all serum electrolytes (*except calcium*, Fig. 3-3). One of these is potassium. So renal failure can lead to hyperkalemia.

 – A *decrease in flow rate* in the distal nephron can lead to a perceived high concentration of potassium in the nephron, thus inhibiting further secretion of potassium into the nephron. This in turn can lead to hyperkalemia. *Hypovolemia or effective volume depletion* (congestive heart failure, cirrhosis) can result in a low distal flow rate.

 – *Hypoaldosteronism*. Since aldosterone is the hormone responsible for potassium secretion, a *decrease* in aldosterone can cause hyperkalemia. Aldosterone secretion from the zona glomerulosa of the adrenal cortex is stimulated by angiotensin (which is stimulated by renin secretion by the juxtaglomerular apparatus of the kidneys). Hypoaldosteronism can result from a *decrease in aldosterone* or a *decrease in the response to aldosterone* (for more on hypoaldosteronism see Chapter 5).

• *Intracellular to extracellular shifts*: pseudohyperkalemia, acidosis, insulin deficiency or resistance, beta-blockers.

 – *Any process that leads to breakdown of cells can cause hyperkalemia*, since these broken cells release their potassium when they lyse. Common causes include crush injuries or other major trauma, rhabdomyolysis, and tumor lysis after chemotherapy. This elevated potassium from cell breakdown can also explain a very common cause of elevated potassium on laboratory blood work: the blood cells in the blood draw lyse, releasing their potassium. This situation is called *pseudohyperkalemia* since the serum potassium is not really elevated, the elevated [K⁺] is just an artifact of the blood draw. When unsure whether the hyperkalemia is real or an artifact, one draws another sample of blood to recheck the [K⁺].

 – *Acidosis*. Acidosis (too much acid, i.e., high [H⁺] = low pH) and alkalosis (too much base/not enough acid, i.e., low [H⁺] = high pH) are discussed in the next section. One way to compensate for an aberrancy in acid/base status is by exchanging K⁺ for H⁺. The body is willing to tolerate shifts in potassium in an attempt to restore acid/base homeostasis.

Fig. 3-17. Shifts of K⁺ and H⁺ in acidosis and alkalosis. In *acidosis*, there is too much H⁺ in the blood. H⁺ moves from the blood into the cells in exchange for K⁺, which moves from the cells to the blood to maintain electroneutrality. This can lead to hyperkalemia. Alternatively, in *alkalosis*, there is not enough H⁺ in the

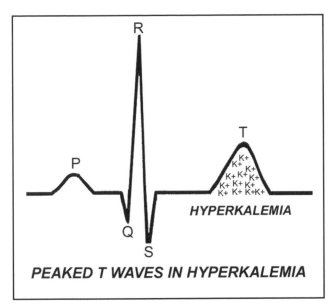

PEAKED T WAVES IN HYPERKALEMIA

Figure 3-18

blood, so the cells release H⁺ into the blood in exchange for K⁺, which enters the cells from the blood. This can lead to hypokalemia.

– *Insulin deficiency or resistance* (e.g., diabetes mellitus) can also lead to hyperkalemia. *Insulin causes K⁺ entry into cells.* A way to remember that insulin causes K⁺ to move into cells is simply to remember its action on glucose. Insulin causes glucose entry into cells. So just think of *in*sulin as something that moves things *in*to cells. Therefore, insulin deficiency or resistance can decrease the ability to move K⁺ into cells, resulting in hyperkalemia.

– Like insulin, *catecholamines also cause K⁺ entry into cells*. Therefore, blocking catecholamines with *beta-blockers* (used in the treatment of hypertension and heart disease) can decrease the ability to move K⁺ into cells, resulting in hyperkalemia.

Fig. 3-18. Peaked T waves in hyperkalemia. Why does hyperkalemia matter? The body expends a large proportion of its energy running the Na⁺/K⁺ pump, which pumps Na⁺ out of cells and K⁺ in. This pump maintains the electrical system that allows for cardiac, neural, and muscular function. If the extracellular potassium begins to rise, the electrical potential across these membranes is altered, and this can affect their function. A worrisome outcome of hyperkalemia is cardiac dysfunction. On EKG, hyperkalemia first manifests as peaked T waves, and can lead to ventricular fibrillation, which can be fatal. Cardiac complications can be prevented with the administration of calcium (usually administered as calcium gluconate), which stabilizes the cardiac membrane. Mnemonic: imagine a peaked T wave as being peaked because it is a mountain of K⁺.

Hypokalemia

Fig. 3-19. Causes of hypokalemia.

Hypokalemia is logically caused by all of the opposites of what caused hyperkalemia. Serum potassium concentration can decrease secondary to three basic mechanisms:

• *Decreased intake*

• *Increased loss* (renal or GI)

• *Movement of K⁺ from the blood into cells*

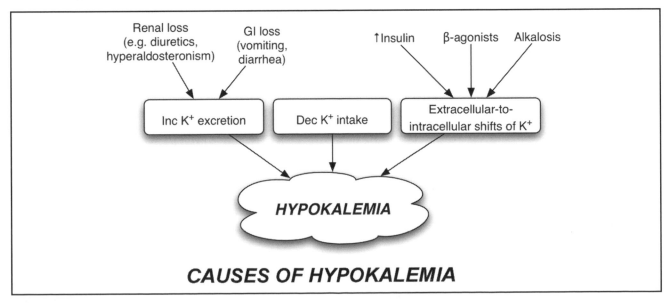

CAUSES OF HYPOKALEMIA

Figure 3-19

- **Decreased intake.** Since the body has many mechanisms of K⁺ regulation (aldosterone, insulin, catecholamines), a potassium-deficient diet alone very rarely causes hypokalemia, although it could be a contributing factor.

- **Increased loss: renal vs. GI.**

  - *Renal loss of K⁺* can occur due to an increased distal flow rate. A very increased rate washes away potassium, making the lumen of the nephron appear to be lacking in potassium, which in turn causes increased potassium secretion. This results in hypokalemia in the blood. Renal losses of K⁺ due to this increased flow rate are commonly seen in *diuretic therapy*. Renal loss of K⁺ can also be induced by *hyperaldosteronism*. Causes of hyperaldosteronism include adrenal adenomas or carcinomas that secrete aldosterone.

  - *GI losses* such as vomiting and diarrhea can lead to potassium loss. Some of this loss is direct, i.e., potassium is lost in the vomit and diarrhea. Vomiting can also result in *indirect* urinary loss of K⁺. Let's go through the indirect K⁺ loss step by step. What happens when one vomits? One loses lots of *acid* from the stomach. If vomiting causes acid loss, an *alkalosis* will remain behind in the serum. This is because H⁺ loss leaves behind an excess of the base HCO_3^-. This excess HCO_3^- eventually makes it to the kidneys, and thus the tubule lumen has more negatively charged ions than usual. One way of compensating for that is secreting the positive ion K⁺ into the lumen. So vomiting can lead to increased loss of K⁺ in the urine, resulting in hypokalemia.

- **Extracellular to intracellular shifts.** Insulin *excess*, *beta agonist* treatment (e.g., albuterol for asthma), and *alkalosis* can all lead to hyp**o**kalemia (see Fig. 3-19). Contrast this with insulin deficiency/resistance, beta-blockers, and acidosis leading to hyp**er**kalemia (see Fig. 3-16). Insulin excess can occur secondary to insulin therapy or an insulin-secreting tumor (*insulinoma*). When treating diabetic ketoacidosis, a complication of diabetes, one uses insulin to reduce blood sugar and restore euglycemia. Because this will also cause a shift of K⁺ into cells, risking hypokalemia, the patient is simultaneously given IV potassium chloride.

Fig. 3-20. Summary of factors affecting serum potassium concentration.

- *Catecholamines (sympathetic nervous system) promote K⁺ entry into cells* via beta receptors. Beta-blockers can cause hyperkalemia, and beta agonists can cause hypokalemia.

- *Insulin also causes K⁺ entry into cells.* Insulin deficiency or resistance can cause hyperkalemia, and insulin excess can cause hypokalemia.

- *Aldoste**R**o**N**e causes **R**eabsorption of **Na⁺** and secretion of K⁺.* Hyp**o**aldosteronism can cause hyperkalemia, and hyp**er**aldosteronism can cause hypokalemia.

- *Distal flow rate in the nephron* is another determinant of K⁺ metabolism. A low distal flow rate can cause hyperkalemia, and a high distal flow rate can cause hypokalemia.

- *Acid/base status affects potassium concentration.* Acidosis can cause hyperkalemia, and alkalosis can cause hypokalemia.

Note from figure 3-20: *Decreases* in pH, aldosterone, catecholamines, insulin, and distal flow rate can cause hyp**er**kalemia. *Increases* in pH, aldosterone, catecholamines, insulin, and distal flow rate can cause hyp**o**kalemia.

Acid/Base Pathophysiology

The blood pH is the negative of the logarithm of the hydrogen ion concentration in the blood:

$$pH = -\log [H^+]$$

Normal blood pH is around 7.4. An increase in blood pH is called alkalemia, and a decrease is acidemia. Acido-*sis* and alkal*osis* occur when the aberration of pH is large enough to be pathologic. Since pH is the *negative* log of the H⁺ concentration in solution, the pH goes *down* as the [H⁺] rises (i.e., more acid). On the other hand if the [H⁺] falls (i.e., more basic), the negative log of [H⁺] becomes more positive, and the pH *increases*.

Acid-base status in the serum is maintained by the following equilibrium:

$$HCO_3^- + H^+ \rightarrow H_2CO_3 \rightarrow CO_2 + H_2O$$

In acute acid-base disturbances, shifts in this equilibrium can partially buffer changes in pH away from 7.4. Over time, other more substantial compensation is necessary through the organs that regulate HCO_3^-, CO_2, and H⁺. What organs regulate these molecules? The lungs are responsible for blowing off CO_2 (which is a by-product of various metabolic reactions). The kidneys regulate bicarbonate (HCO_3^-). Most bicarbonate is reabsorbed in the proximal tubules, and a little is reabsorbed in the distal tubules.

The kidneys and lungs are the main generators of (and compensators for) acid/base disturbances, but the GI tract also handles acids and bases. Vomiting and diarrhea can thus also lead to acid/base abnormalities. Acid (H⁺) concentration is higher in the stomach since the stomach secretes acid to digest proteins. Base

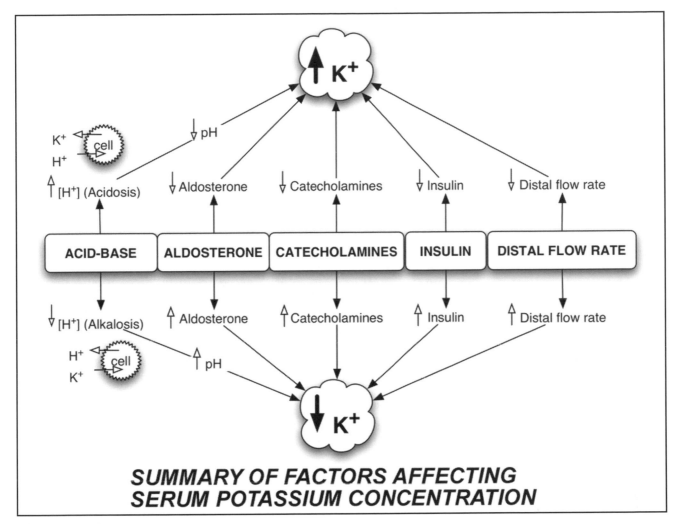

SUMMARY OF FACTORS AFFECTING SERUM POTASSIUM CONCENTRATION

Figure 3-20

(HCO_3^-) concentration is higher in the duodenum and distally because it is secreted from the pancreas into the duodenum to neutralize the stomach acid. So vomiting leads to acid loss (leaving a basic environment behind, which can cause alkalosis), and diarrhea leads to base loss (leaving an acidic environment behind, which can lead to acidosis).

The basic principles of acid/base pathophysiology are as follows:

- If the cause of an acidosis or alkalosis is respiratory, *the kidneys will compensate.*

- If the cause of an acidosis or alkalosis is renal, *the lungs will compensate.*

- The lungs cause disturbances via CO_2. CO_2 increases in respiratory acidosis; CO_2 decreases in respiratory alkalosis.

- The kidneys cause disturbances via HCO_3^-. HCO_3^- elevation via increased retention (or decreased excretion) can result in alkalosis; HCO_3^- decrease via increased excretion can cause acidosis.

- The lungs *compensate for a metabolic disturbance* by doing to CO_2 whatever the kidneys did to HCO_3^-. For example, in a metabolic alkalosis, HCO_3^- rises, so the lungs *retain* CO_2 to compensate.

- The kidneys *compensate for a respiratory disturbance* by doing to HCO_3^- whatever the lungs did to CO_2. For example, in a respiratory alkalosis, CO_2 decreases, so the kidneys *decrease* HCO_3^- (i.e., increases secretion of HCO_3^-) to compensate.

Fig. 3-21. Henderson-Hasselbach equation. The last two points above can be understood in terms of the Henderson-Hasselbach equation. First, remember that log 1 = 0. So if the ratio of [HCO_3^-] to [CO_2] is 1, the log of the ratio will be zero, and the pH will equal pK

$$pH = pK + \log \frac{[HCO_3^-]}{[CO_2]} \qquad \text{To maintain stable pH, } \log \frac{[HCO_3^-]}{[CO_2]} \text{ should} = 0$$

$$\therefore \frac{[HCO_3^-]}{[CO_2]} \text{ should} = 1. \text{ If one is disturbed, the other compensates by going in the same direction.}$$

THE HENDERSON-HASSELBACH EQUATION

Figure 3-21

(equilibrium pH). If either $[HCO_3^-]$ or $[CO_2]$ is significantly increased or decreased, the ratio of the two will change from 1. Since this ratio is added to the pK to give pH, a change in the ratio will change the pH. The goal of compensation is always to *maintain* this ratio at 1 so as to keep pH unchanged. So if the concentration of either CO_2 or HCO_3^- goes up, the compensation is that the other goes up. If the concentration of either CO_2 or HCO_3^- goes down, the compensation is that the other goes down. For example, in metabolic alkalosis, the cause is elevated HCO_3^-, so to compensate (i.e., return the ratio to close to 1) the lungs must *raise* CO_2. In respiratory alkalosis, the cause is decreased CO_2, so to compensate (i.e., return the ratio to close to 1) the kidneys must *decrease* HCO_3^- (i.e., excrete more HCO_3^-). *So the compensating organ always compensates by making the substance it controls (i.e., HCO_3^- for the kidneys, CO_2 for the lungs) go in the **same** direction as the abnormality-causing substance.*

If you understand the basic mechanism by which respiratory acidosis occurs both physiologically and biochemically, you can easily figure out the rest of the acid/base disturbances. This goes for any individual disturbance: learn one well and you can deduce the other three.

Respiratory Acidosis

Fig. 3-22A. Respiratory acidosis. This is an acidosis caused by elevated CO_2. Looking at the chemical reaction at the bottom of fig. 3-22, if the CO_2 is high, the system moves towards equilibrium by *running the reaction toward the right,* thus generating H^+. This increase in H^+ leads to acidosis.

If the lungs cause an aberration, the kidneys will compensate (and vice versa). If the H^+ is high, how could the kidneys buffer that? By retaining HCO_3^-, the kidneys give the blood a buffer that can "soak up" the H^+ generated by the lungs and thus restore a normal pH. So CO_2 rises $\rightarrow$ equilibrium shifts $\rightarrow$ H^+ rises $\rightarrow$ acidosis $\rightarrow$ kidneys try to buffer by *increasing* HCO_3^-. So in a respiratory acidosis, pH is low, CO_2 is high, HCO_3^- is high.

What causes respiratory acidosis? That is, how could one end up with *too much CO_2*? There must be either *over-production of CO_2, increased inspiration of CO_2,* or *decreased expiration of CO_2.* How could these occur? Overproduction occurs in hypercatabolic states (e.g., malignant hyperthermia). Increased inspiration could occur if there is increased concentration of CO_2 in the inspired gas mixture. Decreased expiration of CO_2 is the most common cause of respiratory acidosis. Why would the lungs have trouble expiring? *Obstruction* (foreign object, tumor, or obstructive lung disease), *damage to the lungs or chest wall* (e.g., pneumothorax), or a *problem with the muscles of respiration or their neural input.* Damage to the neural input can occur in the central nervous system (e.g., brainstem infarct, opiate suppression of respiratory drive), the peripheral nervous system (Guillain-Barré), or the respiratory muscles (e.g., myasthenia gravis).

Respiratory Alkalosis

Fig. 3-22B. Respiratory alkalosis. While respiratory acidosis occurs from elevated CO_2, respiratory *alkalosis* is caused by *increased expiration* of CO_2. This decrease in CO_2 drives the reaction in fig. 3-22 in a way that attempts to create more CO_2 to maintain equilibrium. This is accomplished by the combination of HCO_3^- and H^+, thus *decreasing* H^+ (which *raises* pH). If the lungs cause the pH to be high, the kidneys can compensate by getting rid of HCO_3^-, the body's own base, thus making things less basic. So CO_2 decreases $\rightarrow$ equilibrium shifts $\rightarrow$ decreased H^+ $\rightarrow$ alkalosis $\rightarrow$ the kidneys try to get rid of base (HCO_3^- decreases). So in respiratory alkalosis, pH is high, CO_2 is low, and HCO_3^- is low.

How could one end up with decreased CO_2? The only way is by breathing it off too rapidly, i.e., hyperventilating. Hyperventilation can be induced by a physiological drive for more oxygen if there is hypoxemia. Examples include high altitude and anemia. Hyperventilation can also be drug-induced (e.g., salicylates)[9], pain/anxiety-induced, stroke-induced, or in-

---

[9] Salicylate toxicity can cause respiratory alkalosis and metabolic acidosis.

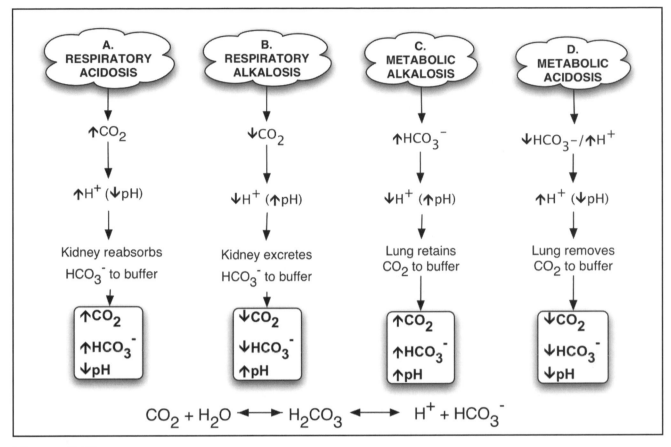

Figure 3-22

duced by pulmonary pathology (e.g., pulmonary embolus can lead to hyperventilation).

Asthma can cause respiratory acidosis *or* respiratory alkalosis. Initially, an asthma attack causes hyperventilation, which can result in respiratory alkalosis. As the obstruction becomes severe and the respiratory muscles fatigue, CO_2 retention occurs, resulting in respiratory acidosis.

Metabolic Alkalosis

Fig. 3-22C. Metabolic alkalosis means that there is an alkalosis not caused by the lungs. *For a metabolic alkalosis to occur [H+] must be decreased* (which would leave behind excess base) *or [HCO3−] must be increased.*

H+ Decrease:

- *Renal loss* of H+. *Aldosterone causes acid secretion.* (Aldoste**R**o**N**e causes **R**eabsorption of Na+, and secretion of K+ and H+). So hyperaldosteronism can lead to increased acid secretion, leaving behind a basic environment and thus alkalosis.

- *Shift of H+ into cells.* Recall that H+ and K+ can be exchanged across cell membranes to restore acid-base balance at the expense of disturbing K+ balance. The reverse situation can also occur: hypokalemia causes some K+ to leave cells in an attempt to correct the hypokalemia and it does this in exchange for H+, which enters the cells. Pulling H+ out of the serum leaves behind a more basic environment. Hypokalemia can be caused by diuretics, hyperaldosteronism, etc., as discussed above.

- *Vomiting* (loss of H+ in vomited stomach acid)

HCO3− Increase:

- *Increased intake* (e.g., iatrogenic bicarbonate infusion)

- *Loss of acid* (leaving behind a relative surplus of HCO3−), e.g., hyperaldosteronism

- Volume depletion (*contraction alkalosis*): if fluid with a low bicarbonate concentration is lost, this leads to an increase in bicarbonate concentration, which can cause alkalosis. This can happen from over-diuresis, for example.

How would the lungs compensate for a metabolic alkalosis? If HCO_3^- is too high, what would the lungs want to do to CO_2? There are two ways to think about this. One way is to remember that when CO_2 is high in the lungs, this causes an acidosis. Thus, to compensate for an alkalosis elsewhere, the lungs must try to bring things back to normal by going "in the acid direction" by retaining CO_2. Another way to think about this is in terms of the Henderson-Hasselbach equation: the compensating molecule must do the same thing that the aberrant molecule did. Here HCO_3^- is elevated, so CO_2 must rise to compensate. So in metabolic alkalosis, pH is high, HCO_3^- is high, and CO_2 is high.

Metabolic Acidosis

Fig. 3-22D. Metabolic acidosis is caused by *HCO_3^- decrease* or *acid increase*. The latter is often caused by *addition of another acid to the serum*. The lungs compensate for metabolic acidosis by decreasing CO_2 (i.e., by blowing off more CO_2). So in metabolic acidosis, pH is low, HCO_3^- is low, and CO_2 is low.

One must determine whether a metabolic acidosis is due to bicarbonate loss or acid gain. Bicarbonate loss can be caused by diarrhea or some renal problem leading to HCO_3^- wasting. The main causes of acid gain are usually grouped under the mnemonic MUDPILES (methanol, uremia, diabetic ketoacidosis, paraldehyde, isoniazid or iron, lactic acid, ethylene glycol, salicylates).

The anion gap. Aside from a history or lab chemistries that point toward an increased level of any of these substances, there is also a calculation based on a few ion concentrations that can distinguish between acid gain vs. bicarbonate loss. This calculation uses *serum* ion concentrations, and is known as the *anion gap*:

$$Na^+ - [Cl^- + HCO_3^-] \text{ or } Na^+ - Cl^- - HCO_3^-.$$

This calculation is essentially the *main extracellular cation minus the main extracellular anions*.

Normally, Na^+ is about 140, Cl^- is about 108, and HCO_3^- is about 24. This would give an anion gap of 8. *If the anion gap is higher than 10 - 12, this must mean that the sum of Cl^- and HCO_3^- is decreased* ***and another acid is present***. A logical question is: "But if one loses bicarbonate *without* addition of some other acid, shouldn't that cause an increased anion gap too? That is, if there is diarrhea or a renal problem causing HCO_3^- loss, wouldn't this also increase the anion gap since one of the things being subtracted (HCO_3^-) is now much lower?" Actually, due to various exchange transporters, when there is HCO_3^- loss, there tends to be an *increase* in serum chloride. This leads to maintenance of a normal anion gap in situations where HCO_3^- is decreased. So *an elevated anion gap means that some other acid is present in serum* that increases the gap (MUDPILES). *A normal anion gap metabolic acidosis means that bicarbonate loss is occurring secondary to either diarrhea or a renal problem*.

Urine anion gap. If there is metabolic acidosis and the anion gap is *normal*, one must distinguish between a renal problem and diarrhea (the latter may be obvious clinically: i.e., the patient is having diarrhea). In a normal anion gap metabolic acidosis, one looks at the *urine anion gap*. The urine should have an equal balance of positive and negative ions, namely $Na^+ + K^+ + NH_4^+$, should equal Cl^- concentration:

$$[Na^+] + [K^+] + [NH_4^+] = [Cl^-]$$

Since it is easiest to measure Na^+, K^+, and Cl^-, one can rearrange the equation to:

$$[Na^+] + [K^+] - [Cl^-] = -[NH_4^+]$$

The negative sign before NH_4^+ does *not* refer to the charge; it is just a result of the algebraic solution to the first equation. The kidneys have various ways of secreting acid in an attempt to maintain normal pH, and one of those is the secretion of H^+ bound to NH_3, which is NH_4^+. If an acidosis is created by diarrhea, and the kidneys are functioning normally, it will try to secrete that excess acid in the form of NH_4^+. This will make the equation ($Na^+ + K^+ - Cl^-$) very *negative*. (A very negative value means a *high* $[NH_4^+]$ because of the negative sign on the NH_4^+ in the equation.)

On the other hand, if the kidneys are responsible for the acidosis, that must mean they are not working properly, and thus *not* appropriately secreting NH_4^+. In this scenario, the $Na^+ + K^+ - Cl^-$ will be closer to zero or even positive. Thus, if the urine anion gap is very negative, we know the kidneys are working properly and secreting acid (in the form of NH_4^+), and thus the source of the acidosis is not renal, but most likely diarrhea. If the urine anion gap is close to zero or positive, the kidneys are not appropriately responding to the acidosis by secreting NH_4^+, and thus the kidneys are the source of the acidosis (*renal tubular acidosis*). *The urine anion gap is only useful in the setting of a non-anion gap metabolic acidosis*. If there is an anion gap in the serum, the urine anion gap calculation is meaningless.

Renal tubular acidosis (RTA) can be caused by a variety of conditions that lead to *decreased* hydrogen ion excretion. This results in acidosis. Normally, the kidneys' defenses against acidosis are reabsorbing base (HCO_3^-) or excreting acid in the urine. The kidneys can secrete excess acid in the form of NH_4^+ (NH_3 carrying an acidic H^+) and $H_2PO_4^-$ (HPO_4^{2-} carrying an acidic H^+).

The three types of RTA are type 1, type 2, and type 4. [10]

Types 1 and 2 RTA are classified by where along the tubule the defect occurs: Type 1 occurs in the distal nephron (mnemonic: D**1**stal), Type 2 occurs in the proximal nephron (mnemonic: pro**2**imal). Type 4 is hypoaldosteronism (mnemonic: hypoaldoste**4**onism).

Type 1 RTA (Distal). In Type 1 RTA, impaired H+ secretion in the distal nephron occurs secondary to a genetic defect of ion transporters, in association with autoimmune diseases, or from drug toxicity. If the collecting ducts do not adequately secrete acid, what do you think the *urine* pH will be? Basic. This basicity of the urine can lead to formation of kidney stones. So remember D**1St**al: Type 1 = Distal, **St** for **st**ones)

Type 2 RTA (Proximal) is a defect in bicarbonate reabsorption. Therefore, HCO_3^- (bicarbonate) in the urine will be elevated. This can occur from drug toxicity, as a genetic defect, or as apart of Fanconi's syndrome. Fanconi's syndrome[11] is proximal tubule dysfunction, which can be hereditary, or secondary to renal damage from proteins (multiple myeloma, amyloidosis), drugs (e.g., chemotherapy agents, aminoglycosides), or toxins (e.g., heavy metals).

One might expect that the urine in Type 2 RTA should be basic like Type 1 RTA since one is wasting bicarbonate in the urine, but the story is a bit more complicated. As bicarbonate is wasted, the plasma level of bicarbonate decreases. In fact, HCO_3^- level becomes so low that when it arrives at the proximal tubule, it does *not* exceed the kidneys' (reduced) reabsorptive capacity. So because of the low level of bicarbonate in the circulation due to the initial defect, in the end one does not end up with that much bicarbonate in the urine. The low level of bicarbonate that is left from the initial wasting is small enough that it can be reabsorbed. This low level of bicarbonate thus cycles through the system, maintaining the same level. What would happen if the patient with Type 2 RTA was given an IV bicarbonate injection? *Now* the reabsorptive capacity would be overwhelmed, bicarbonate would be wasted in the urine, and the urine would become alkaline with a high bicarbonate concentration. To treat an acidosis, one gives some bicarbonate to neutralize the acid. *In Type 2 RTA, this bicarbonate therapy will lead to alkalanization of the urine*, a *serum bicarbonate less than expected* (because now the diminished renal reabsorptive capacity is being overwhelmed), and a *high urine bicarbonate* (also because of the overwhelmed reabsorptive capacity of the kidneys).

Type 4 RTA is hypoaldosteronism. Why would this cause metabolic acidosis? Remember that aldosterone is responsible for stimulating H+ secretion (aldoste**RoNe** causes **R**eabsorption of Na+ and secretion of K+ and H+). So a low level of aldosterone will lead to decreased H+ secretion, which can result in an accumulation of H+ in the blood (acidosis). What other electrolyte abnormalities would you expect? If aldosterone is low, Na+ reabsorption and K+ secretion will both decrease. So hyperkalemia and hyponatremia can be present in hypoaldosteronism. What causes hypoaldosteronism? Aldosterone comes from the adrenal cortex, so *adrenal insufficiency* is one cause. What stimulates aldosterone? The renin-angiotensin-aldosterone axis. *Decreased renin secretion* (e.g., hyporeninemic hypoaldosteronism, which can come from any cause of renal failure, most often diabetic nephropathy) or *decreased angiotensin* (e.g., caused by an ACE inhibitor) can lead to decreases in aldosterone levels.

Overall Algorithm for Acid/Base Disturbance Diagnosis

First, look at the pH. 7.4 = normal. Decreased pH = acidosis, elevated pH = alkalosis. Then look at either CO_2 or HCO_3^-.

- If there is *acidosis* and *CO_2 is elevated*, this must be *respiratory acidosis* (if CO_2 is *decreased,* this must be *metabolic* acidosis: the decreased CO_2 is the respiratory compensation).

- If there is *acidosis* and *HCO_3^- is decreased,* this must be *metabolic acidosis* (if HCO_3^- is *elevated,* this must be *respiratory* acidosis: the elevated HCO_3 is the renal compensation).

- If there is *alkalosis* and *CO_2 is decreased*, this must be a *respiratory alkalosis* (if CO_2 is *elevated,* this must be a *metabolic* alkalosis: the elevated CO_2 is the respiratory compensation).

- If there is *alkalosis* and *HCO_3^- is increased* this must be a *metabolic alkalosis* (if HCO_3^- is *decreased,* this must be a *respiratory* alkalosis: the HCO_3^- decrease is the renal compensation).

Fig. 3-23. Determining the cause of metabolic acidosis. If there is a metabolic acidosis, calculate an anion gap using *serum* concentrations ($Na^+ - [Cl^- + HCO_3^-]$). If the anion gap is elevated (greater than or equal to 10-12), extra acid (i.e., MUDPILES) must be present. If the anion gap is normal, there is either diarrhea or renal tubular acidosis (RTA). To distinguish between these two, use the *urine* anion gap. $Na^+ + K^+ - Cl^- = -(NH_4^+)$. If it is very negative, the kidneys are appropriately secreting NH_4^+ in response to acidosis, and

---

[10] The term "type 3" is no longer in use. Some sources say that what was once referred to as type 3 is now thought to be a variant of type 1, while others say type 3 referred to a combination of types 1 and 2.

[11] Note: This is different from Fanconi's *anemia*, which is an autosomal recessive disease of the bone marrow leading to pancytopenia.

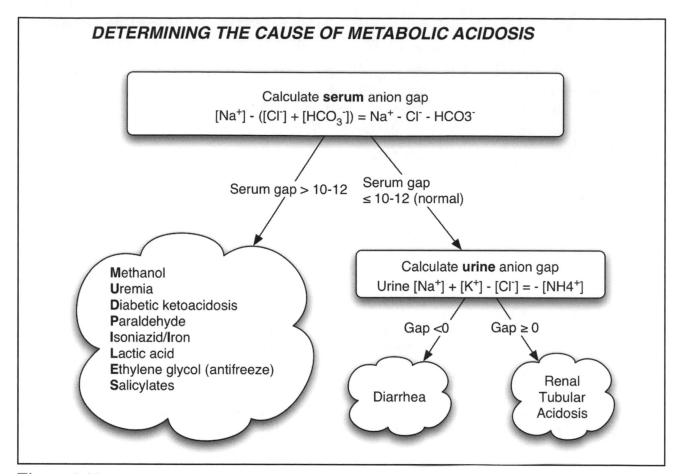

Figure 3-23

the cause must be diarrhea (hopefully you got that on the history). If it is positive or zero, the kidneys are *not* appropriately secreting NH_4^+, and thus the problem is intrinsic to the kidneys, i.e., RTA. If it is RTA with a basic urine, this is most likely Type I (distal) or Type 4 (hypoaldosteronism). If the urine is not basic but becomes so with bicarbonate therapy, this is more likely type 2 RTA (proximal). If the RTA is accompanied by hyperkalemia, type 4 is more likely.

CHAPTER 4. THE GASTROINTESTINAL SYSTEM

ANATOMICAL OVERVIEW

The GI tract is a muscular tube from the mouth to the anus with different regions specialized for different digestive functions. These regions are the esophagus, stomach, small intestine, and large intestine. The liver and pancreas are accessory organs that produce substances that aid digestion, amongst numerous other functions.

Since the GI tract is a muscular tube specialized for digestion and/or absorption, the potential types of pathology are:

- Problems with the muscle or its innervation

- Obstruction of the tube (e.g., foreign objects, tumors)

- Deficient digestion and/or absorption, which can be due to:
  - A problem with an enzyme or its secretion
  - A problem with an absorptive surface of the GI tract (e.g., inflammatory bowel disease or bacterial overgrowth)

- Problems with the blood vessels/blood supply (e.g., esophageal varices, mesenteric ischemia, GI bleeding)

Fig. 4-1. Overview of GI function and pathology.

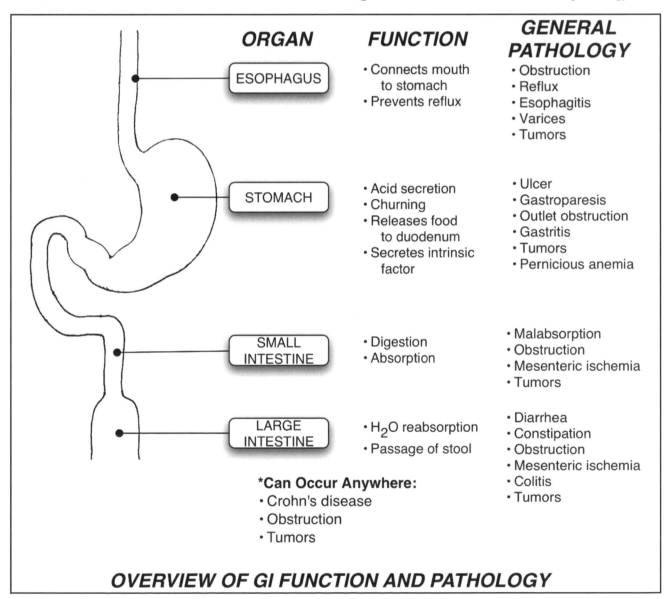

OVERVIEW OF GI FUNCTION AND PATHOLOGY

Figure 4-1

In *any region* of the GI tract, abnormalities of the *blood supply*, *inflammation*, and *tumors* can occur.

- *Blood supply abnormalities*
  - Upper or lower GI *bleeding*
  - *Ischemia* due to loss of blood supply, e.g., secondary to thrombosis or atherosclerosis (*mesenteric ischemia*)

- *Inflammation*
  - Esophagitis
  - Gastritis
  - Colitis
  - Crohn's disease

- *Tumors*:
  - Esophageal cancer
  - Gastric cancer
  - Small bowel tumors
  - Colon cancer

The following are *region-specific* GI-tube-related pathologies:

- The *esophagus* is a tube that transports food from the mouth to the stomach and prevents motion in the opposite direction. Deficiency of transport can be secondary to *obstruction*. A problem with preventing motion back from the stomach can lead to *reflux*.

- The *stomach* produces acid (to break down food) and intrinsic factor, which binds vitamin B12. Excess acid secretion can be associated with *ulcer* disease; *loss of intrinsic factor* results in decreased B12 absorption (pernicious anemia). The stomach also churns food and sends it to the small intestine; paralysis (*gastroparesis*) and *outlet obstruction* are the corresponding pathologies of these two functions.

- The *small intestine* continues digestion and begins absorption of substances from the gut to the bloodstream. *Malabsorption* and *obstruction* can occur in the small intestine.

- The *large intestine* reabsorbs water from the luminal contents, stores undigested food, and passes this undigested food to the outside world as stool. Pathology of the large intestine can result in *diarrhea* or *constipation*. *Obstruction* can also occur in the large intestine.

DISEASES OF THE ESOPHAGUS

No digestion or absorption occurs in the esophagus; it is simply a muscular tube that transports food from the pharynx to the stomach by coordinated muscular contraction. So what could interfere with this transport or the coordinated muscular function it requires?

- *Obstruction*

- *Dysfunction of the muscle or its innervation*

- *Outpouchings (diverticula)* that prevent the food from going where it is supposed to go

- Inability to prevent stomach contents from re-entering the esophagus (gastroesophageal reflux disease: GERD)

Obstruction

What can cause a blockage? From the inside of the esophagus, a foreign object, an esophageal tumor, rings and/or webs can all cause obstruction. From the outside, think about the anatomical location of the esophagus: the posterior mediastinum, just behind the trachea. So lung cancer or enlarged lymph nodes (e.g., secondary to metastasis or tuberculosis) can obstruct the esophagus from the outside.

Patients with esophageal obstruction typically have trouble swallowing (*dysphagia*). This can feel like trouble getting the food down, pain in the chest (sometimes presenting like angina), or in some instances, regurgitation of *undigested* food. (The food is undigested since it has not yet made it to the stomach). If the stenosis is from a tumor, for example, first this dysphagia would be for solid foods and then, as the tumor grows and further encroaches on the lumen, dysphagia for liquids can occur.

Muscle

Any muscle could fail in one of two ways: it could *fail to contract* or *fail to relax*. Failure of muscle to contract or relax could be due to a muscle itself or secondary to a problem with the nervous system that controls it.

Let's review the sympathetic and parasympathetic nervous systems with regard to the gastrointestinal system. The sympathetic system is for fight/flight, and the parasympathetic system is for rest/digest. Thus, the parasympathetic system tells the GI tract to do things related to digestion: *squeeze* to pass food down and *open* the lower esophageal sphincter to allow food to pass to the stomach. If parasympathetic input is compromised, the esophagus will have decreased peristalsis and be unable to relax the lower esophageal sphincter to allow passage of food to the stomach.

Failure to Contract

Esophageal dilatation can occur in scleroderma and other connective tissue diseases, as well as in Chagas disease (infection with *Trypanasoma cruzi*). These diseases cause damage to the collagenous architecture of the esophageal wall.

Failure to Relax

Spasm can occur diffusely throughout the entire esophagus, appropriately named *diffuse esophageal spasm*. Some patients get an occasional spasm while others may have spasms every time they swallow. This can present as chest pain that mimics angina.

Failure to Contract and Relax: Achalasia

In achalasia, the lower esophageal sphincter remains constricted and is unable to relax. Although achalasia means failure to relax, later in the disease there is also failure to constrict: the lower two thirds of the esophagus lose the ability to peristalse. As food travels down the esophagus and gets stuck before the stomach, the esophageal walls get stretched, leading to dilatation of the esophagus proximal to the unrelaxable lower esophageal sphincter. The constricted sphincter and proximal dilation classically resemble a "bird's beak" on barium swallow imaging. Do you expect that achalasia is caused by a problem of the sympathetic or the parasympathetic nervous system? Peristalsis and relaxation of the lower esophageal sphincter are both processes necessary for digestion. The parasympathetic nervous system is responsible for stimulating these processes. In achalasia, a poorly understood process destroys postganglionic parasympathetic neurons of the esophagus.

Diverticula

Diverticula are outpouchings of the esophagus. If there is distal obstruction, the proximal portion of the esophagus tries to out-squeeze the obstruction, and this weakens its walls over time. This could cause *pulsion diverticula* proximal to the obstruction. (Diverticula can also occur in the large intestine by a similar mechanism). Esophageal diverticula can also be caused by *traction*, which is usually due to adjacent lymph nodes (most commonly from tuberculosis) that pull on the esophagus. Diverticula can also occur congenitally.

A *Zenker's diverticulum* lies just behind the upper esophageal sphincter. It is an out-pouching of the lumen that causes food and drink to get stuck there instead of continuing down. Because the food remains stuck there, patients with a Zenker's diverticulum may regurgitate undigested food. If regurgitated food is *undigested* it has obviously not made it to the stomach. If the regurgitated food appears *digested*, it must be coming from *below* the gastro-esophageal junction, and thus *cannot* be the result of a Zenker's diverticulum.

Reflux

Gastroesophageal reflux disease (GERD) is the most common disorder of the esophagus. The lower esophageal sphincter normally prevents food from coming back into the esophagus from the stomach. Reflux refers to the backwash of stomach acid up through the lower esophageal sphincter, which literally burns the esophageal mucosa (*esophagitis*). Why would this happen? The sphincter could be incompetent or distorted (for example, in a *hiatal hernia*, the lower esophageal sphincter slides above the diaphragm). Alternatively, the stomach could be creating excessive back-pressure, which could overcome the lower esophageal sphincter barrier. Why would there be increased stomach pressure? Impaired emptying of the stomach is one possibility, e.g., secondary to obstruction or gastroparesis (poor gastric motility).

GERD can be painful (e.g., heartburn, sour taste in the mouth, chest pain) and it is typically worse when bending over or when lying down after eating. This is because if the lower esophageal sphincter is incompetent or if there is a hiatal hernia, bending over or lying down will allow stomach contents to spill back through to the esophagus. Over time, acid reflux can damage the esophagus, leading to *Barrett's esophagus*, a premalignant condition (of metaplasia from squamous epithelium to columnar) that predisposes to esophageal *adenocarcinoma*.

Other Causes of Esophagitis

In addition to being caused by GERD, *esophagitis* (inflammation of the esophagus) can be caused by medications (e.g., chemotherapy), radiation, Crohn's disease, and infection. Infectious esophagitis occurs only very rarely in otherwise healthy individuals, but is much more common in immunocomprised patients (e.g., patients with HIV or hematologic malignancy). In immunocompromised patients, Candida, herpes simplex virus (HSV), and mycobacteria can cause esophagitis.

Esophageal Cancer

There are two types of esophageal cancer, *adenocarcinoma* and *squamous cell carcinoma*. GERD-induced Barrett's esophagus predisposes to adenocarcinoma; smoking and alcohol predispose to squamous cell carcinoma. Both can present as dysphagia secondary to obstruction from the tumor, and can also cause respiratory symptoms if the trachea is compressed or invaded by the tumor. Treatment involves surgery, chemotherapy, and/or radiation.

Esophageal Varices

Esophageal varices are dilations of esophageal veins, usually caused by liver disease/portal hypertension (see Fig. 4-12). Since dilated vein walls are more fragile, and since these varices are under high pressure, they can rupture, causing esophageal bleeding. If a varix bleeds, and the patient vomits blood, what should this bloody vomit look like? In an acute bleed, the blood should be undigested (i.e., still red) since it has not had time to make it to the stomach. This is in contrast to the *digested* blood that is vomited from more slowly bleeding gastric or duodenal ulcers in the stomach and duodenum, which is much darker (appearing like *coffee grounds*). Massive bleeding from gastric or duodenal ulcers can also cause bright red blood in the vomit, since the massive bleeding does not have time to be digested (see Fig. 4-9).

DISEASES OF THE STOMACH

The stomach churns food, produces acid to break food down, lets this digested food out (through the pyloric sphincter) to the duodenum for further digestion/absorption, and produces intrinsic factor, which aids in the absorption of B12. Because of the acid secretion necessary for digestion, the protection offered by the gastric mucosal lining is essential. Stomach pathologies include:

- Disruption to mucosal protection and/or excess acid production (associated with *ulcer*)

- Loss of intrinsic factor, leading to decreased B12 absorption (*pernicious anemia*).

- *Outlet obstruction* preventing release of digested food to the duodenum

- Loss of churning action (and/or loss of propulsion through the pylorus) (*gastroparesis*)

- Gastritis (inflammation of the stomach)

- Gastric cancer

Peptic Ulcer Disease

Peptic ulcers can occur in the stomach (*gastric ulcers*) or in the duodenum (*duodenal ulcers*).

Fig. 4-2. Regulation of gastric acid secretion. The parietal cells of the stomach secrete acid by pumping H^+ into the stomach lumen in exchange for K^+. This mechanism is stimulated by gastrin, histamine, and acetylcholine, and inhibited by somatostatin, prostaglandins, secretin, and VIP (vasoactive intestinal peptide). The mucous cells secrete a mucosal protective layer, and this secretion is mediated in part by prostaglandins.

Fig. 4-3. Causes of ulcer formation. There are two basic pathophysiological causes of ulcer formation: *decreased mucosal protection* and *increased acid production*. Infection with *Helicobacter pylori* is one of the most common causes of ulcer. *H. pylori* leads to ulcer formation by *both* of these mechanisms: the bacterium damages the mucosal lining and creates an inflammatory process that leads to increased acid secretion.

Decreased Mucosal Protection

Prostaglandins *increase* mucus secretion in the stomach. Molecules within the prostaglandin family

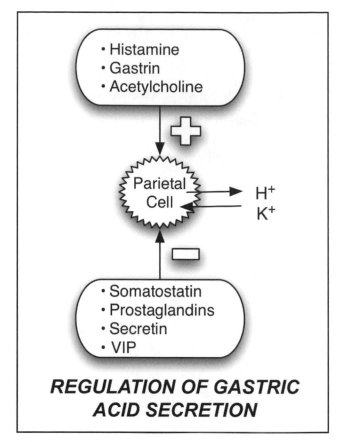

REGULATION OF GASTRIC ACID SECRETION

Figure 4-2

(arachidonic acid, COX, etc.) also mediate inflammation and pain. Non-steroidal anti-inflammatory drugs (NSAIDs) block these pain/inflammation pathways, but in so doing, also decrease mucus secretion in the stomach. Thus, prolonged NSAID use can cause ulcers. The COX-2 inhibitors (e.g., celecoxib, rofecoxib) selectively block the pain pathway and interact less with COX-1 (which is involved in stomach mucus secretion). This leaves mucosal protection in the gut relatively intact, so COX-2 inhibitors have fewer GI side effects. Tobacco and alcohol can also decrease mucosal protection, predisposing to ulcer formation.

Stress ulcers occur during severe physiologic stress, e.g., during shock (due to sepsis, burns, hemorrhage, etc.). Under such stress, the decrease in stomach perfusion can lead to decreased mucosal protection, which can result in ulcer formation. Therefore, many hospitalized patients are prophylactically placed on anti-ulcer medications since they may be subjected to various physiologic stresses during hospitalization.

Increased Acid Secretion

Recall that the hormone gastrin, secreted by the G cells of the stomach, stimulates acid secretion. In

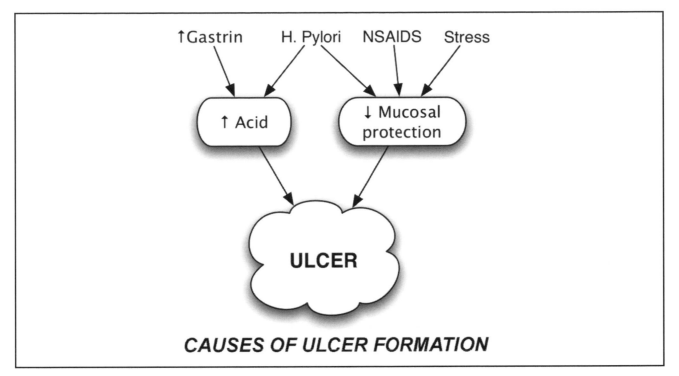

Figure 4-3

Zollinger-Ellison syndrome, a pancreatic tumor called a *gastrinoma* secretes gastrin. The increase in gastrin secretion by the gastrinoma leads to increased acid production, causing ulcers. Consider the diagnosis of Zollinger-Ellison syndrome in patients with multiple ulcers at different sites. This diagnosis can be proved by marked elevation in serum gastrin and by elevation of serum gastrin in response to *secretin*.

Fig. 4-4. Secretin Test. How does this secretin test work? Secretin is a hormone normally produced by the small intestine when food arrives from the stomach. Secretin stimulates the pancreas to secrete bicarbonate, which neutralizes the duodenal contents. Normally secretin *inhibits gastrin secretion*. If there is a pancreatic gastrinoma, secretin injection will paradoxically *increase* serum gastrin. A positive secretin test (i.e., elevation of serum gastrin in response to secretin) is diagnostic for Zollinger-Ellison Syndrome.

Symptoms and Signs of Peptic Ulcer Disease

Ulcers can cause pain (see Fig. 4-5), nausea, vomiting (with red blood or digested blood; digested blood can look like "coffee grounds"), tarry stools (melena), and changes in appetite. Severe ulcer disease can lead to *perforation* of the duodenal or gastric wall. Perforated ulcers can present as acute abdominal pain with air under the diaphragm visible on X-ray. Emergency surgery is necessary for repair of a perforated ulcer.

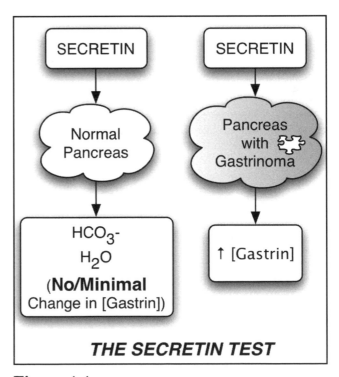

Figure 4-4

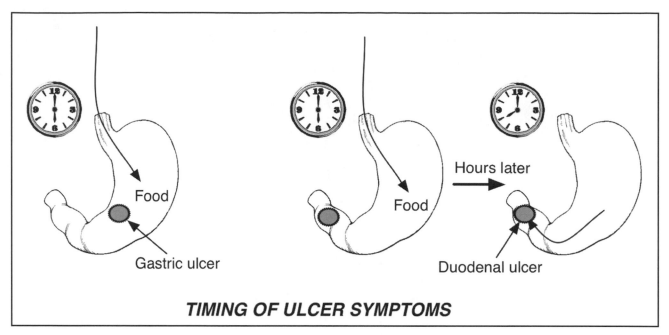

TIMING OF ULCER SYMPTOMS

Figure 4-5

Timing of Ulcer Symptoms

Fig. 4-5. Timing of ulcer pain. Ulcers can form in the duodenum and/or in the stomach. In which site would ulcer pain get worse immediately after eating and in which site would this pain occur somewhat later? What happens when food arrives in the stomach? First, acid is secreted and the food is churned around before anything else happens. Since acid secretion in the stomach will exacerbate the pain of any denuded area of mucosa (i.e., an ulcer), it should make sense that eating causes pain in gastric ulcers. It is not until later after a meal that the food is passed into the duodenum. At that time, the acidic gastric contents could irritate a duodenal ulcer, if one is present. So duodenal ulcer pain typically occurs much later after a meal. Although these are "classic" presentation patterns, ulcer pain can have a variety of relationships to eating patterns across patients. Many exceptions to the above patterns can occur, and thus *endoscopy* is often necessary to make a definitive diagnosis.

Gastric ulcers should *always* be biopsied to rule out gastric cancer, since gastric cancer may ulcerate and thus appear similar to a peptic ulcer on endoscopy.

Ulcer Treatment

Fig. 4-6. Ulcer treatment. Since increased acid secretion and/or decreased mucosal protection can cause ulcers, treatments include drugs that *neutralize acid,* *prevent acid from being secreted, increase mucosal protection,* or *eradicate H. Pylori.*

To *neutralize acid,* we simply use base. Examples include antacids such as magnesium or calcium salts (i.e., milk of magnesia, Tums tablets).

To *decrease acid production,* one can either directly decrease production by the parietal cell itself or decrease/block the chemicals that stimulate the parietal cell. To directly affect acid secretion one must block the H^+/K^+ pump in the parietal cells; the proton pump inhibitors such as omeprazole or pantoprazole work in this way. To decrease *stimulation* of the parietal cells, one can block histamine; the H2 blockers (e.g., ranitidine) block the H2 receptors on parietal cells. The H2 receptors are the receptors to which histamine binds to stimulate acid release. One can also surgically sever the branches of the vagus nerve (cranial nerve X) that provide the parasympathetic input that stimulates acid-secreting cells (*vagotomy*).

Another type of treatment approach *increases the mucosal defense* of the lining, either by providing a mucus-like substance or by increasing mucus production. *Sucralfate* forms a viscous gel in the stomach and helps to form a protective barrier. How could you increase mucus production? Remember that prostaglandins are partially responsible for increased mucosal secretion. *Misoprostol* is a synthetic prostaglandin that increases mucosal secretion and protects against ulcer formation.

Antibiotics are used to treat *H. pylori.*

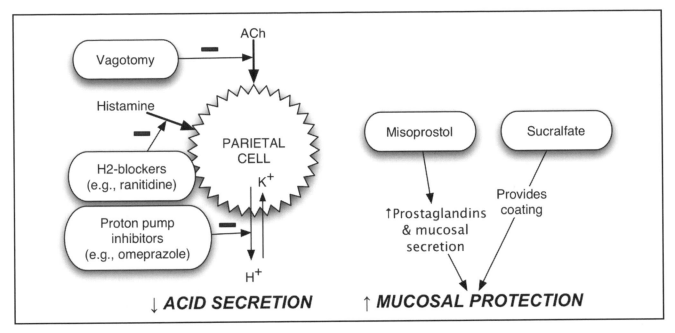

Figure 4-6

Other Causes of Gastritis

In addition to *H. pylori*, NSAIDs, and severe physiologic stress, the following may also cause gastric inflammation (*gastritis*): alcohol, radiation, other infectious agents, Crohn's disease, and reflux of bile and/or pancreatic secretions.

Loss of Intrinsic Factor

The parietal cells of the stomach produce intrinsic factor. Intrinsic factor binds B12, facilitating its absorption. Pernicious anemia (*autoimmune gastritis*) is a condition in which antibodies form against the parietal cells, leading to loss of intrinsic factor. Without intrinsic factor, B12 cannot be absorbed, which can lead to anemia. This condition, its pathophysiology, and its diagnosis are discussed in the anemia section of the hematology chapter (Chapter 6).

Obstruction

To pass food to the duodenum, the pyloric sphincter must be patent and the stomach must squeeze the food through it. How could the pyloric sphincter become obstructed? As with the esophagus (in fact, with the whole GI tract), whenever there is obstruction, it can occur from the inside or from the outside. For the pyloric sphincter, from-the-inside obstruction can occur from a foreign body, a gastric polyp, or gastric cancer; from-the-outside obstruction can be caused by a pancreatic tumor. Additionally, the pylorus can become scarred shut by acid in peptic ulcer

disease or by ingestion of a caustic substance. In *congenital pyloric stenosis*, the baby is born with a hypertrophied pylorus. Surgical opening of the sphincter is usually necessary in babies with congenital pyloric stenosis.

What would the symptoms be if the stomach is squeezing against a closed pylorus? Well, where else can the gastric contents go...but backward? Thus, vomiting is a chief complaint. Early satiety and abdominal distension can occur as well. *Congenital pyloric stenosis* can present as a palpable olive-like mass on exam (the hypertrophied sphincter) and visible waves of peristalsis as the stomach tries in vain to overpower the stenosis.

Gastroparesis

Gastroparesis is paralysis of the stomach. The stomach is under the control of the enteric nervous system. Parasympathetic input to the stomach comes from the vagus nerve (cranial nerve X). A problem with the parasympathetic nerves to the stomach can lead to decreased stomach muscle activity and gastroparesis. Nerve dysfunction here can be due to damage to the nerve itself or a blockage of neural transmission to the stomach. Nerve damage can be secondary to diabetic neuropathy or other neurological diseases. Since *all parasympathetic nerves release acetylcholine at their synapses*, drugs that block acetylcholine can cause gastroparesis. Additionally, any drug that decreases gastric motility (e.g., narcotic analgesics) can result in gastroparesis.

Gastric Cancer

Gastric cancer is more common in people of Asian descent. Many of the causes of gastritis also predispose to development of gastric cancer (e.g., *H. Pylori* infection, pernicious anemia, radiation). Most commonly, gastric cancer is adenocarcinoma, though MALT (mucosa-associated lymphoid tissue), GI stromal tumor (GIST), and leiomyosarcoma (smooth muscle tumor) can also occur in the stomach. Symptoms and signs (e.g., nausea/vomiting, early satiety, GI bleed) generally occur late in the course of the disease, so prognosis is often relatively poor by the time the tumor is discovered. Surgery may be supplemented with radiation and/or chemotherapy for treatment.

DISEASES OF THE SMALL INTESTINE

As with any portion of the GI tract, *inflammation* (e.g., Crohn's disease), *tumors, obstruction,* and *bleeding* are possible in the small intestine. The main function of the small intestine is absorption, and the corresponding pathology is *malabsorption*.

Malabsorption

Fig. 4-7. Causes of malabsorption. Any defect in digestion/absorption can lead to malabsorption. Let's review the main steps and their potential corresponding pathologies. Food is churned and broken down in the stomach and arrives in the small intestine. This stimulates release of cholecystokinin (CCK) and secretin by the duodenum, which cause the gall bladder to release bile and the pancreas to release HCO_3^- and digestive enzymes (e.g., chymotrypsin), which further digest the food. The digested products are then absorbed across the intestinal membrane, further metabolized by cells of the gut wall, and passed to the bloodstream. Any problem along this path can lead to malabsorption. Causes of malabsorption can be attributed to either problems with *digestion* or problems with *absorption*.

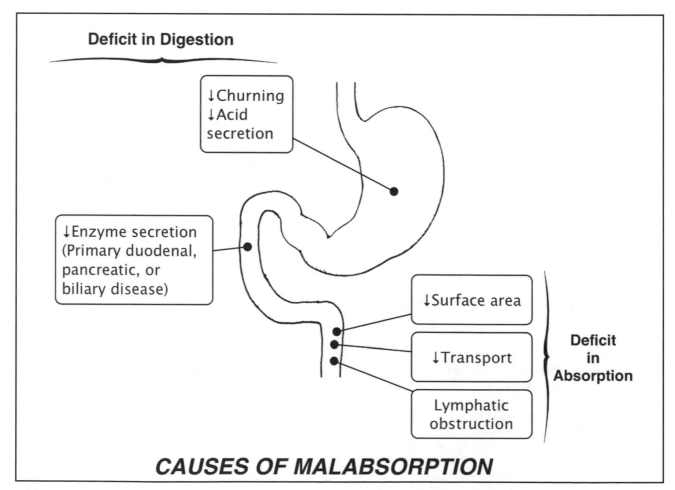

Deficit in Digestion

↓Churning
↓Acid secretion

↓Enzyme secretion (Primary duodenal, pancreatic, or biliary disease)

↓Surface area

↓Transport

Lymphatic obstruction

Deficit in Absorption

CAUSES OF MALABSORPTION

Figure 4-7

Problems with Digestion

A defect in *digestion* can occur secondary to:

- *Failure of stomach acid secretion or churning* (See Gastroparesis)

- *Failure of enzyme secretion into the gut lumen*
  - Pancreatic insufficiency or failure causes a decrease in secretion of digestive enzymes.
  - Liver disease or gall bladder obstruction leads to decreased bile acids.
  - Duodenal resection leads to loss of cholecystokinin secretion and thus secondarily to reduction in pancreatic and gall bladder secretion of digestive agents.

- *Failure or decrease of an enzyme* (e.g., lactase deficiency leading to lactose intolerance)

Problems with Absorption

A defect in absorption can occur secondary to:

- *Reduced surface area*
  - Resection of bowel
  - Damage to the absorbing mucosa (Crohn's disease, parasitic infection, drugs, radiation, sprue[1])

- *Biochemical aberrations in transport/intracellular metabolism* (e.g., abetalipoproteinemia)

- *Obstruction of the lymphatics/lacteals* (e.g., by tumor)

Obstruction

As with the rest of the GI tract, the small intestine can become *obstructed*. Causes of small bowel obstruction can include: adhesions from a prior surgery, small bowel tumors (these are extremely rare), nearby tumors in other organs (e.g., pancreas), gallstones, hernias, and inflammatory changes (e.g., Crohn's disease). *Complete* small bowel obstruction is a surgical emergency; *partial* small bowel obstruction can usually be managed by prohibiting oral intake, using nasogastric tube decompression, and administering IV fluids.

Small Bowel Tumors

Small bowel tumors are extremely rare. Pathologically, these may be benign adenomas, lipomas, and leiomyomas, or malignant adenocarcinomas, lymphomas, carcinoids, GI stromal tumors (GIST), or sarcomas. Small bowel tumors can cause bleeding and/or obstruction,

potentially resulting in nausea, vomiting, abdominal pain, weight loss, and/or fatigue.

DISEASES OF THE LARGE INTESTINE

As with any region of the GI tract, *tumors* (e.g., colon cancer), *inflammation* (e.g., ulcerative colitis, Crohn's disease), *obstruction* (most commonly due to colon cancer), and *bleeding* can occur in the large intestine. The functions of the large intestine are delivery of stool to the outside and some water and sodium reabsorption. Failure of the first can lead to *constipation*, while problems with the second can lead to *diarrhea*. Constipation can occur for either of two reasons: the muscles are not squeezing appropriately, or there is some sort of obstruction (tumor, or otherwise). *Irritable bowel syndrome* (abdominal pain, diarrhea, and/or constipation with unknown etiology) may be due to problems with regulation of gastrointestinal muscular activity; the pathophysiology has not yet been fully elucidated.

Hirschprung's Disease

Hirschprung's disease is a cause of constipation in children. In Hirschprung's disease, neural crest cells fail to migrate to the distal portion of the colon during development. The bowel dilates massively proximal to this denervated stretch of colon (hence the other name for this disease: aganglionic megacolon). Although Hirschprung's disease often presents as failure to pass meconium in infancy, the presentation can be later in childhood if the disease is less severe. Hirschprung's should thus be ruled out as a cause of chronic constipation in children. Treatment is surgical.

Diverticula

If a person's diet is low in fiber, the formation of hard stools can create extra squeezing work for the large intestine. Over time this excessive squeezing can weaken the walls of the large intestine, leading to diverticula. Most typically this occurs in the descending colon (which lies on the left side of the body). Diverticula can lead to lower GI bleeding and/or pain, classically in the left lower quadrant (*diverticulosis*). Diverticula can also become inflamed (*diverticulitis*).

What sits next to the descending colon? The bladder. In severe diverticulosis, the diverticula can rupture and adhere to the bladder, even creating a communication between the two. This *colovesical fistula* can cause *pneumaturia* (air in the urine) and *fecaluria* (feces in the urine).

---

[1] There are two types of sprue: celiac sprue and tropical sprue. *Celiac sprue* (a.k.a. non-tropical sprue, gluten-sensitive enteropathy) is caused by a reaction to gluten, a component of wheat. The reaction leads to inflammation of the small intestine mucosa and subsequent malabsorption. The condition improves when gluten is no longer consumed. *Tropical sprue* is endemic to tropical areas; the infectious agent that causes it is unknown.

Diarrhea

Fig. 4-8. Causes of diarrhea. What could cause too much fluid to end up at the end of the large intestine? *Excess secretion*, *decreased absorption*, or *presence of some substance that increases osmolarity of the colonic contents*. For example, a patient with lactose intolerance lacks adequate lactase enzyme. Thus, lactose, which should have been broken down and absorbed in the small intestine, remains in the large intestine. Since this increases the solute concentration of the intraluminal fluid compared with the cellular fluid around it, water is naturally drawn into the lumen.

What else could cause excess secretion or decreased absorption? The bacterium *Vibrio cholera* has a toxin that activates adenylate cyclase. This leads to *activation* of transporters that increase Cl^- and K^+ secretion (into the lumen from the cells) and *inhibition* of one of the luminal electrolyte transporters that is responsible for Na^+ absorption (from the lumen into the cells). This excess Na^+, K^+, and Cl^- in the lumen increases luminal osmolarity, which results in an osmotic gradient that draws in water, leading to diarrhea. *E. coli* can also produce toxins that affect the various transporters, leading to decreased absorption of Na^+ and/or increased secretion of K^+ and Cl^-. Other bacteria (e.g., *Shigella, Salmonella, Campylobacter, Bacillus*) and some viruses (e.g., rotavirus, Norwalk virus) cause diarrhea by direct damage to the intestinal wall. This damage also affects these transporters, resulting in over-secretion and/or decreased absorption.

A rare cause of diarrhea is *pancreatic cholera,* where a tumor (usually in the pancreas) secretes vasoactive intestinal peptide (VIP). Normally, VIP secretion inhibits gastric secretion, relaxes gut musculature, and increases pancreatic bicarbonate secretion. Excess VIP increases adenylate cyclase activity in the large intestine, which results in increased secretion and

decreased absorption as described above. This condition is also known as *VIPoma, Werner-Morrison syndrome*, or *WDHA* (watery diarrhea, hypokalemia, and achlorhydria).

Colon Cancer

Colon cancer (adenocarcinoma) is one of the most common cancers. Genetic predisposition to colon cancer occurs in people with a strong family history or genetic syndromes such as hereditary nonpolyposis colorectal cancer (HNPCC) and familial adenomatous polyposis (FAP). Colon cancer can present with symptoms including abdominal pain, lower GI bleeding (often occult), changes in bowel habits (timing, amount, shape of stools), and/or intestinal obstruction. Because colon cancer is so common, regular screening after age 50 using fecal occult blood testing, flexible sigmoidoscopy, barium contrast X-ray, and/or colonoscopy is recommended. Treatment involves surgery, chemotherapy, and/or radiation.

Colitis

Inflammation of the colon (*colitis*) can occur secondary to infection, ischemia, drugs (e.g., antibiotics), radiation injury, or inflammatory bowel disease (see below). Symptoms/signs can include changes in bowel patterns, abdominal pain, and/or lower GI bleeding.

INFLAMMATORY BOWEL DISEASE (IBD): CROHN'S DISEASE AND ULCERATIVE COLITIS

The underlying etiology of these disorders has not yet been fully elucidated. From the name *ulcerative colitis*, it should be clear that the primary feature of this disease is ulceration in the colon. In fact, aside from the occasional occurrence of backwash ileitis, *ulcera-*

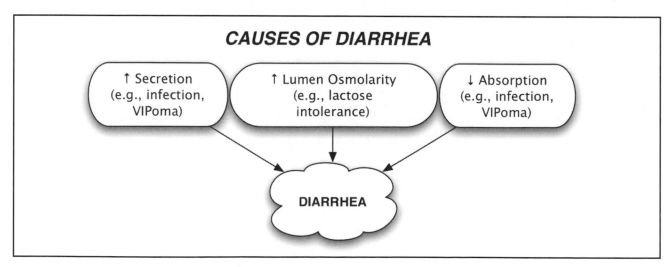

Figure 4-8

tive colitis is limited to the colon. Because of the ulceration, blood in the stool is a common presenting symptom. *Crohn's disease*, on the other hand, can occur *anywhere* along the GI tract, from mouth to anus.

Mnemonic: **Cr**ohn's **cr**osses boundaries. Crohn's disease can occur from mouth to anus, and causes transmural inflammation (crossing histologic boundaries) and fissures (boundary-crossing tears). Crohn's disease's effects on the small intestine can lead to malabsorption and B12 deficiency anemia (because damage to the terminal ileum decreases B12 absorption).

A number of associated findings can occur in inflammatory bowel disease, including aphthous ulcers (canker sores in the mouth), sclerosing cholangitis (inflammation of the bile ducts), skin findings (pyoderma gangrenosum, erythema nodosum), and/or eye findings (iritis, scleritis). IBD can also increase colon cancer risk.

UPPER AND LOWER GI BLEEDING

Fig. 4-9. Localizing GI Bleeding. When a patient vomits blood or has blood in the stool, the most likely location of the bleeding can be deduced from the history. Let's begin with bloody vomit. If the bleeding is *above* the gastroesophageal junction (GEJ), this blood is *not* digested and should appear bright red in vomit (e.g., bleeding esophageal varices). If the bleeding is coming from the stomach or lower, the blood will have been digested, and this makes it much darker. This results in the classic "coffee grounds" vomit typically found with a bleeding gastric or duodenal ulcer. A massive rapid-onset bleed from an ulcer can also cause bright red blood in the vomit, if the bleed is so large and/or rapid that the blood does not have time to be digested.

As for bleeding from the rectum, bright red blood (*hematochezia*) also means that the blood has come

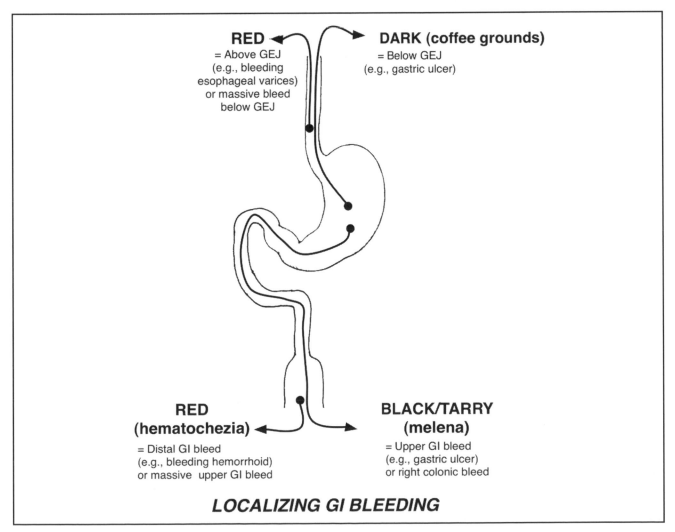

LOCALIZING GI BLEEDING

Figure 4-9

from a source relatively near to the site of exit, since it has not been digested, e.g., bleeding hemorrhoids, bleeding colon cancer, bleeding diverticula. If there is an upper GI bleed (e.g., a bleeding ulcer), stools will typically be described as black and tarry (*melena*) since the blood has come from higher up in the GI tract and has thus been digested. Summary: *Red blood from mouth or anus indicates a source close to the site of bleeding whereas dark, digested blood indicates a more remote source.* These are broad generalizations: If there is a sudden onset of massive bleeding below the gastroesophageal junction, the blood will not have had time to be digested and can appear as bright red blood in the vomit or stool. Also, lower GI bleeding can appear as *melena,* if the blood remains in the GI tract long enough before being excreted (e.g., bleeding from the right colon).

DISEASES OF THE LIVER

Overview of Liver Function

The hepatic portal vein drains the gut's venous system, carrying absorbed nutrients to the liver. The liver performs many metabolic functions. For example, the liver provides much of the glucose during fasting (via gluconeogenesis and glycogenolysis), detoxifies various substances, stores glycogen, and produces bile, as well as various proteins and lipids.

What would happen if the liver failed?

- *Decrease in detoxification reactions*, resulting in accumulation of toxic substances in the blood, which can lead to hepatic encephalopathy

- *Decrease in gluconeogenesis*, which can cause fasting hypoglycemia

- *Decrease in protein production*, which can decrease clotting factor production, increasing the risk of bleeding

- *Failure of the liver to secrete conjugated bilirubin or failure to conjugate it*, which can cause jaundice

Bilirubin and Jaundice

Fig. 4-10. Bile metabolism and causes of jaundice. Bile emulsifies fats in the GI tract, facilitating their absorption. Bile is produced in the liver and then drains through the intrahepatic biliary system into the extrahepatic biliary tree. One component of bile is bilirubin, a product of the breakdown of old (or damaged) red blood cells. When red blood cells break down, unconjugated (indirect) bilirubin forms in the circulation. *The liver conjugates this bilirubin, thus producing **conjugated (direct) bilirubin**.* The conjugated bilirubin is secreted into the bile. *Jaundice*, where the sclerae and skin turn yellow, occurs due to an increase in either conjugated or unconjugated bilirubin in the circulation.

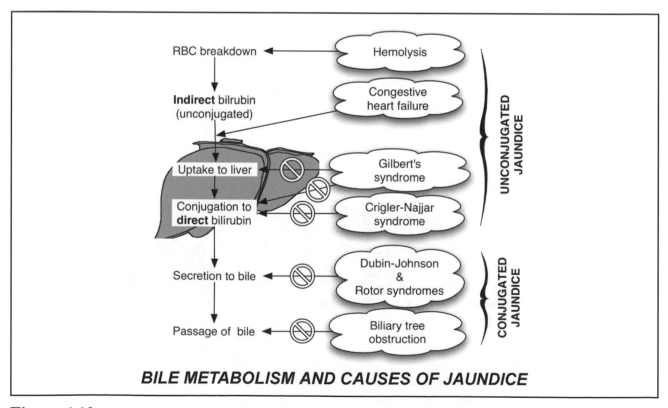

BILE METABOLISM AND CAUSES OF JAUNDICE

Figure 4-10

For *unconjugated (indirect) bilirubin* to increase, there must be either *increased production* of bilirubin, *decreased uptake* of bilirubin by the liver, or *decreased conjugation* of bilirubin by the liver. Since bilirubin comes from the breakdown of old or damaged red cells, any cause of hemolytic anemia would lead to *increased production* of bilirubin. This increase can exceed the liver's capacity to conjugate, leading to an elevation of unconjugated bilirubin. Congestive heart failure reduces blood flow to the liver, which can decrease delivery of bilirubin for conjugation, resulting in unconjugated jaundice. Decreased uptake and conjugation can also occur secondary to two genetic syndromes: *Crigler-Najjar* and *Gilbert's*. Mnemonic: In **C**rigler-**N**ajjar syndrome patients **can**not **con**jugate bilirubin. In **G**ilbert's syndrome, patients can't **g**et the bilirubin into the liver (decreased uptake) and cannot conjugate it.[2]

What about increases in *conjugated* bilirubin? If the elevation of bilirubin is largely conjugated, this means that the bilirubin has made it into the liver and conjugation has occurred. What would cause a backup of conjugated bilirubin in the blood? Either the liver does not accomplish the final step of secreting the bilirubin into the bile ducts, or the biliary tree is obstructed. *Any disease that can damage the liver can decrease the liver's ability to secrete bilirubin* (e.g., toxin-induced hepatic failure or infectious, alcoholic, or autoimmune hepatitis). Any obstruction in the biliary tree can cause a backup of conjugated bilirubin. The site of obstruction can be intrahepatic (e.g., cancer, granuloma, primary biliary cirrhosis) or extrahepatic (e.g., stones, stricture, cancer). Dubin-Johnson and Rotor syndromes are genetic defects that impair secretion of bilirubin into the bile.

Jaundice is not the only color change when there is elevated bilirubin in the circulation due to obstruction. Excess pigment that arrives in the urine leads to dark (tea-colored) urine.[3] Lack of bile pigment making it to the GI tract (secondary to the obstruction) leads to lack of this pigment in the stool *(clay-colored stools)*. Bile salt deposits in the skin lead to severe itching *(pruritis)*.

Liver Function Tests

AST, ALT, and Alkaline Phosphatase

AST (aspartate aminotransferase) and ALT (alanine aminotransferase) are two liver enzymes involved in metabolic reactions. Alkaline phosphatase is mainly present in the cells of the bile ducts. In liver disease, the liver cells release AST and ALT into the circulation.

When the biliary tree is obstructed, the cells of the bile ducts release alkaline phosphatase ("alk phos").[4] Mnemonic: alk ph**os** = **o**bstruction. In long-standing obstruction, the AST and ALT may begin to rise as well, though typically the rise is far less dramatic than that of the alkaline phosphatase. Similarly, alkaline phosphatase can be mildly elevated in liver disease, but the AST and ALT are generally elevated to a much greater extent. Obstruction can be due to various pathologies of the biliary tract (e.g., stones, inflammatory disease, cancer). Although AST, ALT, and alkaline phosphatase are commonly referred to as "liver function tests," they do *not* measure liver *function*. Rather, they are markers of *injury* to hepatocytes (AST and ALT) or the bile ducts (alkaline phosphatase).

Bilirubin, Albumin, and Prothrombin Time

Bilirubin, albumin, and prothrombin time are measures of liver *function*. *Bilirubin* is discussed above as a measure of the liver's ability to perform enzymatic and metabolic function(s) such as conjugation of unconjugated bilirubin and secretion of conjugated bilirubin (see Fig. 4-10). Since secretion of bilirubin is the rate-limiting step in this process, *conjugated (direct) bilirubin* is often elevated in liver disease.

Albumin and *prothrombin time* assess the liver's synthetic function. Albumin is a serum protein synthesized by the liver, so albumin level measures the liver's capacity for protein synthesis. Thus, albumin level can *decrease* in liver disease. Decreased serum albumin can also occur in inflammatory diseases, severe trauma, malnutrition, and diseases causing proteinuria (e.g., nephritic syndrome).

Prothrombin time measures function in part of the clotting cascade (see Fig. 6-10). Since the liver synthesizes most of the coagulation factors, deficient clotting (and hence *elevated* prothrombin time) can result from liver disease. Specifically, prothrombin time assesses the extrinsic pathway of the clotting cascade, namely factor VII. Since factor VII is rapidly degraded, measuring the integrity of the extrinsic pathway by prothrombin time is a good marker of the liver's synthetic capacity. Prothrombin time can also be elevated with anticoagulant therapy (e.g., coumadin) and vitamin K deficiency.

Elevated prothrombin time is more associated with *acute* liver disease, while a decrease in albumin is generally associated with *chronic* liver disease.

[2] Both Crigler-Najjar and Gilbert's syndromes are associated with mutations in uridinediphospho-glucuronate glucuronosyltransferase (UGT), an enzyme that participates in conjugation. In Crigler-Najjar this enzyme is extremely reduced or absent, whereas in Gilbert's it is only mildly reduced. Thus, Gilbert's is a much milder disease, and may even be asymptomatic.

[3] Dark urine from jaundice only occurs when the bilirubin is conjugated. This is because unconjugated bilirubin is not water-soluble and thus does not end up in the urine. So although any elevation of bilirubin (conjugated or unconjugated) can lead to jaundice, it is only when the elevation is predominantly conjugated (i.e., from a failure to secrete bilirubin or biliary obstruction) that the urine can become dark.

[4] Elevated alkaline phosphatase can also come from bone breakdown.

In summary, elevated AST and ALT indicate liver *injury* and elevated alkaline phosphatase can suggest *biliary obstruction*. *Increased* conjugated bilirubin, *decreased* serum albumin, and/or *increased* prothrombin time can all indicate decreased liver *function*.

Diseases of the Liver Parenchyma

Causes of liver disease include: viral hepatitis, toxin-induced liver disease (e.g., drugs, alcohol), hepatic steatosis, autoimmune liver disease, hemochromatosis, Wilson's disease, alpha-1 antitrypsin deficiency, and hepatic neoplasia. Any liver disease can lead to jaundice and elevation of liver enzymes. Any of these diseases can also eventually lead to *cirrhosis*, which is scarring of the liver parenchyma. Cirrhosis can cause an elevated pressure/resistance to blood flow and thus *portal hypertension*. Cirrhosis (or any of its causes) can also increase the risk of hepatic cancer (*hepatocellular carcinoma*).

Viral Hepatitis.

Fig. 4-11. Viral hepatitis.

Drug Reactions can be acute (adverse reaction to a drug or overdose) or chronic (i.e., from sustained use).

Fatty Liver (*hepatic steatosis*) can occur secondary to alcohol abuse (*alcoholic liver disease*) or in patients with no history of alcohol use (*non-alcoholic fatty liver disease*). Alcoholic liver disease typically produces mild elevations of AST:ALT, classically in a 2:1 ratio. Additionally, GGT (gamma- glutamyltransferase) is typically elevated in alcoholics. Non-alcoholic fatty liver (also known as *nonalcoholic steatohepatitis - NASH*) is a condition in which liver disease develops with the same histological pattern as in alcoholic liver disease despite *lack of significant alcohol consumption*. There is some association with obesity and diabetes.

Figure 4-11 Viral Hepatitis

TYPE	TRANSMISSION	CLINICAL	SEROLOGY
Hepatitis A	• Fecal-oral	• Acute viral hepatitis: fever, jaundice, and a painful enlarged liver – 1% develop fulminant hepatitis – Never becomes chronic	• Anti-HAV IgM = Active disease • Anti-HAV IgG = Old; no active disease protective against repeated infection
Hepatitis B	• Blood transfusion • Needle sticks • Sexual • Across the placenta	• Acute viral hepatitis • Fulminant hepatitis: severe acute hepatitis with rapid destruction of the liver • Chronic hepatitis (10%) – Asymptomatic carrier – Chronic persistent hepatitis – Chronic active hepatitis • Coinfection or superinfection with – Hepatitis Delta Virus (HDV) *Complications:* • Primary hepatocellular carcinoma • Cirrhosis	• HBsAg = Disease (Acute or Chronic) • Anti-HBsAg = immunity: provides protection against repeat infection • IgM anti-HBcAg = New infection • IgG anti-HBcAg = Old infection • HBeAg = High infectivity • Anti-HBeAg = Low infectivity (sAg = surface antigen, cAg = core antigen, eAg = envelope antigen)
Hepatitis C	• Blood transfusion • Needle sticks • Sexual • Across the placenta	• Acute viral hepatitis – 50% will get chronic hepatitis – 20% will develop cirrhosis – Increased risk of developing primary hepatocellular carcinoma	• Screening: anti-HCV antibodies
Hepatitis D	• Blood transfusion • Needle sticks • Sexual • Across the placenta	• Coinfection: HBV and HDV are acquired at the same time, and cause an acute hepatitis. Anti-HBV antibodies help cure infection. • Superinfection: HDV infects a patient with chronic hepatitis B who cannot manufacture Anti-HbsAg antibodies. *Complications:* • Fulminant hepatitis • Cirrhosis	• Serology is not very helpful since detectable titers of IgM and IgG anti-HDV are present only fleetingly.
Hepatitis E	• Fecal-oral	• Hepatitis (like hepatitis A)	

Modified from Gladwin and Trattler: *Clinical Microbiology Made Ridiculously Simple*, MedMaster 2004

Autoimmune Hepatitis. Like many other autoimmune diseases, autoimmune hepatitis tends to affect women predominantly and can be associated with other autoimmune conditions (e.g., arthralgia, rash, thyroid disease). Anti-smooth muscle antibodies are associated with autoimmune hepatitis.

Hemochromatosis is an autosomal recessive disease that results in an abnormally high amount of iron in the blood. This can lead to iron deposition in the heart, causing restrictive cardiomyopathy. Iron deposition in the liver can result in cirrhosis. Iron accumulation in the pancreas can cause diabetes. The skin can become bronze, since iron can be deposited there as well (hence the nickname "bronze diabetes" for hemochromatosis). Deposition in the pituitary can also occur. It is thought that hemochromatosis is far more common than previously imagined. Therefore, some clinicians would argue that a mild elevation of liver enzymes (AST /ALT), even in a healthy patient, should warrant a work-up for hemochromatosis. The work-up assesses transferrin saturation and ferritin, which will both be elevated in hemochromatosis. Genetic testing and liver biopsy to measure iron can confirm the diagnosis.

In ***Wilson's disease***, another autosomal recessive disease, there is decreased copper excretion, leading to deposition of copper in the liver (which can lead to cirrhosis), brain (which can cause movement disorders), and/or the eyes (which can result in a Kayser-Fleischer ring). *Low serum ceruloplasmin* (the serum protein that carries copper) and *increased urinary copper* are the classic lab findings in Wilson's disease.

Liver biopsy demonstrating excess copper can confirm the diagnosis.

Alpha-1 antitrypsin deficiency. Deficiency of this enzyme in the lungs can lead to (panlobular) emphysema, while deficiency of this enzyme in the liver can lead to cirrhosis. A low alpha-1 antitrypsin level in the serum and genetic testing (phenotyping) are necessary for diagnosis.

Hepatic Neoplasm may be benign or malignant. Malignant tumors may be primary or metastatic. Any of these may cause right upper quadrant pain and constitutional symptoms (fever, malaise, weight loss). An enlarged liver or palpable mass may be present on physical exam. Rupture of a tumor can lead to acute abdominal pain. *Benign hepatic adenoma* is more common in women and often secondary to oral contraceptive use. Risk for *hepatocellular carcinoma* is increased by various carcinogens (e.g., aflatoxin) as well as anything that causes cirrhosis (e.g., alcohol, hemochromatosis, hepatitis B and C infection). Elevated alpha-fetoprotein (AFP) is often seen with hepatocellular carcinoma. Metastases to the liver are more common than primary hepatocellular carcinoma in the United States. Treatment involves surgery, chemotherapy, and radiation.

Disease of the Liver Vasculature: Portal Hypertension

Fig. 4-12. Hepatic portal system and sites of origin of portal hypertension. The hepatic portal vein brings blood to the liver from the gut. The portal venous system branches extensively within the liver, and these

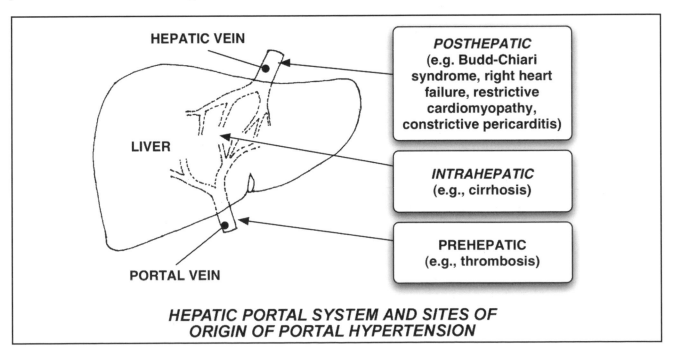

HEPATIC PORTAL SYSTEM AND SITES OF ORIGIN OF PORTAL HYPERTENSION

Figure 4-12

branches rejoin to form the hepatic vein, which joins with the inferior vena cava. Thus, the hepatic venous system can be divided into 3 regions: *prehepatic* (the portal vein), *intrahepatic* (the portal venous system within the liver itself), and *post-hepatic* (the hepatic vein). *Portal hypertension*, an increase in pressure in the hepatic vascular system, can result from pathology at any of these sites:

• *Prehepatic*: The portal vein can be thrombosed.[5]

• *Intrahepatic*: Any liver disease that causes cirrhosis can cause changes in the vascular system leading to portal hypertension.

• *Posthepatic*:
  – The hepatic vein can be thrombosed (*Budd-Chiari syndrome*).
  – The hepatic vein connects to the inferior vena cava, so resistance to flow in this system can also increase portal pressure (e.g., secondary to right heart failure, restrictive cardiomyopathy, or constrictive pericarditis).

What are the consequences of hepatic venous system obstruction? An acute event (like thrombosis of the portal or hepatic vein) can lead to acute liver failure. However, many of the more chronic causes of cirrhosis result in a slower emergence of portal hypertension, which can lead to *ascites* (fluid in the abdomen) and *varices* (venous dilatation).

Ascites

Cirrhosis-induced portal hypertension is the most common causes of ascites, though ascites can also result from infection, malignancy, and nephrotic syndrome. A sample of ascites fluid can be extracted (*paracentesis*) and studied to diagnosis the cause of ascites. A large number white blood cells in the fluid indicates inflammation or infection; cultures can be performed to search for specific organisms. Cytology can be performed to look for malignant cells. The *serum-ascites albumin gradient* (SAAG) can help determine if the etiology is portal hypertension or not. SAAG is measured by subtracting the albumin concentration in the ascites fluid from the albumin level in the serum. Fluid in portal hypertension tends to be relatively dilute, and thus has a *lower* albumin concentration than ascites fluid in infection or malignancy. Thus, the *SAAG tends to be higher in portal hypertension than in other causes of ascites* (since a smaller number is being subtracted from the serum albumin concentration). Generally, in portal hypertension, SAAG > 1.1 g/dl, and in other causes of ascites, SAAG < 1.1 g/dl.

Varices

A large amount of blood flows through the portal system to the liver. If this system is blocked for any reason, the blood needs to find a way back to the heart, and so it reverses flow back down the portal system into other veins to do so. These veins include the splenic vein, umbilical vein, hemorrhoidal veins, and esophageal/gastric veins. These veins are not accustomed to handling such large blood volume and they dilate (*varices*). The backup into the spleen causes it to enlarge. The enlarged spleen starts overdoing its job (*hypersplenism*), which causes an increased removal of blood elements and can lead to anemia. The umbilical veins can sometimes be seen on physical exam as a *caput medusa* (varicose veins around the navel). The enlarged hemorrhoidal veins around the anus can present as *hemorrhoids*.

The esophageal and gastric venous dilatations (*varices*) can rupture, causing a massive (and often lethal) bleed. Bleeding varices require immediate intervention using vasoconstrictive drugs to reduce flow to the varices (e.g., vasopressin or octreotide), endoscopic sclerotherapy (burning the varices), or endoscopic ligation (putting rubber bands around the varices). If the patient survives, beta-blockers can be used to reduce portal pressure, reducing the risk of variceal rupture. The classic scenario in which to suspect bleeding varices is an alcoholic patient who comes to the emergency room vomiting blood.

Another way to reduce pressure in varices is by surgical shunting. Shunts give the blood a path of lesser resistance so as to reduce pressure on varices, in an attempt to prevent their rupture. A shunt can be placed from the hepatic portal vein to the inferior vena cava, or from the splenic vein to the renal vein, or a transjugular intrahepatic portosystemic shunt (TIPS) can be placed linking the hepatic portal vein to the hepatic vein directly.[6] Although shunts reduce flow to varices, much of the blood that normally passes through the liver now gets back to the heart *without* undergoing the myriad of chemical reactions that normally occur in the liver. As discussed above, the liver is a major metabolic and detoxification center. If liver failure decreases detoxification reactions, or if a shunt allows circumvention of the liver, toxic chemicals can affect the brain, resulting in delirium (*hepatic encephalopathy*).

DISEASES OF THE GALL BLADDER AND BILE DUCTS

Fig. 4-13. Biliary tree anatomy. The intrahepatic biliary system in the liver gives rise to the right and left hepatic ducts, which fuse to form the common hepatic duct. The common hepatic duct joins the cystic

---

[5] There are many possible causes of thrombosis, including any cause of a hypercoagulable state (see Chapter 6).

[6] The "jugular" part of the name is because the shunt is placed through catheters inserted into the jugular vein.

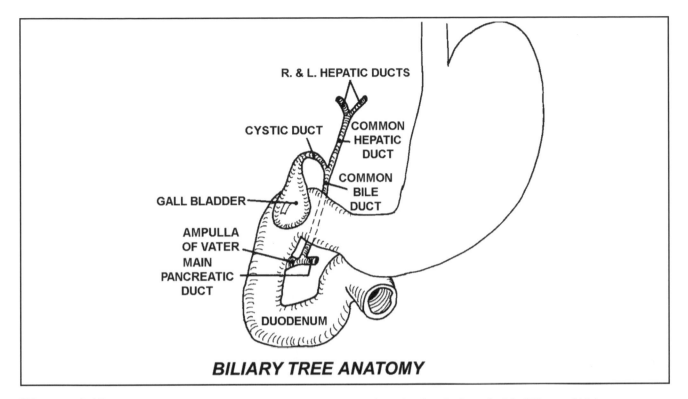

BILIARY TREE ANATOMY

Figure 4-13. Modified from Goldberg: *Clinical Anatomy Made Ridiculously Simple*, MedMaster 2004

duct (which leads to the gall bladder) to form the common bile duct, which usually unites with the pancreatic duct at its entry into the duodenum. The liver constantly produces bile, which is then stored in the gall bladder. Upon arrival of partially digested food in the duodenum from the stomach, cholecystikinin (CCK) is released. This stimulates contraction of the gall bladder and release of bile, which emulsifies fats for absorption.

What could go wrong with bile ducts? Since we're dealing with tubes, obstruction is one possibility. Obstruction prevents bile from making it to the duodenum, and this can lead to decreased fat breakdown, causing fat malabsorption. Obstruction also leads to backup of bile/bilirubin, leading to jaundice and potentially to liver damage. Remember that in *o*bstruction, alk ph*o*s is typically elevated. Ultrasound of the biliary system can look for stones or dilation of the ducts (which would suggest distal obstruction).

How could the biliary system become obstructed? *Obstruction by a gallstone* or *tumor, inflammation/scarring* of the biliary tree, and *biliary atresia* are the most common causes of biliary obstruction.

Gallstones (Cholelithiasis)

Normally, stones should not form in the biliary system, as long as concentrations of all components nec-

essary for bile synthesis are in the appropriate equilibrium. The two main components are (1) pigment from bilirubin breakdown and (2) cholesterol. Excesses of either of these components can lead to stone formation, causing black stones or cholesterol stones, respectively. Excess pigment can occur secondary to hemolysis (e.g., in sickle cell disease). Excess cholesterol occurs in the classic "female, fat, forty, fertile" scenario. Another type of pigment stone, *brown stones*, can form from the products of bacterial metabolism in biliary infection. Predisposition to gallstones formation also occurs when there is excessive stasis in the gall bladder.

Large gallstones that stay in the gall bladder are not as bad as they sound; they simply stay there since they are too big to pass into the cystic duct or common bile duct. If the stones are small enough to pass into the *cystic duct*, but get stuck before the common bile duct, this is *choledocholithiasis* and can lead to *cholecystitis* (inflammation of the gall bladder). The obstruction of a tube is painful because the proximal tube (and in this case the gall bladder) squeezes to try to push the obstruction away (a similar phenomenon occurs with kidney stones passing into the ureters, bowel obstruction, etc.). This leads to intermittent crampy pain, classically in the right upper quadrant.

The stone can also pass into the *common bile duct* and obstruct it. This not only affects gall bladder outflow but *liver* bile outflow as well. This can lead to jaundice.

The stone can pass all the way to the entrance of the duct at the duodenum, where it joins the pancreatic duct. This can obstruct the pancreatic duct and is one of the most common causes of pancreatitis.

The stone can pass into the duodenum and obstruct it, leading to *gallstone ileus*.

Cancer of the Bile Ducts (Cholangiocarcinoma)

Cholangiocarcinoma can obstruct the bile ducts, leading to jaundice. Cholangiocarcinoma is associated with parasitic infection (e.g., *Clonorchis sinensis*) of the liver, primary sclerosing cholangitis, and toxins. Gallstones also predispose to development of gall bladder cancer. Gall bladder cancer can present just as does cholecystitis, but is often asymptomatic and discovered incidentally upon removal of the gall bladder for cholelithiasis. The treatment of cholangiocarcinoma involves surgery, radiation, and chemotherapy.

Inflammatory Diseases of the Biliary System

Primary Biliary Cirrhosis is an autoimmune disease in which the autoimmunity is directed at the intrahepatic biliary ducts. The result is scarring and obstruction of these ducts. Remember that obstruction leads to elevated alk phos. Antimitochondrial antibodies are associated with primary biliary cirrhosis. Primary biliary cirrhosis predominantly affects women.

Primary Sclerosing Cholangitis is a disease of the larger bile ducts. In contrast to autoimmune hepatitis, primary biliary cirrhosis, and many other autoimmune diseases, primary sclerosing cholangitis predominantly affects men. *Primary sclerosing cholangitis is associated with inflammatory bowel disease, usually ulcerative colitis.* (Remember the rhyme/chant "sclerosing cholanGItis, ulcerative coLItis, sclerosing cholanGItis, ulcerative coLItis…."). Bile duct cancer (*cholangiocarcinoma*) risk is elevated in primary sclerosing cholangitis.

Biliary Atresia

Biliary atresia is inflammation and obliteration of the extrahepatic biliary system in the neonate. It presents as jaundice and can lead to cirrhosis severe enough to require liver transplantation if not detected early. Treatment is surgical; the *Kasai procedure* removes the obliterated ducts and reconnects the duodenum to the liver to normalize the flow of bile. The post-opera-

tive proximity of the gut environment to the liver can result in infection (*ascending cholangitis*).

DISEASES OF THE PANCREAS

The pancreas has two main functions, endocrine and exocrine. The endocrine portion regulates blood glucose via glucagon and insulin (see Chapter 5). The exocrine function is the production and release of digestive enzymes (trypsin, chymotrypsin, lipase, amylase) and bicarbonate into the duodenum (first portion of the small intestine). If there is a problem with the pancreas' ability to make or secrete its digestive enzymes, malabsorption can occur. In cystic fibrosis, for example, thickened secretions clog the pancreas, leading to inability to secrete its digestive enzymes. The resulting malabsorption can give rise to floating, foul-smelling stools. For more on cystic fibrosis, see Chapter 2.

As with any organ, the pancreas can become inflamed (*pancreatitis*) or develop cancer.

Pancreatitis

Pancreatitis is an inflammation of the pancreas. The two most common causes of pancreatitis are alcohol and gallstones. When a gallstone lodges in the distal bile duct at its entrance to the duodenum, the anatomy is such that this can also obstruct the distal pancreatic duct. Pancreatitis generally presents as mid-epigastric pain radiating to the back. Analogous to the liver's release of AST and ALT when injured, and the bile ducts' release of alkaline phosphatase when damaged, the pancreas releases *amylase* and *lipase* when affected, so these levels can be elevated in pancreatitis.[7] Other causes of pancreatitis, aside from alcohol and gallstones, include drugs, hypercalcemia, scorpion bite, and hereditary pancreatitis syndromes.

Pancreatic Tumors

Pancreatic cancer. Due to the anatomical location of the pancreas (adjacent to the bile ducts), a cancerous growth within it can obstruct the bile duct, leading to jaundice. So pancreatic cancer should be part of the differential diagnosis of jaundice.

Other pancreatic tumors include *gastrinoma* (see Zollinger-Ellison Syndrome), *insulinoma* (see hypoglycemia in Chapter 5), *VIPoma* (see diarrhea), *glucagonoma*, and *somatostatinoma*. Glucagon normally increases blood sugar. In glucagonoma, excess glucagon secretion leads to hyperglycemia. A rash called *necrolytic migrating erythema* is commonly found in patients with glucagonoma. Somatostatin normally inhibits production of GI hormones and secretions. Excess somatostatin secretion in somatostatinoma

---

[7] Amylase can also be elevated if there is a salivary gland tumor (salivary amylase).

causes inhibition of pancreatic enzymes (leading to malabsorption, diarrhea, and hence weight loss), decreased insulin secretion (causing diabetes mellitus), and decreased gall bladder activity (which can cause gallstones).

APPROACH TO ABDOMINAL PAIN

Abdominal pain is a common complaint in the emergency room and office. Before we deal with the questions, physical exam, and lab tests that you would use to solve a case of abdominal pain, let's answer the following questions: What structures are in the *abdomen,* and how can these things cause *pain*? With any type of pain, think about what is in/near the region of interest and what might cause any of these things to be painful.

What is in the abdomen? The *GI system* (stomach, small intestine, large intestine, liver, gall bladder, pancreas), the *urinary system* (kidneys, ureters, bladder), the *reproductive system* (females: ovaries, uterus; males: embryologically, the testes descend from the abdomen, and can refer pain to the abdomen), the *spleen,* the *blood supply* to all of these organs from the *abdominal aorta* and its branches, and the *abdominal wall*.

The next question is: How can each of these be painful? We can divide the abdominal contents into *tubes* (gut, fallopian tubes, bile duct, ureters), *solid organs* (liver, pancreas, spleen, ovaries, kidneys), and *blood vessels*.

What can make tubes hurt? One cause is obstruction. What can obstruct these tubes? Kidney stones can obstruct ureters; gallstones can obstruct bile ducts. The GI tract can also become obstructed. Appendicitis is usually due to obstruction from a fecolith or hypertrophy of lymph tissue in the appendix. A common cause of bowel obstruction is adhesions/scarring from previous abdominal surgery (e.g., gynecologic procedures). Other causes of obstruction include tumors (of the GI tract or adjacent organs), hernia (if a loop of bowel gets stuck in the hernia opening and obstructs itself), and volvulus (twisting of the intestine around itself).

What could get stuck in the fallopian tubes? Any female patient of reproductive age with abdominal pain needs a pregnancy test. Pregnancy itself can cause abdominal pain, but so can a tubal (ectopic) pregnancy, when the pregnancy inappropriately implants in the fallopian tube or elsewhere in the abdomen. What else might obstruct the fallopian tubes? Pelvic inflammatory disease (PID) is an infection of the female reproductive organs that often presents as lower abdominal pain (common culprits are gonorrhea and chlamydia). So pus or abscess (tubo-ovarian abscess) can also obstruct tubes.

What is another way a tube can get obstructed besides getting something stuck in it or against it? One way is *torsion*: the gut, the fallopian tube/ovary, and the testicle/spermatic cord can all twist around themselves, leading to intense pain.

Why is obstruction painful? Any obstructed tube builds up pressure behind it. This squeezing of the tube against resistance leads to the phenomenon of cramping. Additionally, torsion or herniation can lead to ischemia of the tube in question.

Tubes can also cause pain if they *perforate*. For example, a gastric or duodenal ulcer can perforate, as can ischemic bowel or a diverticulum.

Infection or *inflammation* of any tube can also cause pain.

What can make the solid organs hurt? Any organ with a tumor (benign or malignant) can cause pain due to stretching of the organ's capsule or pressure on adjacent structures (although not all tumors cause pain). Anything that could cause inflammation/swelling could be painful.

Causes of inflammation in abdominal organs include:

* Bowel: inflammatory bowel disease, gastritis, colitis

* Liver: hepatitis (e.g., viral, autoimmune, or alcoholic hepatitis)

* Pancreas: pancreatitis (many potential causes including, most commonly gallstone obstruction of the pancreatic duct and alcoholism)

* Kidney: infection (e.g., pyelonephritis)

* Spleen: infarction (e.g., in sickle cell)

* Ovaries: cysts, tumors, torsion, or ectopic pregnancy

How could the blood supply cause pain? Ischemia/infarction is quite painful. We have already mentioned that ischemia/infarction can occur due to obstruction (e.g., secondary to torsion or hernia). An embolus in an abdominal vessel, vasculitis, or a hypercoagulable state can cause *mesenteric ischemia* (ischemia and potential infarction of a region of gut). If a patient complains of abdominal pain, vasculitis or a hypercoagulable state might not be first on your list in a differential diagnosis, but if it turns out that either of these is present in the past medical history, this would certainly cause you to re-juggle your list of possible etiologies. An abdominal aortic aneurysm can also cause abdominal pain.

What can cause pain in the abdominal wall? Trauma, prior surgery, herpes zoster (shingles), hernia, or a focus of endometriosis on the abdominal wall can also cause abdominal pain.

To review, in the abdomen, we have the GI, urinary, and reproductive systems, the spleen, and the blood supply which branches off the aorta: tubes, solid organs, and blood vessels. The differential diagnosis for abdominal pain comes from realizing that tubes can get obstructed, perforated, inflamed, or infected; solid organs can get inflamed, infected, or develop a neoplasm; and blood vessels can have an aneurysm or lead to ischemia/infarction.

Referred pain. Pain afferents from the viscera often share spinal cord synapses with sensory afferents from other parts of the body. Thus, when the viscera scream in pain, their scream may sound to the brain like some other part of the body screaming. In the classic heart attack scenario, the patient can have referred pain in the jaw or down the left arm. Abdominal viscera also refer pain. Appendicitis classically begins as peri-umbilical pain, which migrates to the right lower quadrant. The peri-umbilical pain is *referred pain*. The later right lower quadrant pain signifies peritoneal irritation in that specific location.

The diaphragm is innervated by the phrenic nerve ("C 3, 4, and 5 keep the diaphragm alive"). Diaphragmatic irritation thus refers pain to the sites of somatic innervation of C 3, 4, 5, namely the shoulder blades. So pain in the region of the right shoulder blade can signify gall bladder disease.

The testicles descend from the abdomen during development, and thus abdominal pain can be referred pain from the testicles (e.g., testicular torsion, see Ch. 9).

Associated symptoms. In addition to pain, abdominal organ dysfunction can produce other symptoms and signs. Recall the various responsibilities of the liver: bilirubin conjugation, protein manufacturing, detoxification reactions, etc. Thus, phenomena such as jaundice, decreased albumin, elevated bilirubin, and/or coagulation dysfunction (due to decreased clotting factor production) with concomitant abdominal pain could help make a diagnosis of some hepatic problem. Blood or pus in the urine or in the stool or from the vagina could indicate renal, GI, or gynecologic cause of abdominal pain, respectively. Vomiting can result from obstruction or gastroenteritis (which might have accompanying fever and/or diarrhea). Vomiting blood that is red vs. vomiting blood that is digested (coffee grounds) can suggest the source of bleeding (if it is red blood, it is more likely to be above the gastroesophageal junction, e.g., bleeding varices; see Fig. 4-9). Fever can be due to an infection (pelvic inflammatory disease, pyelonephritis, gastroenteritis, acute hepatitis) or any other inflammatory process.

Diagnosis of Abdominal Pain

History

Fig. 4-14. The four quadrants. The abdomen is typically divided in the left upper quadrant (LUQ), left lower quadrant (LLQ), right upper quadrant (RUQ), and right lower quadrant (RLQ). The structures in each of these regions are as follows.

In all quadrants: bowel
Bilateral posterior: kidneys/ureters
Midline, posterior: aorta
Upper midline (posterior): pancreas, aorta
Lower midline, anterior: uterus, bladder
Bilateral: ovaries, kidneys, ureters
LUQ: stomach, gastroesophageal junction, spleen
LLQ: descending colon (common site of diverticula), left ovary/fallopian tube
RUQ: liver, gall bladder, bile duct
RLQ: appendix, right ovary/fallopian tube

The *diaphragm* lies just above the abdomen, and the lungs and heart lie just above the diaphragm. *An inferior myocardial infarction or lower lobe pneumonia can thus present as abdominal pain.*

The most likely cause(s) of pain in any given region are those related to the organ(s) that are in that region, so asking the patient "Where does it hurt?" is a good place to start.

Severity/quality. We mentioned above that causes of pain in the abdomen are obstruction of tubes, inflammation, infection, or tumor of solid organs, and ischemia or infarction secondary to alteration in blood supply. How would these types of pain differ? In obstruction, what is painful is not so much the blockage but the proximal squeezing of the tube trying to squeeze the obstruction away. How would this feel? Typically squeezing leads to *cramping pain.* Commonly, patients with a ureteral stone writhe and cannot get comfortable as a result of this cramping.

Solid organ pain (e.g., from tumor, infection, inflammation) is generally more constant. It can be sharp or dull, but there is typically no squeezing or cramping sensation.

If the pain is unrelated to eating or bowel movements, and tends to occur with postural changes and/or tensing of the abdominal wall muscles, the *abdominal wall* may be the site of pathology.

Timing. Alteration in the blood supply (such as that due to an embolus) is typically sudden in onset, whereas a tumor characteristically has a more insidious time course.

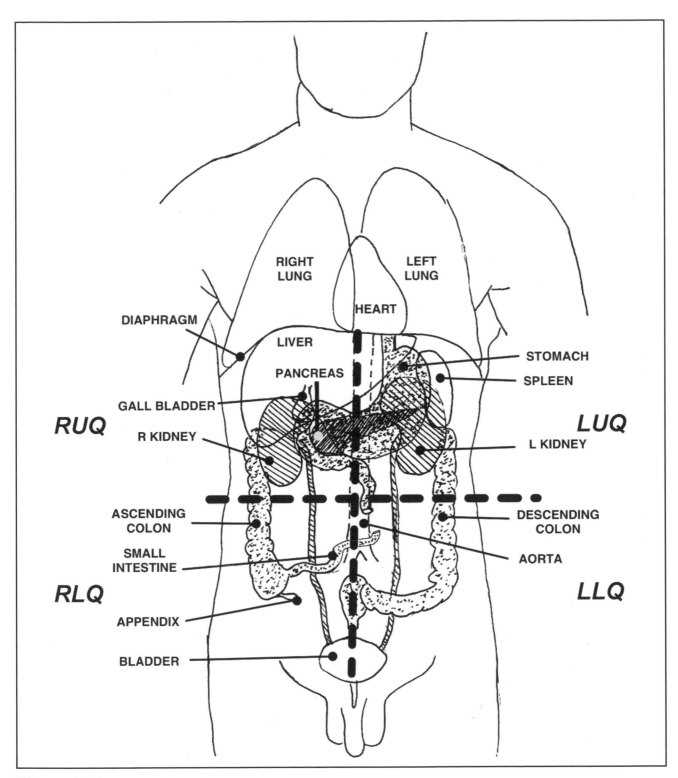

Figure 4-14

Examples:

- A 50-year-old man has "boring" pain in the center of the upper abdomen, radiating through to the back.

  What's there? Pancreas, stomach, part of the small intestine, the inferior border of the heart, and the aorta. So your initial differential should include pancreatitis, ulcer, obstruction, inferior myocardial infarction, and aortic aneurysm. If you now find out that the patient is an alcoholic, this would increase the likelihood of pancreatitis or ulcer. Labs (e.g., elevated amylase, lipase) would favor pancreatitis, and imaging can help you to zero in on a diagnosis.

- A 45-year-old woman has crampy RUQ pain after finishing dinner.

  What's there? The liver and the gall bladder. What could cause cramps? Obstruction of a tube. This is the classic presentation of a gallstone ("fat, forty, fertile female"). Although this story is classic for gall bladder disease, remember that *right next to the upper quadrants are the lower lung fields.* So if the case were a 45-year-old woman with RUQ pain, fever, and cough, a chest X-ray would be necessary to evaluate the possibility of pneumonia.

- A young boy has periumbilical pain for 3 hours and now complains of pain in the RLQ.

  A classic story for appendicitis, but what else is there? Referred pain from a torsed testicle could also cause RLQ pain, though it would also typically present with sudden pain and swelling of the scrotum.

- A 75-year-old man has LLQ pain.

  This is the classic story for diverticulitis, but if it were a woman, what else is there? Left ovary/tube, so ovarian neoplasm would also be on the list. The time course, type of pain, etc., would be key to narrowing down this differential.

- A 30-year-old woman has severe RLQ pain.

  What's there? Appendix, ovary, fallopian tube. So appendicitis, ovarian torsion, ruptured ovarian cyst, ectopic pregnancy, and pelvic inflammatory disease are all possibilities. Physical, labs, and imaging can help to distinguish among them.

The point of presenting these brief vignettes is to demonstrate an important point: upon hearing the chief complaint, and thinking about the anatomy and physiology of the abdominal organs, a differential begins to form in your mind. That differential will serve to guide your history, physical exam, and diagnostic work-up to arrive at the diagnosis.

Physical Exam

Observation. Is the patient writhing in pain (e.g., some kind of obstruction of some tube)? Is the patient lying absolutely still (e.g., peritonitis)? Is the abdomen distended (e.g., ascites or obstruction of a tube causing proximal dilation)? Does the patient look diaphoretic, pale, clammy (e.g., bleeding or myocardial infarction)? Does the patient have caput medusa or other evidence of dilated veins (e.g., liver disease)? Is the patient vomiting? Is the vomit bloody? Is the blood in the vomit digested (i.e., looks like coffee grounds and thus comes from the stomach or lower, e.g., bleeding ulcer) or undigested (bright red and thus likely from above the gastroesophageal junction, e.g., bleeding varices)?

Obviously, observation is important in assessing the severity of the situation: Do you need to stabilize this patient before taking a history?

Auscultation. High-pitched sounds and/or absence of bowel sounds can both be due to obstruction (imagine the obstructed bowel not making any noise or air squeaking by the obstruction). The renal artery or aorta can be occluded by atherosclerosis and can create bruits.

Palpation. Which quadrant is painful? Is the pain on deep palpation or light touch? Rebound pain (which occurs when withdrawing one's hands from the abdomen) and guarding (spontaneous contraction of the abdominal musculature) indicate peritoneal inflammation (*peritonitis*). This can occur in pelvic inflammatory disease, appendicitis, or with ruptured bowel. Is there a pulsating mass (abdominal aortic aneurysm)?

Pelvic exam can help to determine if pelvic inflammatory disease or any of the gynecologic causes discussed above are producing the abdominal pain.

Percussion. A lot of air makes a hollow sound; fluids and solids make dull sounds. So a lot of air (e.g., in a dilated bowel proximal to an obstruction) would give a tympanitic sound. Fluid (e.g., ascites) would be dull. Because the liver is solid and dull, you can percuss out its size. It may be enlarged in any cause of cirrhosis, if there is tumor in the liver (primary or metastatic), or if there is congestion secondary to portal hypertension or right-sided heart failure.

Laboratory Tests

- A high *WBC count* can indicate an infectious/ inflammatory process (e.g., acute appendicitis, pelvic inflammatory disease). Of course, there are many other reasons for WBC count to be elevated (see Chapter 6). However, in the case of abdominal pain, a high WBC with LLQ pain, for example, could be diverticulitis, and a high WBC count with RLQ pain could be appendicitis. Colitis can also present with abdominal pain and an elevated WBC count.

- *AST/ALT* can be elevated in any disease of the liver. Remember that AST and ALT are usually disproportionately higher than alkaline phosphatase if due to liver disease (e.g., hepatitis) as opposed to biliary tract obstruction. AST and ALT can be elevated in obstruction if the obstruction is bad enough to start damaging the liver, but alkaline phosphatase will be elevated to a much greater degree.

- *Alkaline phosphatase.* Alk ph*o*s is elevated in *o*bstruction of the biliary tree (e.g., stones, cancer). Remember that alkaline phosphatase can also come from bone.

- *Bilirubin.* Unconjugated bilirubin can be elevated in hemolytic anemia, congestive heart failure, Crigler-Najjar syndrome, and Gilbert's syndrome. Conjugated bilirubin can be elevated in any liver disease, biliary obstruction (which can be secondary to a tumor, a gallstone, or inflammatory disease of the biliary system), Dubin-Johnson syndrome, or Rotor syndrome.

- *Serum albumin* decreases in liver disease (and also in inflammatory disease, severe trauma, and/or nephrotic syndrome).

- *Prothrombin time* increases in liver disease.

- *Amylase* and *lipase* are classically elevated in pancreatitis. Amylase can also be high with certain salivary gland tumors.

Imaging and Endoscopy

- *Abdominal X-rays* can identify dilated loops of bowel in obstruction and some types of kidney stones and gallstones. Administration of contrast (e.g., barium) can allow for a more detailed view of possible obstructions or peristaltic dysfunction.

- *Ultrasound* can be used to examine the gall bladder and biliary tree (for dilatation and stones), the ovaries and fallopian tubes (for cysts, ectopic pregnancies, etc.), or the appendix (for appendicitis).

- *Abdominal MRI* and *CT* scanning can be used to look for malignancy, inflammatory changes, or causes of obstruction.

- *Upper endoscopy* can be used to examine the esophagus and stomach for causes of ulcer, sources of bleeding, tumors, or varices. Biopsies can be obtained during endoscopy and varices can be ligated or sclerosed.

- *Lower endoscopy* can be used to examine the colon for sources of bleeding, tumors, and to obtain biopsies to examine neoplastic growths and/or sites of inflammation/infection.

- *Percutaneous transhepatic cholangiography* (PTC) and *endoscopic retrograde cholangiopancreatography* (ERCP) can be used to assess intrahepatic ductal dilatation (e.g., secondary to primary biliary cirrhosis, liver tumor, etc.).

CHAPTER 5. THE ENDOCRINE SYSTEM

GENERAL PRINCIPLES

Fig. 5-1. The hypothalamic-pituitary-target gland axis. The hypothalamus produces *releasing hormones,* which stimulate the pituitary to release *stimulating* hormones. The stimulating hormones stimulate target organs (e.g., the adrenal, thyroid, gonads) to secrete their hormones. For example, the hypothalamus secretes thyroid hormone releasing hormone (THRH), which stimulates the thyrotroph cells of the anterior pituitary to secrete thyroid-stimulating hormone (TSH). TSH stimulates the thyroid gland to release thyroid hormone (T4 and T3).

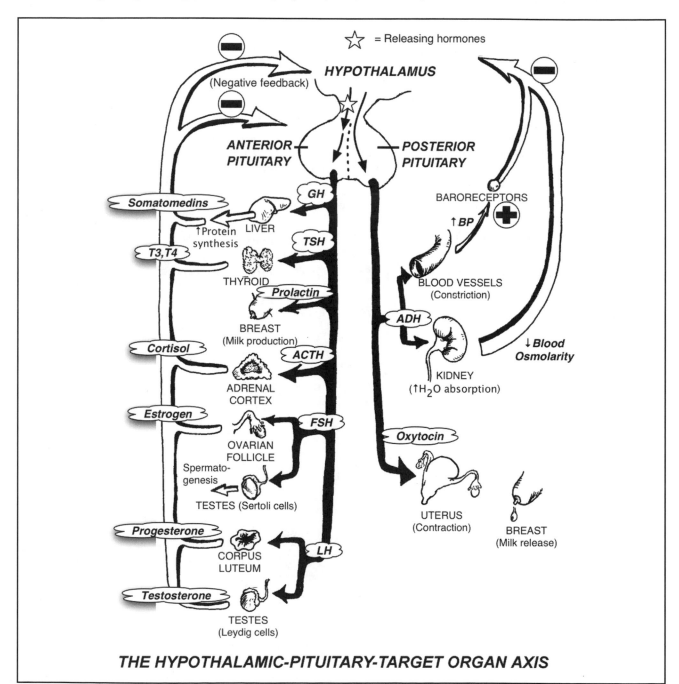

Figure 5-1. Modified from Goldberg: *Clinical Physiology Made Ridiculously Simple*, MedMaster 2004

The prolactin system is an exception to the above in that it is an *inhibitory* system: hypothalamic dopamine *inhibits* prolactin release from the anterior pituitary.

Fig. 5-2. Negative feedback. At each level of the hypothalamic-pituitary-target organ axis there is *negative feedback* from each step on the previous ones. This prevents over-secretion of any hormone. A commonly used analogy is that of a thermostat. If the house is cold, the thermostat senses this drop in temperature and turns on the heat. Of course, if the heat stayed on indefinitely, the house would get too hot. So at a certain equilibrium temperature, the thermostat senses that the right point has been reached and the heat goes off again. This is negative feedback. It is called "negative" because the feedback turns the system *off*. For example, thyroid hormone (T4 and T3) secreted by the thyroid exerts negative feedback on the hypothalamus and pituitary, decreasing their secretion of TRH and TSH, respectively. The concept of negative feedback is extremely important in understanding both the physiology of endocrine disorders and the lab tests used in their diagnosis.

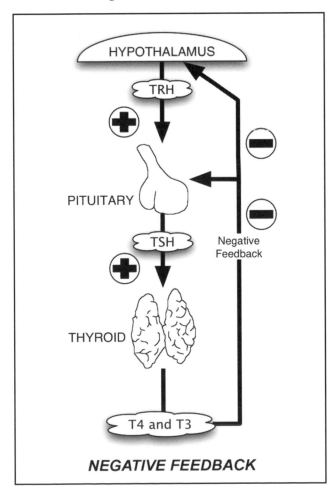

NEGATIVE FEEDBACK

Figure 5-2

Endocrine diseases are generally divided into hyper- states (states of increased hormone secretion) and hypo- states (states of decreased hormone secretion).

Increased hormone secretion or action could occur because:

1. The target gland (e.g., thyroid) over-secretes due to pathology directly affecting it (a *primary disorder*). In a primary hyper- disorder, the concentration of the hormone secreted by the target gland will be high, but the *stimulating hormone* concentration (from the pituitary) will be low due to increased negative feedback from the hyperactive target gland.

2. The pituitary/hypothalamus over-stimulates the target gland (a *secondary disorder*). In a secondary hyper- disorder, both target gland hormone and stimulating hormone levels will be high.

3. There is some *ectopic* site of hormone production. For example, struma ovarii (an ovarian tumor) can secrete thyroid hormone, small cell lung cancer can secrete adrenocorticotropic hormone (ACTH), squamous cell carcinoma of the lung can secrete parathyroid hormone-related protein (PTHrP), etc.

4. The target hormone receptors could be hyperactive (i.e., some genetic mutation).

Decreased hormone secretion or action could occur because:

1. There is a congenital or acquired problem of the target gland, (a *primary disorder*). In a primary hypo-disorder, there will be low target hormone level and high stimulating hormone level, because of *loss* of negative feedback from the hypo-active target gland.

2. The pituitary does not secrete enough stimulating hormone (a *secondary disorder*). In a secondary hypo- disorder, there will be decreases in both target gland hormone and stimulating hormone levels.

3. The hypothalamus does not secrete enough releasing hormone (a *tertiary disorder*).

4. The hormone is defective. This would cause high hormone levels, but the function that is supposed to be initiated by the hormone will *not* occur. This should be correctable by exogenous injection of the hormone.

5. The receptors of the target organ do not respond. Again, there will be high stimulating hormone levels because the organ producing the hormone is trying to get the target organ to respond. *However*, this time the target organ will *not* respond to exogenous hormone stimulation. An example is *nephrogenic* diabetes insipidus, which is discussed in Chapter 3.

With each endocrine organ, ask yourself: What hormone does this organ secrete? What stimulates it to do so? (Another hormone? A certain metabolic state?) What would happen if this organ were over-secreting? Under-secreting? How would these states affect the various hormone levels in the negative feedback loop? How will this affect laboratory diagnosis?

THYROID

The thyroid secretes thyroid hormone (T4 and T3),[1] which regulates various aspects of metabolism. Thyroid hormone secretion is stimulated by TSH secretion from the pituitary. TSH secretion is stimulated by THRH from the hypothalamus (Fig. 5-2). The following are discussed here: *hyperthyroidism* (increased thyroid hormone secretion), *hypothyroidism* (decreased thyroid hormone secretion), *thyroiditis* (thyroid inflammation), and *thyroid nodules and neoplasia*.

Hyperthyroidism

There are three general mechanisms by which hyperthyroidism can occur:

1. The thyroid over-secretes thyroid hormone (*primary hyperthyroidism*) e.g., toxic nodule, Graves' disease.

2. The pituitary over-stimulates the thyroid to secrete thyroid hormone (*secondary hyperthyroidism*), e.g., a pituitary tumor.

3. Some exogenous source of thyroid hormone exists, e.g., struma ovarii (an ovarian tumor).

Fig. 5-3A-B. Primary and secondary hyperthyroidism. The end result in situations 1-3 above would be the same: *hyperthyroidism* (elevated thyroid hormone). The pathophysiology, however, is different. In the first instance, *primary* hyperthyroidism, the thyroid over-secretes due to some problem *involving the gland itself*. In the second situation, *secondary* hyperthyroidism, the gland secretes excessively because *the pituitary causes it to do so*.

One needs only one laboratory value to distinguish between primary and secondary hyperthyroidism. Which one? Thyroid hormone increases in both cases so that is not helpful (unless the diagnosis of hyperthyroidism itself is in question). Think about negative feedback: If the thyroid itself were to secrete lots of hormone "without being told to," this would increase negative feedback on the pituitary, which would _____ [2] TSH secretion. *So in **primary** hyperthy-*

roidism, the TSH will be **low**. If the hyperthyroidism is secondary, i.e., caused by the over-secretion of TSH by the pituitary, the TSH will be *high*. So TSH is the key to distinguishing between primary and secondary hyperthyroidism.

Causes of Hyperthyroidism

Causes of hyperthyroidism include *toxic nodules, Graves' disease, pituitary tumor, amiodarone toxicity,* and *struma ovarii*.

A *toxic nodule* is a thyroid nodule that becomes independent of the pituitary and secretes excess thyroid hormone.

Graves' disease is an autoimmune disorder that causes hyperthyroidism. In autoimmune disorders, the body produces antibodies against some part of itself. In Graves' disease, the autoantibodies bind to the TSH receptors in the thyroid and *act just like TSH*, stimulating the thyroid to release thyroid hormone. Graves' disease can have some additional clinical features that distinguish it from other causes of hyperthyroidism: *Graves' ophthalmopathy* (inflammation of extraocular muscles and periorbital tissue leading to bulging of the eyes, called *proptosis* or *exophthalmos*), *pretibial myxedema*[3] (non-pitting edema on the anterior knee), and, in some cases, associated autoimmune disorders (e.g., vitiligo, pernicious anemia). Graves' disease is the most common cause of hyperthyroidism.

Other causes of hyperthyroidism include a *pituitary tumor that secretes TSH* (i.e., secondary hyperthyroidism), *amiodarone toxicity*,[4] and *struma ovarii*, an ovarian tumor that secretes thyroid hormone. What would you expect to happen to TSH in struma ovarii? No matter what the source, elevated thyroid hormone will increase negative feedback on the pituitary and hence decrease TSH. So TSH will be low in struma ovarii.

Symptoms and Signs of Hyperthyroidism

Any disease of the thyroid can cause it to enlarge (*goiter*).

What does thyroid hormone *do*? Most generally, thyroid hormone "stimulates," and so a *hyperthyroid* person has many *hyper*active signs/symptoms, e.g., high metabolism (weight loss), tachycardia (sometimes even atrial fibrillation), dyspnea, heat intol-

---

[1] Most of the thyroid hormone secreted is T4. Although a small amount of T3 is made in the thyroid, most T3 comes from peripheral conversion of T4 to T3.

[2] decrease

[3] Note: The term *myxedema* by itself often refers to the condition of hypothyroidism (e.g., "myxedema coma" is a coma induced by severe hypothyroidism). *Pretibial myxedema* is actually a type of edema found in Graves' disease, which causes hyperthyroidism.

[4] Amiodarone is an anti-arrhythmic drug that can cause hyperthyroidism or hypothyroidism. To remember that this drug affects the thyroid, notice the **iod** in its name? Am**iod**aranoe contains **iod**ine in its structure, and that **iod** should make you think of the thyroid.

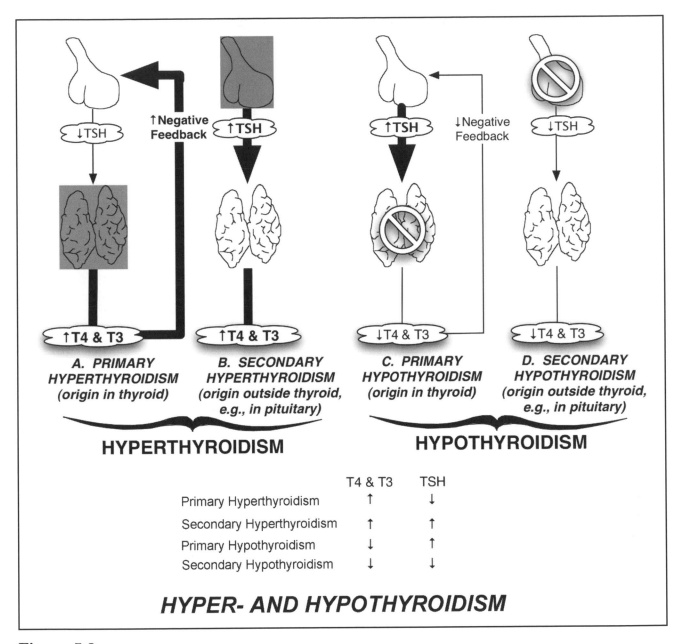

HYPER- AND HYPOTHYROIDISM

	T4 & T3	TSH
Primary Hyperthyroidism	↑	↓
Secondary Hyperthyroidism	↑	↑
Primary Hypothyroidism	↓	↑
Secondary Hypothyroidism	↓	↓

Figure 5-3

erance, hot skin, increased appetite, tremor, nervousness, etc.

Diagnosis of Hyperthyroidism

Clinically, ophthalmopathy, pretibial myxedema, diffuse goiter, and/or thyroid bruit (rushing sound over thyroid on auscultation) will point toward a diagnosis of Graves' disease, though Graves' disease can be present with *none* of these signs. The laboratory test to assess primary vs. secondary hyperthyroidism is TSH; TSH will be low in primary hyperthyroidism (e.g., Graves') but high in secondary hyperthyroidism. In

Graves' disease, in addition to low TSH, anti-TSH receptor antibodies can be found in the serum in many (but not all) cases.

Treatment of Hyperthyroidism

As mentioned, hyperthyroidism speeds up many physiologic functions. Beta-blockers (e.g., propranolol, metoprolol, or atenolol) can be used for symptomatic relief of tachycardia, anxiety, etc. Beta-blockers are typically used in cases where the hyperthyroidism will resolve spontaneously (e.g., thyroiditis).

In cases of thyroid hormone hypersecretion (e.g., Graves' disease), the treatment goal is to reduce the amount of circulating thyroid hormone. Both *methimazole* and *propylthiouricil* decrease thyroid hormone synthesis, and *propylthiouricil* also reduces peripheral T4 to T3 conversion. In most cases, more definitive treatment is preferable to long-term treatment with anti-thyroid drugs: the thyroid can be removed surgically or destroyed by radioactive iodine (I[131]). Either of these treatments can lead to hypothyroidism.

Hypothyroidism

Fig. 5-3C-D. Primary and secondary hypothyroidism.

Like hyperthyroidism, *hypothyroidism* can also be due to either primary thyroid dysfunction or secondary to pituitary dysfunction. In either case, the thyroid hormone level is *low*, by definition. If the thyroid itself is the root of the problem and is not producing any thyroid hormone, this *decreases* negative feedback on the pituitary. So in *primary* hypothyroidism, the TSH level will be *elevated*. In secondary hypothyroidism, the pituitary is the problem: the pituitary is not secreting an adequate amount of TSH, so the TSH will be low.

Causes of Hypothyroidism

Causes of *primary* hypothyroidism include *congenital thyroid problems, Hashimoto's thyroiditis, drugs that are toxic to the thyroid gland* (e.g., amiodarone), *iodine deficiency, post-surgical damage/removal,* or *radiotherapy* with I[131].

Hashimoto's thyroiditis is an autoimmune disease. The antibodies are directed against thyroid peroxidase (TPO) and thyroglobulin (TG), resulting in a lymphocyte infiltration of the thyroid gland, which causes it to cease functioning partially or entirely. Hashimoto's thyroiditis sometimes occurs with other autoimmune diseases (e.g., diabetes Type 1, vitiligo, prematurely gray hair).

Iodine deficiency causes hypothyroidism because iodine is necessary for thyroid hormone synthesis. Decreased thyroid hormone synthesis decreases negative feedback, increasing TSH production. This elevation of TSH stimulates the thyroid gland to hypertrophy, leading to the goiter associated with iodine deficiency. Iodine deficiency is uncommon in the U.S. due to iodinization of salt, but is more common in other parts of the world (Himalayas, Andes, Alps), where it is referred to as *endemic goiter*.

Secondary hypothyroidism can result from pituitary pathology such as *infection, inflammation, infiltration, hemorrhage,* or *tumor* (either a non-functioning tumor within the pituitary or a brain tumor impinging upon it).

Tertiary hypothyroidism can be caused by hypothalamic under-activity or tumor.

Symptoms and Signs of Hypothyroidism

Hyperthyroidism speeds everything up. Hypothyroidism slows everything down: symptoms of hypothyroidism can include weight gain, cold intolerance, fatigue, weakness, bradycardia, hypoventilation, constipation, myalgias, arthralgias, and/or anemia. Goiter can be present.

Laboratory Diagnosis of Hypothyroidism

Remember that TSH is the key: TSH is elevated in primary hypothyroidism and decreased in secondary hypothyroidism. The above-mentioned serum autoantibodies (anti-TPO and anti-TG) can be present in Hashimoto's thyroiditis.

Treatment of Hypothyroidism

To treat a hypothyroid patient, we restore what is missing: thyroid hormone. Thyroxine is the synthetic form of T4 that is generally used.

Thyroiditis

Thyroiditis, inflammation of the thyroid gland, can cause hyperthyroidism or hypothyroidism as well as thyroid enlargement and/or pain. In addition to Hashimoto's thyroiditis, other causes of thyroiditis include viral infection (*de Quervain's thyroiditis*), radiation, amiodarone, autoimmunity (*subacute lymphocytic thyroiditis*), and delivery of a baby (*postpartum thyroiditis*). NSAIDs, steroids, and/or agents to treat hyper- or hypothyroidism may be used in treatment of thyroiditis.

Thyroid Nodules and Thyroid Cancer

A thyroid nodule can be a neoplasm such as an adenoma (benign) or carcinoma (papillary, follicular, medullary, or anaplastic), but can also be a non-neoplastic entity such as cyst, hyperplasia, or a focal region of thyroiditis. Nodules may be asymptomatic, discovered for the first time on physical exam. Alternatively, nodules can cause symptoms of hyperthyroidism and/or symptoms related to compression of nearby structures such as the trachea (causing cough) or esophagus (causing dysphagia). A definitive diagnosis is made by fine needle aspiration biopsy. Malignant neoplasms are treated surgically, while benign nodules are often observed if they are asymptomatic.

ADRENAL GLANDS

The adrenal glands secrete a number of hormones: aldosterone, glucocorticoids, sex hormones, norepinephrine, and epinephrine. The three zones of the cortex of the adrenal gland, from exterior to interior, are the zona glomerulosa (which secretes aldosterone), zona fasciculata (which secretes glucocorticoids), and zona reticularis (which secretes sex hormones). The adrenal medulla secretes epinephrine.

*Aldoste**R**o**N**e* causes **R**eabsorption of sodium (**Na**+) and secretion of potassium (K+) and hydrogen ion (H+) in the kidneys. What causes aldosterone secretion? The renin-angiotensin-aldosterone system is one way of stimulating aldosterone. Hyperkalemia can also stimulate aldosterone so as to promote K+ secretion in an effort to decrease serum K+. Hyperaldosteronism *is an increase in aldosterone;* hypoaldosteronism *is a decrease in aldosterone.* Increased aldosterone secretion occurs if the adrenal glands themselves hyper-secrete, or if the adrenal glands are stimulated by renin/angiotensin, hyperkalemia, hyponatremia, or hypotension. Decreased aldosterone secretion occurs in adrenal failure, or any of the conditions opposite to those just listed: i.e., decreases in renin/angiotensin, hypokalemia, hypernatremia, hypertension.

Glucocorticoids (e.g., cortisol) have wide-ranging functions. They are stress response hormones that increase blood pressure and gluconeogenesis, and decrease the immune response. Cortisol secretion is stimulated by secretion of ACTH (adrenocorticotropic hormone) from the pituitary. ACTH secretion from the pituitary is stimulated by CRH (corticotropin-releasing hormone) from the hypothalamus. The clinical manifestations of cortisol *elevation* are called *Cushing's syndrome.* Adrenal insufficiency can *decrease* cortisol; primary failure of the adrenal glands or reduced ACTH levels can cause adrenal insufficiency.

The sex hormones are discussed in chapter 9.

Over-secretion of epinephrine occurs in *pheochromocytoma.*

Hyper- and *hypoaldosteronism, Cushing's syndrome, adrenal insufficiency, pheochromocytoma,* and *congenital adrenal hyperplasia* are discussed below.

Hyper- and Hypoaldosteronism

Hyperaldosteronism

Hyperaldosteronism can cause hypernatremia, hypokalemia, and hypertension.

There are two general causes of *hyperaldosteronism:*

1. One or both adrenal glands are hyperactive (*primary hyperaldosteronism*). Causes include adrenal adenoma and adrenal carcinoma.

2. The adrenal glands are over-stimulated to secrete (*secondary hyperaldosteronism*). Causes include hyperkalemia, hyponatremia, and hypotension.

Unlike the thyroid and the cortisol system of the adrenal glands, it is *not* the pituitary gland that tells the adrenal cortex to secrete aldosterone. Recall that aldosterone causes sodium reabsorption (which raises blood pressure) and potassium excretion. *Thus, hyperkalemia, hyponatremia, and hypotension stimulate aldosterone release and can lead to secondary hyperaldosteronism.* In addition to actual hypotension, fluid redistribution leading to effective volume depletion (e.g., congestive heart failure, cirrhosis, nephrotic syndrome) can cause secondary hyperaldosteronism.

If one or both adrenal glands over-secretes (i.e., primary hyperaldosteronism), renin will be *low* since its secretion by the kidneys will be suppressed by negative feedback from the increased aldosterone secretion. In contrast, if the kidneys' secretion of renin is stimulating aldosterone secretion, then this is *secondary* hyperaldosteronism, and the renin *and* aldosterone levels will be elevated. Renin may elevate in response to congestive heart failure, cirrhosis, or volume depletion.

Hypoaldosteronism

Since aldosterone is responsible for sodium reabsorption and potassium excretion, hypoaldosteronism can lead to hyponatremia and hyperkalemia. Hypoaldosteronism can result from a *decrease in aldosterone* or a *decrease in the response to aldosterone.*

- Possible causes of *aldosterone deficiency:*
  - *The renin-angiotensin stimulus for aldosterone is deficient.* In hyporeninemic hypoaldosteronism, renin secretion is diminished by kidney damage due to diabetes, other chronic kidney diseases, or drugs.
  - *ACE inhibitors* prevent angiotensin-stimulated aldosterone release.
  - *The adrenal cortex is not secreting aldosterone* (*adrenal insufficiency*).

- Possible causes of *decreased response to aldosterone:*
  - *Drugs can cause aldosterone resistance*, e.g., spironolactone, a potassium-sparing diuretic that acts by inhibiting aldosterone.
  - *Pseudohypoaldosteronism:* The renal aldosterone receptors are not responsive to aldosterone.

Cushing's Syndrome

Cushing's syndrome refers to a pathological *elevation* of *cortisol*.

Causes of Cushing's Syndrome

Fig. 5-4. Causes of Cushing's Syndrome.

1. *Iatrogenic* (i.e., from long-term treatment with steroids).

2. Primary over-secretion by one or both *adrenal glands* (adrenal adenoma or carcinoma).

3. Over-stimulation of the adrenal glands by an ACTH-secreting tumor in the *pituitary*. This scenario is known as Cushing's *disease*.

4. Over-stimulation of the adrenal glands by an *ectopic ACTH producing tumor*. The most common site of ectopic production is a small cell lung cancer, though other cancers can produce ACTH as well.

Note: Cushing's *syndrome* is any state listed above which creates pathologic hypercortisolism. Cushing's *disease* is the specific case of hypercortisolism resulting from an ACTH-secreting pituitary adenoma.

Symptoms and Signs of Cushing's Syndrome

In Cushing's syndrome any or all of the following can be present: truncal obesity, a moon face, a buffalo hump on the back, easy bruising, purple striae, hypertension, edema, weakness, osteoporosis and/or osteonecrosis, hirsutism, acne, virilization, diabetes, immunosuppression, and/or cognitive effects (anything from mood/affect changes to psychosis).

Diagnosis of Cushing's Syndrome

If the diagnosis of Cushing's syndrome is suspected, one must first confirm that there is indeed elevated cortisol secretion. This can be done by either checking a 24-hour urinary collection for free cortisol, checking the level of cortisol in the saliva in the late evening, or determining if cortisol level suppresses

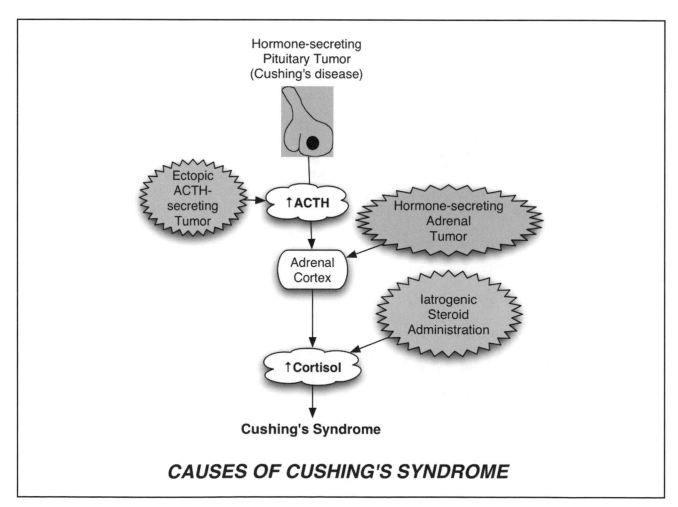

CAUSES OF CUSHING'S SYNDROME

Figure 5-4

normally when exogenous glucocorticoids are given (dexamethasone suppression test, Fig. 5-5). If any of these is present, this suggests Cushing's syndrome, but does not localize the site responsible for the over-production.

If one or both adrenal glands are autonomously hyper-secreting, this hyper-secretion will increase negative feedback on the pituitary and thus ACTH should be low. On the other hand, the combination of *high* ACTH **and** *hypercortisolism* means that something is over-secreting ACTH. This may be the pituitary (Cushing's *disease*) or an ectopic site of ACTH production.

If ACTH and cortisol are both high, one must distinguish between pituitary ACTH secretion and ectopic ACTH secretion. Typically ectopic sites secrete *more ACTH*. It sort of makes intuitive sense that a crazy tumor that is not even part of the endocrine system would secrete far higher levels of ACTH than a mere hyper-functioning endocrine tumor that is simply overdoing it. The ectopic site is, in comparison, going totally nuts.

Localizing Cushing's Syndrome: Pituitary vs. Ectopic

Fig. 5-5. Dexamethasone Suppression Test. The dexamethasone suppression test relies on the principle of negative feedback to localize the source of ACTH. *Normally*, giving the steroid dexamethasone should mimic cortisol and exert negative feedback on the pituitary, *decreasing* ACTH output from the pituitary.

If a *low dose* dexamethasone suppression test does *not* suppress ACTH, this indicates that Cushing's syndrome exists, but does not indicate the source of ACTH over-production. If the pituitary is over-secreting ACTH (Cushing's *disease)* and you give *high dose* steroids, the pituitary should respond to this negative feedback, and ACTH level should decrease. That is, the pituitary still responds to negative feedback, but needs a higher level than normal. *So in Cushing's disease (i.e., pituitary hyper-secretion of ACTH), ACTH level will be suppressed by the high dose dexamethasone suppression test. An ectopic site of ACTH production does not respond to negative feedback,* so failure to suppress the ACTH level with high dose dexamethasone indicates an ectopic source of elevated ACTH.

Metyrapone inhibits cortisol synthesis and can also be used to localize Cushing's syndrome. What would you expect metyrapone to do to ACTH in a *normal* person? If cortisol synthesis decreases, this should *remove* negative feedback, causing an increase in ACTH. A pituitary source of elevated ACTH (Cushing's disease) will respond by increasing ACTH secretion when metyrapone is given. As mentioned above, ectopic sites of ACTH production are generally non-responsive to negative feedback, so ACTH will *not* change in a metyrapone test if the cause of Cushing's syndrome is ectopic ACTH production.

In summary, *when localizing the ACTH source in Cushing's syndrome the pituitary* **does** *respond to negative feedback and ectopic sites* **do not**. The response

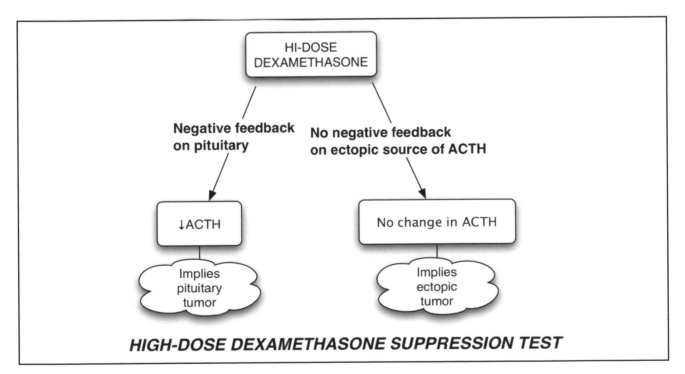

HIGH-DOSE DEXAMETHASONE SUPPRESSION TEST

Figure 5-5

to negative feedback is assessed via ACTH level: If it decreases, that means the secretor was responsive to negative feedback (pituitary); if it does not decrease, that means the secretor was *not* responsive (ectopic).

Inferior Petrosal Sinus Sampling. Sometimes the source of ACTH cannot be determined from these tests, and imaging studies are unrevealing (since pituitary tumors can be extremely small). In inferior petrosal sinus sampling, catheters are threaded up into the petrosal venous sinuses that drain the pituitary. ACTH levels are then measured in the pituitary catheters and from a peripheral vein. A pituitary to periphery ACTH ratio of 2:1 or greater indicates a pituitary adenoma. For additional confirmation, CRH is then administered through the catheter, and ACTH level is measured both in the sinus and simultaneously from a peripheral vein. If the pituitary is over-secreting (Cushing's *disease)*, the level of ACTH in the catheter near the pituitary should have a higher level of ACTH than observed in the periphery (3:1 or greater is diagnostic), since ectopic sites generally do not respond to CRH.

Treatment of Cushing's Syndrome

Cushing's syndrome is treated by the surgical removal (or in some cases radiation) of the offending tumor, or tapering of the glucocorticoid therapy if the Cushing's is iatrogenic.

Adrenal Insufficiency

Adrenal insufficiency can be caused by:

1. Pathology of one or both adrenal glands (*primary adrenal insufficiency*, also known as *Addison's disease).*

2. Lack of ACTH stimulation from the pituitary (*secondary adrenal insufficiency).*

3. Lack of CRH (corticotrophic releasing hormone) from the hypothalamus (*tertiary adrenal insufficiency).*

ACTH stands for adrenocorticotropic hormone, and from the "cort," realize that ACTH predominantly stimulates *cortisol* secretion from the adrenal glands. Aldosterone is regulated largely by concentrations of sodium and potassium as well as the renin-angiotensin-aldosterone axis. Thus, *ACTH (or CRH) deficiency will lead to decreased cortisol with normal aldosterone.*

Fig. 5-6. Primary and secondary adrenal insufficiency. In any cause of adrenal insufficiency, cortisol is low. *If the adrenal gland itself fails (**primary** adrenal insufficiency), **both** cortisol and aldosterone secretion will be affected.* In **secondary (or tertiary)** adrenal insufficiency (decreased ACTH stimulation of the ad-

renal glands), *cortisol secretion decreases, but the renin-angiotensin-aldosterone axis still works.*

Symptoms of adrenal insufficiency can include weakness, fatigue, lightheadedness, weight loss, dehydration, hair loss, vomiting, hypoglycemia, and/or anemia.

Primary Adrenal Insufficiency

Since *both cortisol and aldosterone secretion are affected* in primary adrenal insufficiency, signs/symptoms will reflect both aldosterone *and* cortisol loss. Remember that aldoste**RoNe** causes **R**eabsorption of Na^+ and secretion of K^+ in the kidneys. *Without aldosterone, sodium will be wasted, and potassium will accumulate,* so hyponatremia and hyperkalemia are commonly seen in primary adrenal insufficiency. Sodium wasting can lead to hypotension.

Another characteristic that can be seen in *primary* adrenal insufficiency that is not seen in secondary adrenal insufficiency is *hyperpigmentation*. ACTH and MSH (melanocyte stimulating hormone) have a common precursor, POMC (pro-opio-melanocortin). In adrenal insufficiency, ACTH production is increased due to loss of negative feedback. Because ACTH and MSH share a common precursor, this increased ACTH production will also cause excess MSH to be produced. This results in hyperpigmentation. *Hypotension, hyperkalemia, hyponatremia, salt craving, and hyperpigmentation can help to distinguish primary adrenal insufficiency from secondary insufficiency.*

Causes of primary adrenal insufficiency include:

* *Autoimmune disease*
  - Polyglandular autoimmune syndrome Type 1 (HAM: **h**ypoparathyroidism, **a**drenal insufficiency, **m**ucocutaneous candidiasis)
  - Polyglandular autoimmune syndrome Type 2: (Adrenal insufficiency with either autoimmune thyroid disease or insulin-dependent diabetes mellitus with possible vitiligo, premature ovarian failure, and/or pernicious anemia)

* *Adrenal hemorrhage* (known as Waterhouse-Friedrichsen syndrome if it is secondary to *N. meningitidis*; hemorrhage can also be caused by anticoagulant treatment)

* *Infection* (e.g., tuberculosis, *N. meningitidis*)

* *Tumor metastases* to the adrenal gland

Secondary and Tertiary Adrenal Insufficiency

Pituitary lesions or tumors can lead to *secondary adrenal insufficiency* due to decreased ACTH secretion. Hypothalamic lesions or tumors can cause *tertiary adrenal insufficiency* due to decreased CRH stimulation of ACTH release from the pituitary. Decreased ACTH secretion in either scenario decreases cortisol secretion from the adrenal gland, but the rest of the adrenal still

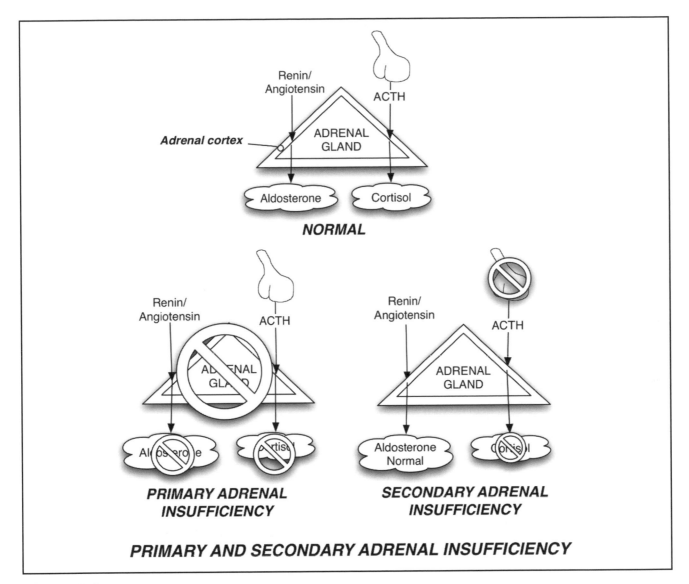

Figure 5-6

functions normally. Thus, there is *no* hyperkalemia in secondary and tertiary adrenal insufficiency.[5]

Adrenal insufficiency can also occur when a patient goes through withdrawal after abrupt termination of steroid treatment. Steroid treatment provides exogenous negative feedback to the pituitary. If steroids are abruptly stopped, the pituitary takes time to recover its function, and during that time, adrenal insufficiency can occur. This is why one never stops steroids abruptly after prolonged treatment, but rather *tapers* them. This is also why patients on steroid treatment who need surgery are often given a stress dose of extra steroids to accommodate the increased stress. Patients on steroids who go for surgery *without* this increased stress dose of steroids lack the ability to increase steroid secretion in response to stress on their own, which may result in adrenal failure.

Diagnosis of Adrenal Insufficiency

It is possible that a patient can have primary adrenal insufficiency without manifesting hyperpigmentation or other distinguishing characteristics. How can one confirm the diagnosis and localize whether the adrenal insufficiency is primary or secondary using laboratory tests? First, if both cortisol *and* aldosterone are low, this suggests primary adrenal insufficiency as discussed above (because the whole adrenal is failing, not

---

[5] Hyponatremia may still occur in secondary adrenal insufficiency because cortisol deficiency can increase ADH secretion. Increased ADH increases fluid retention, diluting serum sodium concentration, which can cause hyponatremia.

merely cortisol secretion). Aldosterone level is not routinely used clinically, but what measurable laboratory findings will *low* aldosterone cause? *Low sodium and high potassium.* Additionally, if ACTH is high, this suggests primary adrenal insufficiency (because of loss of negative feedback from the adrenal on the pituitary).

The ACTH Stimulation ("Cort Stim") Test. If we give some ACTH by injection and it does *not* work (i.e., cortisol level does *not* rise), either the adrenal gland is the problem and cannot respond, *or* there is long-standing secondary adrenal insufficiency, such that the adrenal is slow to respond. To distinguish between these two, a longer dose of ACTH is given (usually 6-8 hours) and in these cases, primary adrenal insufficiency still will *not* respond, whereas secondary adrenal insufficiency finally will (though usually only partially). *So if a cort stim test increases cortisol level, the problem was most likely that the gland was previously being under-stimulated, i.e., secondary or tertiary adrenal insufficiency.* If the cort stim fails to cause a rise in blood cortisol levels, the problem must be the adrenal's inability to respond, i.e., *primary adrenal insufficiency.*

Treatment of Adrenal Insufficiency

Treatment of adrenal insufficiency depends upon its etiology. If cortisol is the only deficient hormone (i.e., aldosterone is fine, which must mean that the insufficiency is *secondary* or *tertiary*), then one replaces cortisol with glucocorticoids, e.g., hydrocortisone with an increased dose for stress (illness, surgery, etc). If the failure also affects aldosterone (i.e., *primary* adrenal insufficiency), then one must replace both cortisol *and* aldosterone. Aldosterone replacement can be accomplished with fludrocortisone.

Pheochromocytoma

A pheochromocytoma is a rare but extremely dangerous cause of hypertension. It is a catecholamine-secreting tumor that most commonly occurs in the adrenal medulla. The catecholamines secreted by the tumor (i.e., norepinephrine/epinephrine) cause vasoconstriction and thus hypertension. Classically, the symptoms are paroxysmal (i.e., they come on once in awhile and then resolve) and include headache, palpitations, sweating, and tremor. The diagnosis can be confirmed by elevated urine levels of catecholamines and their metabolic by-products, called *metanephrines.* Pheochromocytomas are said to follow the "rule of 10s": 10 % are bilateral, 10% are not in the adrenal gland,[6] and 10% are malignant. In other words, most pheochromocytomas are benign, unilateral adrenal tumors. The catecholamines secreted by pheochromo-

cytomas stimulate *both* alpha and beta receptors (alpha=vasoconstriction; beta=vasodilation, tachycardia, bronchodilation). If a beta-blocker is given alone for the tachycardia, the vasodilation of the beta system will be inhibited while the alpha-receptors remain stimulated (by the pheochromocytoma's epinephrine secretion). This can lead to extreme hypertension. *So beta blockade should never be given alone* to a patient with a pheochromocytoma. The drug of choice is phenoxybenzamine, an alpha-receptor blocker. Mnemonic: phenoxy and pheo are similar words. This drug is given to control blood pressure until surgical removal of the tumor.

Congenital Adrenal Hyperplasia

Fig. 5-7. Congenital adrenal hyperplasia is a group of disorders caused by enzymatic defects in adrenal steroid biosynthesis. At first you may ask, "If biosynthesis in the adrenal gland is decreased, why is there *hyper*plasia?" Any of the enzyme defects that can cause congenital adrenal hyperplasia leads to *decreased cortisol synthesis.* Decreased cortisol results in *decreased negative feedback* on the secretion of ACTH. With decreased negative feedback, ACTH level *increases. This elevation of ACTH in the developmental period causes the hyperplasia.* The most common form is a deficiency of 21-hydroxylase, which results in increased androgenic precursors. In females this can lead to menstrual irregularities and hirsutism. If aldosterone production is affected by the biochemical abnormality, what could occur? A loss of aldosterone can lead to hyperkalemia and salt wasting, which can lead to severe hypotension.

MULTIPLE ENDOCRINE NEOPLASIA (MEN)

Patients with MEN develop tumors in multiple endocrine organs. MEN comes in 3 types: MEN 1, MEN 2a, MEN 2b. Mnemonic (see chart): MEN 1, the three Ps: **p**ituitary, **p**arathyroid, and **p**ancreas tumors. To make 2a, *keep* parathyroid tumors and add MTC (medullary thyroid carcinoma) and pheochromocytoma. Then to make 2b, *keep* two (Pheo and MTC) and add marfanoid body habitus.

MEN 1	MEN 2a	MEN 2b
Parathyroid →	Parathyroid	Marfanoid body habitus
Pituitary	*Pheo.* →	Pheo.
Pancreas	*MTC* →	MTC

PITUITARY GLAND

The pituitary lies between the hypothalamus and the target glands in the chain of command of endocrine

---

[6] The most common place a pheochromytoma can occur outside of the adrenal is the organ of Zuckerkandl (a para-aortic component of the sympathetic plexus).

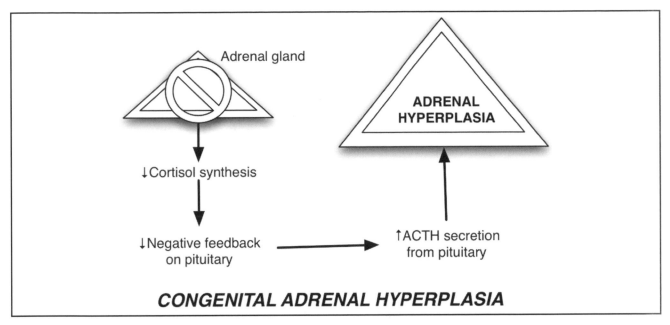

Figure 5-7

function (Fig. 5-1). The anterior pituitary secretes thyroid-stimulating hormone (TSH), adrenocorticotrophic hormone (ACTH), growth hormone (GH), leutinizing hormone (LH), follicle stimulating hormone (FSH), and prolactin. The posterior pituitary secretes oxytocin and ADH (vasopressin).

Anatomically, the pituitary sits beneath the optic chiasm, which is where fibers from both optic nerves (CN II) cross. Thus, pituitary tumors may present with *bitemporal hemianopsia* (loss of the lateral visual field in each eye) because of pressure on the chiasm (see Fig. 7-7).

Diseases of the Anterior Pituitary

Pituitary Adenomas and Hyperpituitarism

Pituitary adenomas are usually benign tumors. They can cause pituitary dysfunction by either oversecreting a hormone or, if quite large, by compressing the pituitary so as to cause hypopituitarism. With the exception of prolactinomas (which often respond to dopamine agonists), radiation or surgical removal of pituitary adenomas is first-line treatment.

ACTH-Secreting Pituitary Adenomas lead to increased cortisol secretion. This is the specific case of Cushing's syndrome known as Cushing's *disease*.

TSH-Secreting Pituitary Adenomas can cause *secondary hyperthyroidism*. What would the labs show? Elevated thyroid hormone and elevated (or inappropriately normal) TSH. (Compare this to *primary hyperthyroidism*, which causes elevated thyroid hormone with *decreased* TSH.)

Growth Hormone Adenomas and Acromegaly. A tumor that secretes growth hormone will make things *big*. The hands, feet, ears, lips, tongue, etc. can all enlarge. However, this enlargement occurs over a long time and may be so insidious as to not be noticed by the patient. Subtle signs like gloves, shoes, and rings not fitting anymore can be clues to the diagnosis. Because of enlargement in the face and hands, snoring, sleep apnea, arthritis, and/or carpal tunnel syndrome can occur.

Growth hormone level itself is not a very reliable diagnostic test because of its pulsatile release. Growth hormone stimulates release of insulin-like growth factor (IGF), so an elevated level of IGF-1 can be seen on laboratory testing with a growth hormone-secreting tumor. Somatostatin inhibits growth hormone, so somatostatin (commercially available as *octreotide*) can be used to shrink these tumors. Surgery is usually necessary for complete cure.

Growth hormone is one of the hormones that counteracts insulin's actions. That is, growth hormone *raises* blood sugar (just like glucagon, cortisol, and epinephrine). If a growth hormone-secreting tumor is suspected, another diagnostic test that can be used is a *glucose challenge test*. If you give a glucose load to a normal patient, what would you expect this to do to growth hormone secretion? If growth hormone *raises* blood sugar, and you give some sugar, this should *decrease* growth hormone secretion in a normal person. Now what would you expect to happen in a patient with a growth hormone secreting-tumor? Well what has happened with all of the other over-secreting tumors when we tried to give them negative feedback?

Usually they do *not* respond at a normal level. So if growth hormone does *not* decrease in response to a glucose tolerance test, this indicates a source of growth hormone that is resistant to negative feedback, most likely a growth hormone-secreting tumor.

LH/FSH-Secreting Tumors. Since the LH and FSH that these tumors secrete are usually *non-functional*, these patients can present with hyp**o**gonadism, contrary to what one might have expected.

Prolactin-Secreting Adenomas. Prolactin is the hormone responsible for milk production. In women, prolactinoma can thus cause *galactorrhea,* which is lactation despite lack of pregnancy (of course one should still be certain by checking a pregnancy test). Prolactin *inhibits* gonadotropic-releasing hormone (GnRH) secretion from the hypothalamus. Decreased GnRH leads to reduced FSH and LH secretion by the pituitary. Elevated prolactin can thus cause diminished libido and irregular menses in women; elevated prolactin can cause impotence, infertility, decreased libido, and sometimes gynecomastia in men.

Hypothalamic-releasing hormones stimulate secretion of most anterior pituitary hormones. Prolactin is an exception: its secretion is under ***inhibitory*** control *of dopamine* secreted by the hypothalamus. That is, dopamine released from the hypothalamus inhibits prolactin release from the anterior pituitary.

Because dopamine normally *inhibits* prolactin-secreting cells, dopamine *agonists* are the first-line treatment for inhibiting the growth of prolactinomas. If dopamine agonist treatment fails, surgical removal is often necessary. When else are dopamine agonists used? To treat dopamine deficiency in Parkinson's disease.

What effects would dopamine *ant*agonists (e.g., for treatment of schizophrenia) have on prolactin? A dopamine *ant*agonist will *release prolactin from its inhibition and thus lead to **increased** prolactin secretion.*

Aside from *dopamine antagonists,* other causes of hyperprolactinemia include:

- *Chest wall injury*, e.g., shingles from herpes zoster, which is thought to activate the same neural pathway that suckling would

- *Hypothalamic lesions*, e.g., a craniopharyngioma, which could decrease dopamine secretion, thus releasing prolactin secretion from its inhibition

- *Decreased clearance of prolactin*, e.g., in renal failure

Hypopituitarism

A pituitary tumor may be metabolically silent, i.e., it may *not* secrete anything. These tumors can cause symptoms because of their growth. Since the pituitary lies beneath the optic chiasm, these patients may have bitemporal hemianopsia (Fig. 7-7). If the tumor is so big that it compresses the pituitary, this could lead to dysfunction of the gland (*hypopituitarism*).

In addition to non-functioning pituitary tumors, various tumors (craniopharyngioma, primary CNS tumors, metastases), radiation, autoimmune diseases (e.g., sarcoidosis), infections (e.g., tuberculosis), infiltrative processes (e.g., hemochromatosis, histiocytosis X), and/or hemorrhage can damage the pituitary, leading to decreased function. *Pituitary apoplexy* is pituitary hemorrhage, which can result from rupture of an adenoma. *Sheehan's syndrome* occurs when peri- or postpartum[7] hemorrhage in the mother results in hypovolemia and subsequent pituitary damage. Though these situations can cause failure of all pituitary function (*panhypopituitarism*), the following are the effects of lack of each individual hormone:

- Loss of ACTH leads to secondary adrenal insufficiency.

- Loss of TSH causes secondary hypothyroidism.

- Loss of GH in a child can result in growth failure, whereas deficiency in adults can lead to fatigue, emotional instability, and/or changes in weight.

- Loss of LH/FSH causes *central hypogonadism*. In children, this can result in pubertal delay; in adults, impotence, menstrual irregularities, infertility, and decreased libido can occur.

Diseases of the Posterior Pituitary

Diabetes insipidus (ADH deficiency) and SIADH (ADH excess) are discussed in the renal chapter (Chapter 3).

THE ENDOCRINE PANCREAS AND GLUCOSE REGULATION

The pancreas has exocrine functions and endocrine functions. The exocrine cells of the pancreas secrete digestive enzymes (trypsin, chymotrypsin, lipase, amylase) and bicarbonate into the duodenum (first portion of the small intestine). The endocrine cells of the pancreas secrete insulin and glucagon, which regulate blood glucose level.

In**sulin** drives glucose ***in*****to** cells. Glu**cagon** is for when glucose is *gone*; it causes release of glucose into the blood for the tissues that need it. Mnemonic: A commercial: "*Is your glucose gone? Get GLUCAGON! Glucagon will RAISE your glucose in a flash!*" Insulin and

---

7 *Peripartum* refers to the time period surrounding the birth of a baby. *Postpartum* refers to the time period after delivery of a baby.

glucagon work in concert to maintain euglycemia, a normal blood glucose concentration. Cortisol, growth hormone, and nor/epinephrine also raise blood sugar levels.

Fig. 5-8. Insulin and glucagon. When there is lots of glucose around, after a big meal for example, insulin is released (from the beta cells of the pancreas). Insulin stimulates glucose uptake into cells and its storage as glycogen (*glycogenesis*), fat, and protein. *Glycolysis* (glucose breakdown for energy) is also stimulated. Since this is a time of plenty, all cells are welcome to have glucose, and since there is a surplus, it can be broken down to make energy (ATP) or stored (as glycogen). Note that *glycogenesis and glycolysis are **both** stimulated by insulin;* the goal of insulin is to *reduce blood sugar levels,* so insulin promotes both glucose storage *and* its breakdown.

Glucagon is secreted during a fast when blood sugar is low. Glucagon *decreases glycolysis* and *increases gluconeogenesis* (glucose formation) *and glycogenolysis* (breakdown of glycogen to release glucose). You may ask, "Wait, if we really need glucose to make energy, why would we be inhibiting glycolysis, the energy-producing process!?" In starvation the goal is to pro-

tect the brain and heart. The goal of glucagon is to *mobilize glucose stores* from the liver so that this glucose can be sent to the brain and heart and used for energy production in those organs.

Diabetes Mellitus

In diabetes mellitus, there is either decreased insulin secretion or insensitivity to insulin. Without insulin's effects, glucose cannot be moved into cells, and *hyperglycemia* (increased blood sugar) can occur.

Type 1 (juvenile-onset) diabetes is believed to result from an autoimmune process that destroys the beta-cells of the pancreas, leading to a loss of insulin production. In Type 2 (adult-onset) diabetes, the underlying pathophysiology is insulin *resistance*. The risk of developing type 2 diabetes is correlated with age, obesity, and family history.[8] Type 2 diabetics increase insulin secretion to compensate for peripheral tissue resistance but

---

[8] Diabetes can also occur in pregnancy (*gestational diabetes*). It is normal in pregnancy for there to be some increased insulin resistance. This keeps the mother's blood sugar high enough to make sure that some glucose gets to the fetus. Exaggeration of this insulin resistance can lead to gestational diabetes.

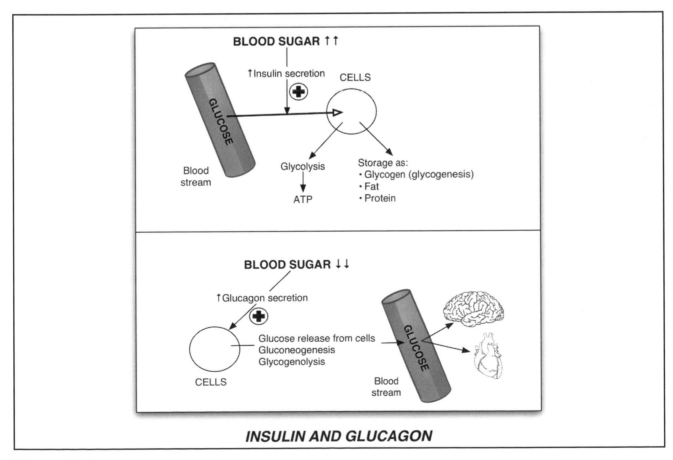

INSULIN AND GLUCAGON

Figure 5-8

eventually this mechanism fails. In some cases, Type 2 diabetics can burn out the pancreas, thus needing insulin replacement just like type 1 diabetics.

Symptoms and Signs of Diabetes Mellitus

Loss of insulin (type 1 diabetes) or insulin resistance (type 2 diabetes) both result in *hyperglycemia*. Hyperglycemia has both short-term and long-term complications. Diabetes is referred to as "starvation in the midst of plenty" since, despite plenty of glucose (hyperglycemia), *this glucose cannot be moved into cells and utilized*. Instead, this glucose stays in the blood and gets excreted by the kidneys. Inefficient use of glucose can lead to weight loss and excessive appetite (*polyphagia*). Elevated blood glucose can predispose to dental caries (cavities) and increased infections such as vaginitis, since increased sugar provides a medium for bacterial growth.

Elevated blood glucose makes the blood hypertonic, creating an osmotic pressure that sucks water into the vascular space. In the short term, the *serum hyperosmolarity* causes *polydypsia* (increased thirst) and *polyuria* (increased urine volume because the hyperosmolarity pulls water into the intravascular space). Extreme hyperglycemia can cause massive fluid shifts. See also hyperosmolar hyponatremia (pseudohyponatremia) in Chapter 3 (Fig. 3-14). This can result in a massive osmotic diuresis (renal water loss) and subsequent hypotension. This is known as a *hyperosmolar nonketotic state* and can lead to coma. A *nonketotic state* is more likely to occur in a type 2 diabetic, since there is still enough insulin to prevent ketosis from occurring. If there is no insulin at all (type 1 diabetes), ketosis can occur. What's ketosis? When starving, the body breaks down fat to satisfy its metabolic needs, and this leads to ketoacid (ketone body) formation. Thus, in severe insulin deficiency, since the body is starving (albeit in the midst of plenty), ketoacids can form in excess (*ketosis*). Diabetic ketoacidosis is a metabolic acidosis. (This is the "D" in MUDPILES. For more on metabolic acidosis, see Chapter 3).

The complications listed above are acute, resulting directly from hyperglycemia and inefficient glucose metabolism. *Chronic* hyperglycemia is detrimental to both the microvasculature and larger vessels. Diabetes is a risk factor for peripheral vascular disease, coronary artery disease, and stroke. Any area with small blood vessels can be affected over time, leading to *retinopathy* (microvascular changes in the retina, which can lead to blindness), *nephropathy* (which can result in renal failure), and/or *neuropathy*.[9] Good

---

[9] Neuropathy from diabetes can be *peripheral mononeuropathy, polyneuropathy*, and/or *autonomic neuropathy*. Consequences of autonomic neuropathy in diabetes can include diabetic gastroparesis (poor stomach motility), postural hypotension, impotence, and/or bowel and bladder problems.

glycemic control substantially reduces the risk of developing these complications.

Diagnosis of Diabetes Mellitus

Clinical features can include polyuria, polydypsia, and/or polyphagia.

The main laboratory abnormality is high blood sugar. The official diagnostic criteria are fasting plasma glucose ≥ 126 mg/dL, random plasma glucose ≥ 200 mg/dL with polyuria and polydipsia, or 2 hours post-glucose tolerance test plasma glucose ≥ 200 mg/dL.

Treatment of Diabetes Mellitus

Fig. 5-9. Diabetes Treatment. If the patient has type 1 (or advanced type 2) diabetes, one must *replace the patient's insulin*. But consider a patient with early type 2 with some insulin resistance but who maintains some insulin secretion. Treatments are targeted to combat high blood sugar, inadequate insulin secretion, and insulin resistance. Thus, treatments function either to *decrease blood sugar, increase insulin secretion*, or *counter insulin resistance*.

How would one decrease blood sugar? Well, where does blood sugar come from? Either from oral intake or from gluconeogenesis, which takes place mostly in the liver. First, we want to reduce the patient's sugar intake, so dietary modification is essential in managing diabetes. If dietary intervention and exercise are ineffective, how else can we decrease blood sugar? *Metformin* is a commonly used diabetic treatment that decreases hepatic gluconeogenesis. A less commonly used drug is *acarbose*, an alpha glucosidase inhibitor that inhibits gut enzymes that normally break down starches to release glucose, thus decreasing glucose available for absorption. What side effects would you expect from such a drug? If you increase the osmolarity of the bowel lumen's contents, then water will be pulled into the gut, leading to diarrhea. This is why acarbose is not used as commonly as metformin.

As for affecting insulin, *sulfonylureas* increase insulin secretion, and *thiazolinediones* decrease insulin resistance.

Hypoglycemia

The main counter-regulatory hormone to insulin is glucagon. Like glucagon, *norepinephrine / epinephrine* (get some sugar for that fight or flight!), *glucocorticoids* (steroid treatment can lead to hyperglycemia/diabetes), and *growth hormone* also increase blood sugar. When blood glucose is low enough to cause epinephrine secretion, the whole "fight or flight" response comes out: anxiousness, diaphoresis, and tachycardia. This causes that shaky, sweaty feeling you get when you skip meals and run around all day.

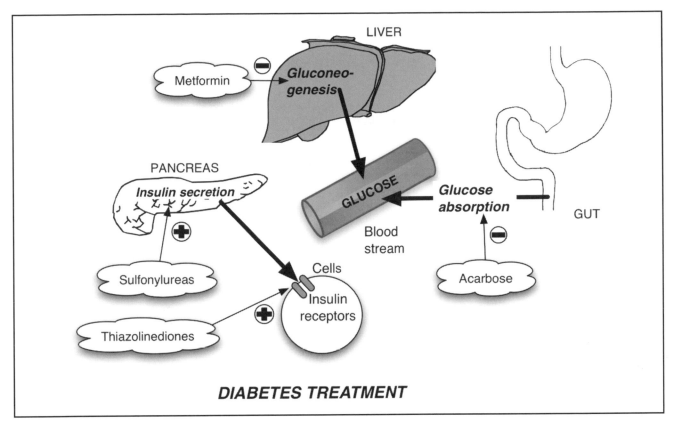

Figure 5-9

Hypoglycemia is defined by **Whipple's triad**: *low plasma glucose, symptoms of hypoglycemia,* and *response to carbohydrates*. The symptoms can be adrenergic (e.g., diaphoresis, weakness, hunger, headache, anxiety) and/or neuroglucopenic (e.g., confusion, slurred speech, coma, seizure). In a normal individual, counter-regulatory hormones have actions that lead to maintenance of blood sugar level. For example, during an overnight fast, the body's counter-regulatory mechanisms (i.e., glucagon-induced gluconeogensis) keep blood glucose levels normal despite lack of glucose intake.

Given the body's regulatory mechanisms, hypoglycemia should not normally occur during a short fast (e.g., between meals). What could cause hypoglycemia? Remember that insulin decreases blood sugar, while glucagon, norepinephrine/epinephrine, cortisol, and growth hormone increase blood sugar. So how could inappropriately low blood sugar occur? Either there must be *excess insulin,* or *decreased counter-regulatory hormones.*

Excess Insulin

Excess insulin can occur with (excessive) *diabetes treatment* or *insulinoma*. What is meant by excessive diabetes treatment is fairly obvious, however "foul play" can also occur, i.e., a non-diabetic taking insulin.

How can you make this diagnosis? Normally when insulin is secreted endogenously, C-peptide is also secreted when proinsulin is cleaved to form insulin. If exogenous insulin is injected, there is no cleavage and hence no C-peptide. Thus, a high insulin level without a correspondingly elevated C-peptide suggests exogenous insulin administration.

An *insulinoma* is an insulin-secreting tumor usually found in the pancreas. If there is an insulinoma, insulin will be normal or elevated *despite hypoglycemia*. (Normally, insulin should be *low* if blood sugar is low.) Since the insulin is endogenous, C-peptide will be elevated with insulinoma.

Decreased Counter-Regulatory Hormones

Decreased glucagon, decreased cortisol (e.g., adrenal insufficiency), or decreased growth hormone (e.g., from hypopituitarism) can cause hypoglycemia. With any endocrine problem, the site of pathology may be either the hormone's secretion or its action. In this case, the hormones could be normal, but there could be *a problem with the actions they are supposed to induce, e.g., gluconeogensis*. A problem with gluconeogenesis could be secondary to liver failure or glycogen storage disease. In these situations, hypoglycemia can occur despite normal hormone secretion.

If acute hypoglycemia is suspected, the reversal of symptoms with glucose administration can help to establish the diagnosis.

Treatment of hypoglycemia is directed at the underlying cause.

CALCIUM, THE PARATHYROIDS, AND BONE

Fig. 5-10. Calcium regulation. The largest calcium store in the body is the bones. Three hormones regulate calcium concentration: parathyroid hormone (PTH), calcitonin, and vitamin D. PTH and vitamin D *raise* blood calcium level; calcitonin *decreases* blood calcium level.

PTH. Located in the neck, the four parathyroid glands secrete parathyroid hormone in response to *low* blood calcium level. PTH secretion is *not* regulated by the pituitary, but by serum calcium concentration. PTH increases blood calcium by:

* *stimulating osteoclasts to break down bone*

* *increasing reabsorption of calcium by the kidneys*

* *increasing conversion of inactive vitamin D to active vitamin D* (which increases calcium reabsorption from the GI tract)

PTH also *decreases reabsorption of phosphate* by the kidneys, leading to its loss in the urine. Why is this important? PTH's action on bone causes release of *both* calcium and phosphate. By decreasing reabsorption of phosphate by the kidneys (and hence increasing excretion), PTH prevents hyperphosphatemia. Thus, PTH causes elevated blood calcium and decreased blood phosphate.

Vitamin D. Vitamin D increases absorption of calcium and phosphate from the gut, increases bone resorption (to release calcium and phosphate into the circulation), and also increases phosphate reabsorption in the kidneys. *So vitamin D increases blood calcium and blood phosphate.* Compare this with PTH, which only increases blood calcium. This distinction becomes important when looking at laboratory tests to diagnose hypercalcemia.

Calcitonin is the antagonist hormone to vitamin D and PTH. Calcitonin decreases blood calcium by using the calcium to build bone, decreasing renal reabsorption of calcium. Calcitonin is secreted by the C cells of the thyroid in response to high blood calcium levels.

Since PTH and Vitamin D increase blood calcium, excess of either hormone can cause hypercalcemia, and decrease of either can cause hypocalcemia. Although calcitonin also affects calcium metabolism, its role is more minor, and so its elevation (e.g., in medullary thyroid cancer) or deficiency do not tend to affect calcium level.

Since calcium is stored in bones and excreted by the kidneys, diseases that affect the bones or the kidneys can cause hyper- or hypocalcemia. Bone breakdown and decreased renal excretion of calcium can lead to hypercalcemia, whereas bone sequestration of calcium ("hungry bone syndrome") and renal failure (see Fig. 3-4) can lead to hypocalcemia. As with other ions, assuming normal renal function and normal hormone activity, it would be difficult to cause an aberrant state of calcium merely by altering intake. However, since vitamin D is responsible for increased calcium absorption from the gut, elevated levels of vitamin D can cause increased absorption of calcium, and malabsorption can decrease calcium absorption from the gut.

Hypercalcemia

Fig. 5-11. Causes of Hyper- and Hypocalcemia. For calcium to be elevated, there must be *increased intake* and/or *absorption* of calcium (mediated by elevated PTH, elevated vitamin D), *decreased excretion* of calcium, or *shifts of calcium from bone into the circulation*.

Specific causes of hypercalcemia include:

* *Increased intake*: excess ingestion from milk and calcium carbonate antacids such as Tums (*milk-alkali syndrome*)

* *Elevated PTH* (hyperparathyroidism)

* *Elevated vitamin D* (lymphoma, granulomatous disease, milk-alkali syndrome)

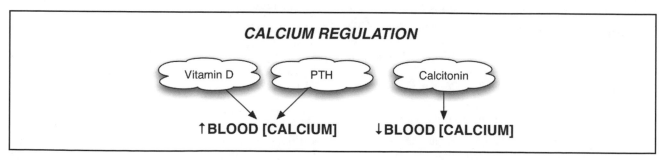

Figure 5-10

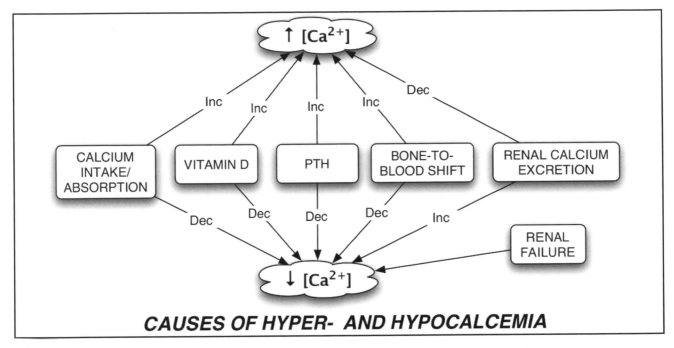

CAUSES OF HYPER- AND HYPOCALCEMIA

Figure 5-11

- *Bone breakdown* (secondary to metastasis to bone, primary bone tumor, multiple myeloma, immobilization, hyperthyroidism)

- *Decreased renal excretion[10]* (thiazide diuretics, lithium)

- *Miscellaneous*
  - *Hypocalciuric hypercalcemia* (which causes both decreased excretion and increased bone resorption, Fig. 5-14)
  - *Paraneoplastic syndrome* (e.g., pheochromocytoma)
  - *Adrenal insufficiency* (Adrenal insufficiency can cause hypovolemia, which can decrease intravascular volume, thus increasing calcium *concentration*. Additionally, glucocorticoids decrease renal calcium reabsorption and increase calcium excretion, so decreased glucocorticoids can cause increased blood calcium.)

Elevated PTH

Primary Hyperparathyroidism is excess secretion of PTH by the parathyroid gland(s). Usually, the underlying pathology is a parathyroid adenoma in one gland, though hyperplasia (growth of all four glands), multiple adenomas in different glands, or parathyroid

cancer are also possibilities. *Increased PTH will raise blood calcium level.*

Lab Findings in Primary Hyperparathyroidism. In primary hyperparathyroidism, serum calcium will be high. In fact, it is often simply an elevated calcium on routine blood screening that raises suspicion for primary hyperparathyroidism. An elevated serum PTH is obviously also present. What about phosphate? Remember PTH's effect on the kidneys: decreased phosphate absorption/increased excretion. So hyperparathyroidism results in a ***low*** serum phosphate and a ***high*** urine phosphate.

Because PTH induces release of calcium from bone, alkaline phosphatase can be elevated, as in any cause of bone breakdown. (Alkaline phosphatase can also be elevated in biliary obstruction.)

What about urine calcium? You might think it would be low since PTH increases renal calcium reabsorption. However, *urine calcium is actually high* in primary hyperparathyroidism because the hypercalcemia in the blood overwhelms the absorptive capacity of the kidneys for calcium. Once this capacity is surpassed, excess calcium spills into the urine.

Another finding in hyperparathyroidism is *increased urinary cAMP*. cAMP is part of many receptor-stimulated second messenger cascades. Mnemonic: PTH is stimulating lots of receptors in the kidneys, which leads to lots of second messenger cascades,

---

[10] Note: renal ***failure*** does *not* cause hypercalcemia. Renal failure results in decreased vitamin D activation, which causes hypocalcemia (See Fig. 3-4).

the effect of which is spilling some excess second messenger into the urine. The real reason for cAMP secretion is far more complex and beyond the scope of this text.

*So in primary hyperparathyroidism: Calcium and PTH are elevated in the **serum**, and phosphate is decreased. Calcium, phosphate, and cAMP are increased in the **urine**.*

Parathyroidectomy is the treatment of primary hyperparathyroidism.

Secondary Hyperparathyroidism. The parathyroid glands are *not* under control of the pituitary. PTH secretion is regulated entirely by calcium concentration. So *secondary hyperparathyroidism is not related to the pituitary* as with other secondary endocrine diseases, but rather to blood calcium concentration: *A decrease in blood calcium causes an increase in PTH secretion.* This can occur secondary to vitamin D deficiency or renal failure (which causes hypocalcemia secondary to decreased vitamin D activation, see Fig. 3-4). Treatment thus involves vitamin D therapy and/or management of renal disease. Note: Secondary hyperparathyroidism is discussed here because it is a cause of elevated PTH. However, secondary hyperparathyroidism it is *not* a *cause* of hyper calcemia; rather, it is a *result* of hypocalcemia.

Tertiary Hyperparathyroidism occurs when secondary hyperparathyroidism *persists inappropriately after the resolution of the renal failure or after renal transplantation.* Parathyroidectomy is often necessary to treat tertiary hyperparathyroidism.

PTH-Related Protein (PTHrP). There are some tumors that secrete a compound known as PTH-related protein (PTHrP). Most commonly, squamous cell lung cancer is the culprit, but breast and kidney tumors can also produce PTHrP. Because PTHrP works just like PTH, calcium will be released from bone, leading to hypercalcemia. However, the resultant high calcium level will *inhibit PTH release* by the parathyroids. Thus, laboratory testing will show increased calcium and a *low* PTH. PTHrP can be measured in the serum to confirm the diagnosis. The other lab findings are the same as those in hyperparathyroidism since the PTHrP functions just like PTH, *except that vitamin D is decreased in PTHrP-related hypercalcemia.*[11] Therefore, in PTHrP-induced hypercalcemia, there is low PTH, low serum phosphate, elevated urinary cAMP, and elevated urine calcium.

[11] The exact reason is not known, but the decreased vitamin D is thought to relate to the PTHrP-induced *hypercalcemia*, not the PTHrP itself.

Vitamin D-Induced Hypercalcemia

Lymphocytes in lymphomas and granulomas (e.g., sarcoid, tuberculosis, etc.) can increase conversion of 25-vitamin D to 1,25-vitamin D (the more active form). This elevation in active vitamin D increases calcium reabsorption, which can lead to hypercalcemia.

Fig. 5-12. Effect of elevated vitamin D on PTH and vice versa. *If vitamin D excess causes hypercalcemia, the elevated calcium will **decrease** PTH level via negative feedback.* Note that the reverse is *not* true: Since PTH actually *increases conversion of vitamin D from the 25-form to the 1,25-form*, vitamin D is actually *elevated* in primary hyperparathyroidism.

Bone Breakdown

PTHrP and lymphomas are not the only ways that malignancy can result in hypercalcemia. Metastases to bone can cause local destruction by their growth, resulting in hypercalcemia. Some hematologic malignancies can produce osteoclast-activating factors (e.g., various cytokines), which can lead to bone destruction. As far as lab findings, this PTH-*independent*, vitamin D-*independent* hypercalcemia will *inhibit both of these hormones, hence **decreasing** their levels in the serum.* The decrease in these hormone levels means there is not much stimulation of their receptors in the kidneys, so urine cAMP will be *low*.

Patients with metastases to bone commonly have bone pain and X-ray and/or MRI findings. Patients with hematologic malignancies may have various aberrancies in their blood cell counts, as well as fatigue, night sweats, and malaise.

Remember that metastases to bone are not the only way to end up with bone destruction and subsequent hypercalcemia. In a diagnostic work-up for hypercalcemia, consider other causes of bone breakdown such as Paget's disease, a disorder of excessive bone formation and breakdown. Prolonged immobilization can also lead to bone breakdown and subsequent hypercalcemia.

Hyperthyroidism can also cause hypercalcemia, because thyroid hormone stimulates osteoclasts, causing bone breakdown.

Fig. 5-13. Summary of hypercalcemia laboratory findings.

Symptoms and Signs of Hypercalcemia

Mild hypercalcemia can be asymptomatic and incidentally noticed on lab testing (this is often how primary hyperparathyroidism is diagnosed). The classic description of hypercalcemia is "stones, bones, abdominal groans, moans and psychiatric overtones," meaning renal stones, bone breakdown, constipation/abdominal pain/pancreatitis, fatigue, weakness, arthralgia, and

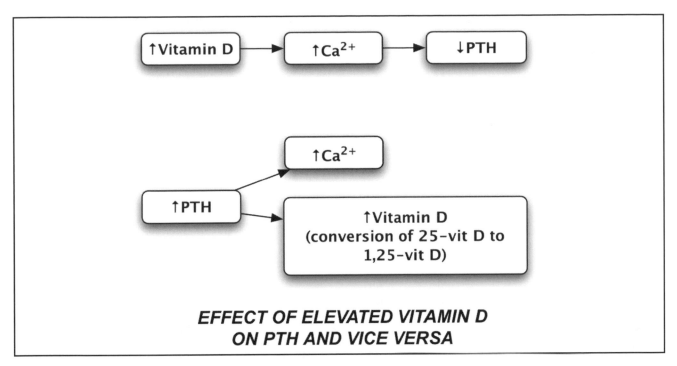

Figure 5-12

	Serum Ca^{2+}	Serum PO_4^{2-}	Urine cAMP	PTH	Vit D
PRIMARY HYPERPARATHYROIDISM	↑	↓	↑	↑	↑
BONE BREAKDOWN	↑	↑	↓	↓	↓
PTHrP	↑	↓	↑	↓	↔/↓
↑ VITAMIN D	↑	↑	↓	↓	↑

SUMMARY OF HYPERCALCEMIA LABORATORY FINDINGS

Figure 5-13

psychiatric disturbances. A shortened QT interval on EKG can also occur. Mnemonic: *Lots* of CALifornians are short QTs (cuties).

Treatment of Hypercalcemia

To decrease blood calcium level, one can *dilute blood calcium* (hydration with IV solutions), *increase calcium excretion* (*loop* diuretics; note: *thiazide* diuretics increase calcium *reabsorption*), *inhibit bone resorption* (calcitonin and bisphosphonates), and/or treat the un-

derlying cause (e.g., surgery for hyperparathyroidism, steroids for granulomatous disease).

Hypocalcemia

Fig. 5-11. Causes of Hyper- and Hypocalcemia. Hypocalcemia can be caused by *decreased intake/absorption* of calcium, *increased excretion* of calcium, *shifts to bone*, or *binding of calcium in the circulation*. The first three of these are mediated by *decreases* in PTH and/or vitamin D.

Specific causes of hypocalemia include:

- *Decreased PTH*
  - *Hypoparathyroidism*
  - *Pseudohypoparathyroidism* (PTH resistance)

- *Vitamin D deficiency* (decreased intake, malabsorption, renal disease, liver disease)

- *Increased excretion* (e.g., Fanconi syndrome: proximal tubule dysfunction leading to loss of calcium and other electrolytes)

- *Shift to bone (hungry bone syndrome)*

- *Binding of calcium*
  - *Hyperphosphatemia* (e.g., rhabdomyolysis)
  - *Pancreatitis* (fats released from pancreas bind calcium)

- *Miscellaneous*
  - *Hypercalciuric hypocalcemia* (increased calcium excretion and decreased bone resorption see Fig. 5-14)
  - *Drugs* (e.g., chemotherapy agents, foscarnet, phenytoin)
  - *Hypoalbuminemia*
  - *Severe/chronic illness (e.g., sepsis)*

Decreased PTH: Hypoparathyroidism and Pseudohypoparathyroidism

Hypoparathyroidism can be caused by:

- *Congenital absence of the parathyroids* (e.g., DiGeorge syndrome is a problem with the third and fourth branchial pouches in which the thymus and parathyroids are absent)

- *Autoimmune destruction of the parathyroids* in rare diseases such as HAM (**h**ypoparathyroidism, **a**drenal insufficiency, **m**ucocutaneous candidiasis) and APECED (**a**utoimmune **p**olyendocrinopathy **c**andidiasis, **e**ctodermal **d**ystrophy)

- *Familial* (i.e., genetic) hypoparathyroidism

- *Surgical damage/removal of the parathyroids,* for example from thyroid surgery

- *Magnesium* (a 2+ ion like calcium), which affects the parathyroids' secretion of PTH; *hypo- or hyper-magnesemia* can lead to hypocalcemia.

- *Infiltrative disease* of the parathyroids (e.g., Wilson's disease)

- *Metastases* to the parathyroids

If calcium *and* PTH are both low, a hypoparathyroid state exists. Alternatively, if calcium is low and PTH is high, one of three scenarios is possible:

1. Vitamin D deficiency is causing the hypocalcemia, and the parathyroids are responding to that hypocalcemia by secreting PTH.

2. PTH itself may be abnormal/non-functional.

3. PTH receptors may be *resistant* to PTH, thus leading to elevated, albeit ineffective PTH. The condition of having receptors that are non-responsive to PTH is known as *pseudohypoparathyroidism.*

Pseudohypoparathyroidism. In pseudohypoparathyroidism, the PTH receptor resistance to PTH is due to mutations in a G protein involved in signal transduction from the PTH receptor. PTH level will be *high*, but to no avail, resulting in hypocalcemia. (A similar scenario occurs in nephrogenic diabetes insipidus, where renal ADH receptors are unresponsive to pituitary ADH.) Patients with pseudohypoparathyroidism type 1a also have *Albright's hereditary osteodystrophy*, which includes features such as short stature, obesity, and round face. Additional manifestations of pseudohypoparathyroidism type 1a are resistance to TSH, gonadotropins, and glucagon. Occasionally, patients will manifest the features of Albright's hereditary osteodystrophy (and have a similar mutation) but maintain PTH-responsive receptors. This condition carries the wonderful name *pseudopseudohypoparathyroidism*, since patients with this disorder have many of the same features seen in pseudohypoparathyroidism, but they are *not* actually hypoparathyroid.

Vitamin D Deficiency

Vitamin D deficiency can result from decreased exposure to UV light, inadequate dietary intake of vitamin D, or malabsorption of vitamin D. Since vitamin D is made in the liver and is activated in the kidneys, liver or renal disease can lead to decreased vitamin D and subsequent hypocalcemia. In children, low vitamin D can lead to problems in growing bone and the growth plate (*rickets*). Vitamin D deficiency in adults results in *osteomalacia* (a decrease in bone density and mineral content causing bone softening).[12]

Hungry Bone Syndrome

After surgical correction of hyperparathyroidism, the bones are suddenly free from the constant breakdown that was being caused by the over-secretion of PTH. The sudden decrease in PTH causes the hungry bones to sequester calcium for re-growth, which can lead to hypocalcemia. This can also occur following thyroid surgery for correction of hyperthyroidism as a response to increased bone breakdown during hyperthyroidism.

---

[12] This is different from *osteoporosis*, where the bones are porous and brittle due to a decrease in bone mass that occurs primarily in the elderly. See Osteoporosis in Bone section below.

Binding of Calcium

Binding of calcium can occur in *hyperphosphatemia*, one cause of which is *rhabdomyolysis*. Rhabdomyolysis is muscle breakdown and can occur secondary to massive trauma/injury, extreme exertion, seizures, drugs/toxins, infections, muscle diseases (e.g., polymyositis, myopathies). Diagnosis of rhabdomyolosis can be confirmed by myoglobin in the urine, and treatment is largely supportive (managing fluids and electrolytes and using diuretics to increase excretion of toxic muscle breakdown products).

Hypoalbuminemia

Since some calcium is bound by albumin, a decreased albumin level can lead to a decreased total calcium level. This is known as "factitious hypocalcemia" because ionized calcium is actually normal. Decreased albumin can occur in malnutrition, liver disease, cirrhosis, nephrotic syndrome, burns, and other major physiological stresses.

Symptoms and Signs of Hypocalcemia

The classic signs of hypocalcemia are tetany, *Chvostek's sign* (tapping over the facial nerve causes a twitch), *Trousseau's sign* (inflating a blood pressure cuff around the arm causes a tetanic spasm of the wrist), circumoral paresthesias, and a *prolonged* QT interval. So high calcium shortens the QT interval; low calcium lengthens the QT interval.

Treatment of Hypocalcemia

In addition to treating the underlying cause, severe acute hypocalcemia can require IV repletion of calcium. Chronic hypocalcemia can be remedied with calcium and vitamin D supplements unless there is significant malabsorption, which would render oral treatments ineffective. In the case of malabsorption, parenteral calcium is sometimes necessary.

Hypercalciuric Hypocalcemia and Hypocalciuric Hypercalcemia

The calcium-sensing receptors (CaSR) on parathyroid cells sense the surrounding calcium level. If calcium is low, the receptors transmit that message to the parathyroids, and the parathyroids respond by *increasing* PTH secretion. If calcium is high, the receptors transmit that message to the parathyroids, and the parathyroids respond by *decreasing* PTH secretion.

The CaSR is also expressed in the nephron. If calcium is low, the CaSR would transmit the message to try to hold on to calcium, decreasing calcium excretion and increasing blood calcium. If there is a high level of calcium, the nephron responds by increasing calcium excretion, reducing blood calcium.

Fig. 5-14. Hypercalciuric hypocalcemia and hypocalciuric hypercalcemia.

In *hypercalciuric hypocalcemia*, the CaSR malfunctions such that it "thinks" there is too much calcium around even when there is not. This leads to *decreased PTH secretion* and *decreased calcium retention* in the nephron. The result is **increased** urine calcium (*hypercalciuria*) and **decreased** blood calcium (*hypocalcemia*).

In *hypocalciuric hypercalcemia*, the CaSR malfunctions such that it "thinks" there is not enough calcium around even when there is. This leads to *increased PTH secretion* and *increased calcium retention* in the nephron. The result is **decreased** urine calcium (*hypocalciuria*) and **increased** blood calcium (*hypercalcemia*).

Diseases of Bone

Bones can become thickened, weakened, fractured, and infected, or they can develop primary or metastatic tumors. Bones are composed of calcium phosphate, so calcium deficiency, vitamin D deficiency, and hyperparathyroidism can weaken bones.

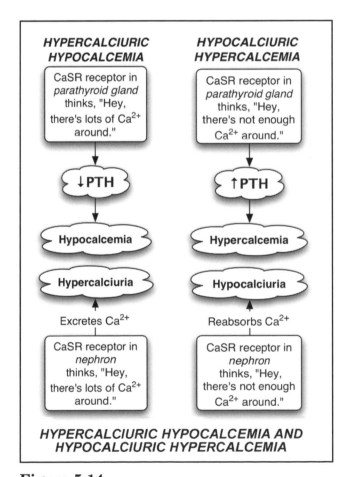

Figure 5-14

Thickened Bones: Osteopetrosis

Normally PTH and calcitonin mediate a dynamic equilibrium between bone formation (by osteoblasts) and bone resorption (by osteoclasts). What might *increase* bone formation? Either increased activity of osteoblasts or decreased activity of osteoclasts.

Osteopetrosis is a genetic disease in which osteoclasts fail to break down bone. A variety of genetic defects can cause osteoclast dysfunction. The uncontrolled bone formation is disorderly, which can predispose to fracture, and these fractures can be difficult to heal. Bony growths can entrap cranial nerves or peripheral nerves. Cranial nerve compression can lead to facial palsy (nerve VII) or deafness (nerve VIII), and peripheral nerve compression can cause carpal tunnel syndrome. Bone pain, osteoarthritis, and osteomyelitis can also occur in osteopetrosis. Impingement of new bone on the bone marrow can compromise hematopoiesis, resulting in anemia, thrombocytopenia, and/or immunosuppression. The disease can present in infants (called *malignant osteopetrosis*) or adults. In infants, bone marrow transplant is the only curative therapy. In adults, in whom the condition tends to be far less severe, surgical treatment is used to correct any nerve compression or arthritis, but treatment of the underlying disease is generally not necessary. In some cases, steroids or vitamin D may be used in treatment.

Weakened Bones: Osteoporosis and Osteomalacia

Osteoporosis is decreased bone mass, which can lead to increased fracture risk. Osteoporosis is common in elderly women (from estrogen deficiency), the elderly in general (senile osteoporosis), and in patients with elevated cortisol (Cushing's, exogenous steroid treatment), chronic diseases, prolonged immobilization, or poor diet (e.g., anorexia nervosa). X-ray demonstrates decreased bone density. Bone density scanning is often used to assess the degree of osteoporosis and fracture risk. Calcium/vitamin D intake and exercise can help to prevent osteoporosis. Estrogen replacement, calcium supplements, bisphosphonates, and calcitonin prevent further progression of osteoporosis. PTH injections can be used to stimulate bone growth.

Rickets/Osteomalacia. In these disorders, vitamin D deficiency leads to a decrease in bone density and mineral content, causing bone softening. Like osteoporosis, this bone weakening leads to a predisposition to fracture. In children, rickets also causes growth plate abnormalities.

Thickened and Weakened Bones: Paget's Disease (Osteitis Deformans)

In Paget's disease of bone, there is repeated bone resorption and bone formation, leading to disorganized, weaker bone. Paget's disease occurs in three phases: a lytic ("hot") phase, an intermediate phase, and a sclerotic ("cold") phase. In the hot phase, some trigger (hypotheses include infectious and genetic possibilities) leads to overactivity of osteoclasts and massive bone resorption. This phase is followed by a compensatory osteoblast response mixed with continued osteolytic activity in which bone is re-formed in a disorganized fashion. In the cold or sclerotic phase, there is continued disorganized bone formation.

This process may occur in any bone and/or multiple bones. Patients may be asymptomatic, but can experience bone pain (including headache if the skull is involved), arthritis, deafness (from bone around cranial nerve VIII and middle ear ossicles), spinal stenosis, fracture, and frontal bossing (enlargement of the forehead). The affected bone is highly vascularized, so it can feel warm to the touch. Extreme cases can thus lead to high output heart failure as the heart struggles to supply the excess vasculature. Paget's can predispose to osteosarcoma. On X-ray, bones may appear hyper-dense, bowed, fractured, or otherwise abnormal. Alkaline phosphatase may be elevated from bone break-down. Although surgery may be necessary to relieve nerve compression, Paget's can be managed with bisphosphonates, which inhibit osteoclast destruction of bone.

Infection of Bone: Osteomyelitis

Infectious agents can reach bone hematogenously from other sites of infection or from contiguous spread during trauma or surgery. Predisposing factors include vascular insufficiency, IV drugs, and immunodeficiency/immunosuppression. *Staph. aureus* is one of the more common causes generally, while *Salmonella* is more common in patients with sickle cell disease. Symptoms include bone pain, fever, chills, and erythema (redness) over the affected bone. X-ray will not demonstrate bony change for several weeks after infection, though soft tissue swelling may be visible early on. CT, MRI, or bone scan may also show changes. Biopsy/aspiration of affected bone can be used for diagnosis and culture to identify the offending organism. IV antibiotics are used to treat the infection, and in some cases surgical debridement is also necessary.

Tumors of Bone

Bone is a common site of tumor metastasis, most commonly in the spine, ribs, and skull, though possible anywhere in the skeleton. In addition, there are several primary bone tumors (e.g., osteosarcoma, osteoblastoma, Ewing's sarcoma). These primary tumors are far less common than metastases to bone and tend to occur in long bones (e.g., femur). A primary or metastatic tumor in bone can cause pain, predispose to fracture, or be asymptomatic, being diagnosed incidentally on X-ray or another radiologic imaging study. Multiple myeloma is a proliferation of plasma cells (terminally differentiated B cells) that occurs most commonly in bone (see Chapter 6).

Note: Whether bone is weakened (e.g., osteoporosis, osteomalacia, or tumor growth) or whether a disease increases bone formation (e.g., osteopetrosis or Paget's disease), *the patient is predisposed to fractures*. This is because the diseases causing increased bone formation often produce *abnormal* architecture of this newly formed bone.

CHAPTER 6. THE HEMATOLOGIC SYSTEM

COMPONENTS OF THE HEMATOLOGIC SYSTEM

The hematologic system includes the red blood cells, white blood cells, platelets, coagulation factors, bone marrow, lymph nodes, and spleen. Red blood cells (RBCs) carry oxygen from the lungs to peripheral tissues, white blood cells (WBCs) are part of the immune system, and platelets and coagulation factors coordinate the formation of clots to prevent bleeding. The bone marrow is the site of formation of new blood elements (*hematopoiesis*) in the adult. The spleen is involved in hematopoiesis in the fetal period and; in adults, the spleen filters out infectious organisms and malformed, damaged, or old red blood cells. The lymph nodes are localized sites of lymphatic tissue, including white blood cells responsible for fighting infection.

Fig. 6-1. Pathology in the hematologic system. *Pathology in the hematologic system can be due to increased or decreased number (or function) of any of its components.*

RED BLOOD CELLS

Red blood cells contain hemoglobin, which carries oxygen to the tissues. RBCs are produced in the bone marrow; erythropoietin (EPO) secretion from the kidneys increases RBC production. *Anemia* is a decrease in RBC number or function. *Polycythemia* is an increase in RBC number.

Too Few RBCs: Anemia

Symptoms and Signs of Anemia

In anemia there is a decrease in the oxygen-carrying capacity of the blood. This occurs secondary to *a decreased number of RBCs* or *a decrease in RBC function* (e.g., a problem with hemoglobin, the molecule that carries oxygen). This results in inadequate oxygen delivery to the tissues. How would the body compensate for this? Hint: What other organs can control oxygen and blood? The heart/circulatory system, the lungs, and the kidneys. How would the heart respond to anemia? In an effort to increase perfusion of the tissues, the heart increases its rate, so *tachycardia* can be one sign of anemia (though tachycardia can occur in many other circumstances as well). If there is not enough oxygen to go around, the most important organs (e.g., the brain) get first dibs, so blood is shunted away from the skin, leading to *pallor*. When the body needs more rapid oxygen delivery to tissues (e.g., during exercise or heavy exertion), there may be *dyspnea* when the lungs and heart struggle to supply the tissues with adequate oxygen. What can the kidneys do? The kidneys can secrete more erythropoietin, to stimulate the bone marrow to produce RBCs.

Symptoms/signs of anemia thus include *tachycardia* (heart trying to pump blood more vigorously to make up for the less "effective" blood), *pallor* (blood shunted away from skin to organs), and *exertional dyspnea*.

Hemoglobin and Hematocrit. Normal hemoglobin concentration is around 13.5-17.5 g/dl for men, 12-16 g/dl for women. Hematocrit is the percent of the blood that is actually RBCs (i.e., not plasma, etc.). A normal hematocrit for a man is about 41-53%, for a woman about 36-46%.

	RBCs	WBCs	Platelets/ Coagulation factors
INCREASE	Polycythemia	Infection Inflammation Malignancy	Hypercoagulable state
DECREASE	Anemia	Immuno-deficiency	Hypocoagulable state

PATHOLOGY IN THE HEMATOLOGIC SYSTEM

Figure 6-1

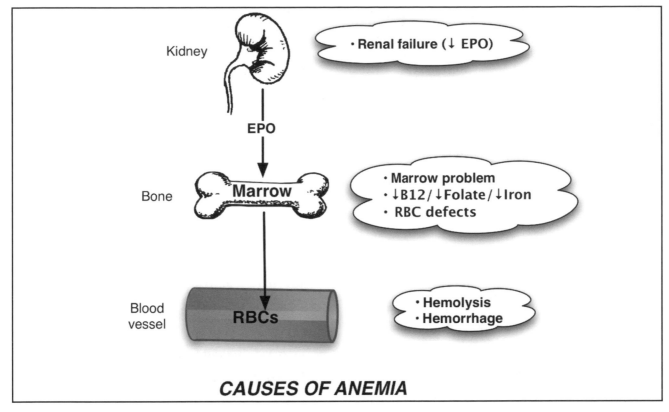

CAUSES OF ANEMIA

Figure 6-2

Causes of Anemia

Fig. 6-2. Causes of anemia. Causes of a decrease in RBC number or function include:

- *Decreased production of RBCs*
  - Secondary to a problem with the bone marrow
  - Secondary to a problem with erythropoietin (EPO), e.g., renal failure
  - Secondary to a lack of raw materials necessary for RBC synthesis: B12, folate, iron

- *Loss of RBCs*
  - From bleeding, obvious (e.g., hemorrhage) or occult (e.g., GI bleed)
  - From destruction (*hemolysis*)

- *Production of defective RBCs* (i.e., a problem with one of the components of the RBC. Though it may not alter RBC number, this will alter RBC *function*, thus leading to anemia).

Decreased Production of RBCs

Bone Marrow Failure, Renal Failure, Aplastic Anemia. In adults, RBCs form in the *bone marrow.* RBC production is stimulated by erythropoietin (EPO), which is secreted by the kidneys. So anemia secondary to *decreased production* of RBCs could result from either a *problem with EPO* secretion or a *problem in the bone marrow.* In renal failure, the kidneys' ability to secrete EPO is diminished, which can result in anemia. If renal failure is the cause of anemia, one would also expect to see electrolyte abnormalities and elevated BUN and creatinine.

What could cause decreased bone marrow production of RBCs? *Infiltrative processes* (e.g., myeloma, leukemia, bone marrow metastases from other cancers), *aplastic anemia*, or *decreased materials necessary for RBC production* (iron, B12, folate).

Aplastic anemia is a loss of hematopoietic cells leading to *pancytopenia* (decrease in all blood cell types). It can be caused by drugs, viruses, or autoimmune processes. Both infiltrative processes and aplastic anemia would cause low levels of WBCs and platelets, in addition to just a decrease in RBCs. If a hematologic malignancy exists in the bone marrow, the number of the malignancy-causing hematologic cell population will be extremely high. Patients with hematologic malignancy may also experience constitutional symptoms such as fever, night sweats, and fatigue.

Iron, B12, and Folate Deficiency. Aside from intrinsic bone marrow disease or renal failure, the bone marrow may simply not have the materials necessary to make functional RBCs, namely *iron, folic acid,* and *B12.* Deficiencies of any of these can cause anemia.

Iron Deficiency Anemia. Iron is necessary for hemoglobin production and function. Hemoglobin gives RBCs their nice red color and full shape, so when there is not much iron around, the result is pale (*hypochromic*), small (*microcytic*) red blood cells. Thus, iron deficiency is a *hypochromic, microcytic* anemia.

Other symptoms, signs, and lab abnormalities in iron deficiency anemia: Patients can have *pica* (craving ice or other non-food objects). Mnemonic: Imagine that the body "knows" it is craving iron and seeks metal-flavored things to munch on. (It is not known why this really happens.) As with any anemia, symptoms/signs such as pallor, tachycardia, and exertional dyspnea may be present. Serum iron will obviously be low.

Fig. 6-3. Ferritin and transferrin (TIBC) in iron deficiency anemia. Ferritin is a protein that stores iron. Most ferritin is found in the liver, spleen, and bone marrow, and some ferritin circulates in the blood. If there is excess iron in the blood, ferritin concentration in the blood increases to bind the extra iron. In iron deficiency, ferritin has no need to come into the blood and bind iron. Thus, *ferritin is low in iron deficiency anemia. Trans*ferrin *trans*ports iron in the blood. Transferrin saturation is typically measured indirectly by assessing the total iron binding capacity (TIBC). What would happen to the binding *capacity* in iron deficiency? It should *increase* since there is not much iron to bind. Another way of saying that there is increased binding capacity is that there is *decreased transferrin saturation. So in iron deficiency, ferritin is low and TIBC is elevated (meaning that transferrin **saturation** is decreased).*

Folate and B12 Deficiency. Folate and B12 are involved in DNA metabolism. If there is inadequate folate and/or B12, the red blood cells do not form properly, and they are released prematurely while they

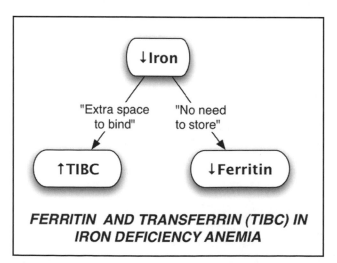

FERRITIN AND TRANSFERRIN (TIBC) IN IRON DEFICIENCY ANEMIA

Figure 6-3

are still big. This leads to a *macrocytic anemia*. Folate and/or B12 deficiency also alters DNA synthesis in *white* blood cells, the result of which can be seen in polymorphonuclear white cells (PMNs) on blood smear. Although PMN nuclei are normally multi-lobed (2-3 lobes), the folate or B12 deficiency leads to *hypersegmentation of PMN nuclei* (i.e., 5-6 lobes). How does one distinguish between folate and B12 deficiency if both lead to macrocytic anemia with hypersegmented neutrophils? One can check B12 and folate levels. Additionally, B12 deficiency can lead to neurological symptoms such as numbness and tingling due to problems with the dorsal columns of the spinal cord. Folate deficiency does not lead to such symptoms.

Why would someone be deficient in folate or B12?

- *Inadequate intake (diet).* Folate is found in leafy vegetables and fresh fruits; deficiency can be seen in alcoholics and in the elderly. B12 is found in liver, muscle, eggs, dairy, seafood, so a strict vegan diet or severe malnutrition can result in B12 deficiency.

- *Increased demand* (e.g., pregnancy, malignancy)

- *Decreased absorption*
  - For either B12 or folate: Secondary to disease of the terminal ileum, which is the final portion of the small intestine (e.g., sprue, Crohn's disease)
  - For B12: Secondary to decreased intrinsic factor (e.g., *pernicious anemia, gastritis*)

- *Drugs* (e.g., methotrexate is a folate antagonist)

In the stomach, parietal cells secrete a protein called *intrinsic factor*, which binds B12 and allows it to be absorbed in the terminal ileum. So a problem with the *production of intrinsic factor* or with the *terminal ileum* could lead to B12 deficiency.

In *pernicious anemia*, autoantibodies are produced against parietal cells, causing a decrease in the production of intrinsic factor. The loss of intrinsic factor results in a loss of B12 absorption. Other gastric diseases that damage the parietal cells can also lead to intrinsic factor deficiency (e.g., autoimmune gastritis).

Two main types of pathology can affect the *terminal ileum*: infection (with bacterial overgrowth) or inflammatory disease (e.g., Crohn's disease or sprue). Surgery that removes a portion of the ileum will also reduce its ability to absorb B12 (because the absorptive surface area is decreased). How could you figure out which one of these causes of B12 deficiency is present? *The Schilling test.*

Fig. 6-4. Schilling test. The Schilling test localizes the site of pathology in B12 deficiency. In this test, a patient gets an intramuscular injection of *non*radioactive B12. This saturates the patient's B12 receptors.

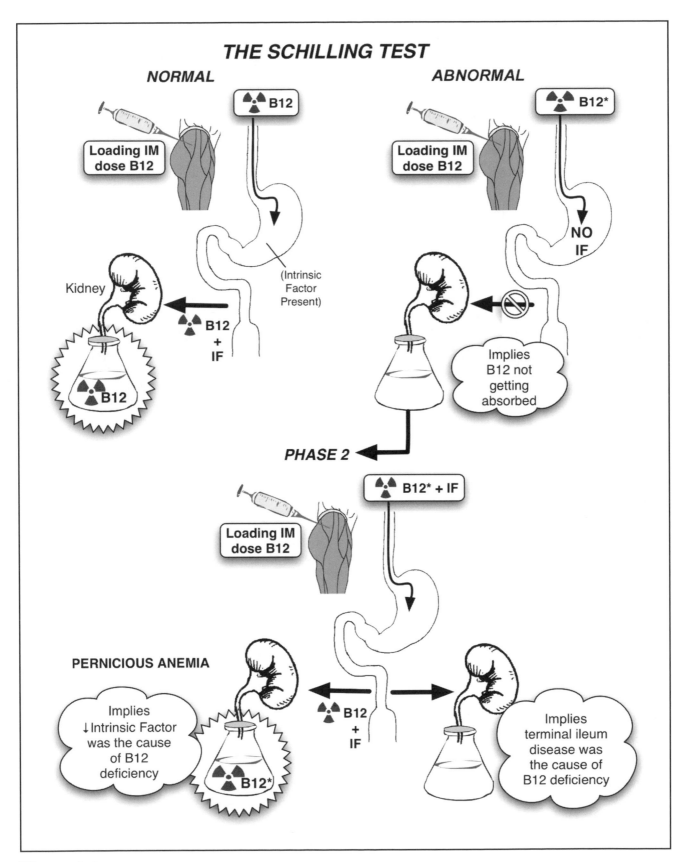

Figure 6-4

The patient then ingests radioactive B12 (shown as B12* in the figure). What would happen in a normal patient (or in a patient who is B12 deficient due to decreased dietary intake)? In such cases, the radioactive B12* should be bound by intrinsic factor (IF) and absorbed in the ileum. If the radioactive B12* is absorbed into the bloodstream, but all of the receptors are saturated (due to that intramuscular injection of B12), the radioactive B12*, now in excess, will be excreted in the urine where it can be measured. So in a *normal* patient, we would expect to see this radioactive B12* in the urine.

In pernicious anemia there is no intrinsic factor. If there is no intrinsic factor, the radioactive B12* *never* gets absorbed, so it never gets into the blood, never makes it to the kidneys, and thus never appears in the urine. So the *lack* of radioactive B12* in the urine indicates *either* pernicious anemia, *or* some other problem with absorption of B12. How would you distinguish between the two? In phase 2 of the Schilling test, everything in phase 1 is repeated, but now the patient is also given intrinsic factor. If the problem is pernicious anemia, exogenous intrinsic factor should correct it, and radioactive B12* should appear in the urine. If there is still no radioactive B12* in the urine on phase 2, we know that intrinsic factor could not fix the problem. Thus, there must be some problem with absorption in the terminal ileum. This can be due to bacterial overgrowth, Crohn's disease, or sprue.

In summary, B12 deficiency can occur secondary to *inadequate intake, lack of intrinsic factor,* or *decreased absorption in the terminal ileum.* The Schilling test determines whether B12 deficiency is secondary to intrinsic factor loss (pernicious anemia) or terminal ileum disease (e.g., Crohn's disease, sprue, bacterial overgrowth).

Increased Loss of RBCs: Bleeding and Hemolysis

Bleeding. Internal or external hemorrhage can lead to anemia. If a patient is overtly hemorrhaging, the cause of the anemia should be relatively obvious. However, a patient with a slowly evolving anemia may be having slow *internal* bleeding. For example, colon cancers can bleed slowly and the blood can blend with the stool, thus covertly disguising blood loss over time.

Hemolysis. Anemia can also be caused by RBC destruction or because of a problem with one of the components of the RBC (membrane, hemoglobin, metabolic enzymes). In fact, in many cases these problems are related: a problem with a component of the RBC changes its shape, causing it to get destroyed or targeted for removal by the spleen. RBC destruction can be caused by external factors (*extracorpuscular defects*) or problems with the RBCs themselves (*intracorpuscular defects*).

Extracorpuscular defects

Autoimmunity (e.g., idiopathic/primary or secondary to lupus or neoplasia), infection (e.g., malaria), drugs (e.g., penicillin, quinidine), a hyperactive spleen, or intravascular trauma from a prosthetic heart valve or a microangiopathic hemolytic syndrome (e.g., disseminated intravascular coagulation, hemolytic uremic syndrome) can all lead to hemolysis. In the case of intravascular trauma, strange-shaped red cells (*schistocytes*) such as "helmet cells" may be seen on blood smear.

Intracorpuscular defects: Problems with RBC components

Fig. 6-5. RBC components and pathologies. The RBC is essentially a sac of hemoglobin; it has no nucleus and no mitochondria. What else does it have? Like all cells, RBCs have membranes and metabolic enzymes. So the three components of the RBC are *hemoglobin, the membrane, and metabolic enzymes.*

Hemoglobin protein is a tetramer composed of 4 subunits: 2 alpha chains and 2 beta chains. Genetic mutations can cause hemoglobin protein to form incorrectly (e.g., sickle cell) or cause inadequate amounts of alpha or beta chains (thalassemia) to be formed, either of which can cause anemia.

Sickle Cell Anemia arises from a mutation in the beta chain of hemoglobin that causes it to malform. When red cells carrying this malformed protein deoxygenate, they adopt a sickled shape, which can both shorten their life span and occlude small blood vessels. This sickling is more likely to occur under times of physiologic stress such as fever, infections, cold weather, etc. The sickling clogs small blood vessels and can cause acute painful crises, acute chest syndrome (ischemia in the lungs), stroke, and renal ischemia. Long-term consequences of sickle cell anemia can include gallstones (from the elevated level of bilirubin caused by hemolysis), asplenia (destruction of the spleen from chronic clogging and infarction), and renal failure.

Thalassemia results from mutations that cause loss of one or both alpha chains or one or both beta chains of the hemoglobin tetramer. The decreased amount of hemoglobin in each cell results in anemia. The anemia is microcytic. Mnemonic to remember that thalassemia is a microcytic anemia: The red cells are small in thalassemia because they don't have much hemoglobin in them. In thalassemia, "target cells" (erythrocytes with a dark spot in their pale centers causing them to look like targets) may be seen. Target cells can also be seen in liver disease, sickle cell disease, iron deficiency, and post-splenectomy.

Membrane. RBCs must squeeze through the tiniest capillaries and thus their ability to "squish" is essential. Properties of the RBC membrane facilitate this

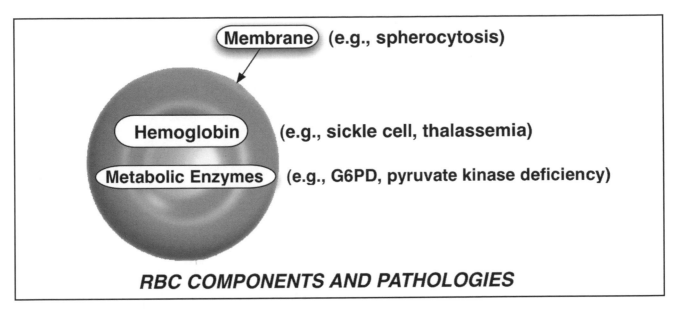

Figure 6-5

squeezing. If abnormalities cause RBC membranes to not be as deformable as they should be, they get stuck in the spleen and destroyed (e.g., *hereditary spherocytosis*).

Metabolic Pathways. The red cell is just a sac of hemoglobin: no nucleus, no mitochondria, only hemoglobin and some enzymes surrounded by a membrane. Since RBCs lack mitochondria, they rely on glycolysis for energy. Two enzyme deficiencies of RBCs are *pyruvate kinase deficiency* and *G6PD (glucose-6-phosphate dehydrogenase) deficiency*. Pyruvate kinase is necessary for glycolysis, and its absence can result in damage and death to the RBCs, causing anemia. G6PD is involved in protecting the RBC against oxidative stress. In patients with a deficiency of this enzyme, oxidative stress (e.g., from infection, certain drugs, fava beans) causes the red cells to be oxidatively damaged beyond their ability to repair themselves, resulting in destruction and anemia.

Though these problems with RBC components represent quite different pathophysiologic entities, the end results are the same: The abnormalities lead to decreased function and/or destruction of RBCs, and subsequent anemia. These pathologies are known collectively as the intracorpuscular defects, defects of the RBC components that lead to hemolysis. Notice that they are all hereditary abnormalities.

Lab Findings in Hemolysis

RBC breakdown produces *indirect bilirubin*. The liver conjugates this bilirubin to form *direct bilirubin*. Jaundice occurs when bilirubin is elevated, either due to an overwhelming amount of indirect bilirubin that the liver cannot conjugate, or due to a problem with the liver or biliary system (see Fig. 4-10). When hemolysis causes red cell breakdown, indirect bilirubin levels can rise beyond the capacity of the liver to conjugate it. This results in jaundice and elevated indirect bilirubin. *Haptoglobin* is a protein in the blood that binds hemoglobin. If there is hemolysis, destroyed RBCs release lots of hemoglobin into the circulation. Thus in hemolytic anemia, ***free*** *serum haptoglobin level is* ***reduced*** since the haptoglobin is bound by hemoglobin (and thus is no longer free). LDH (lactic acid dehydrogenase) is elevated in hemolytic anemia. LDH is a red cell enzyme, and destruction of red cells leads to its release into the circulation. Reticulocyte count is elevated in hemolytic anemia (Fig. 6-6). Summary of findings in hemolytic anemia: increased indirect bilirubin, decreased free haptoglobin, increased LDH, increased reticulocytes, and, if the underlying etiology involves microvascular disease leading to red cell trauma, funny-shaped red cells (*schistocytes*) may be present.

Fig. 6-6. The reticulocyte count. Reticulocytes are immature red cell precursors, and normally account for about 1-2% of the RBCs in circulation. In anemia, the body tries to increase RBC production. In so doing, the number of precursors released prematurely into the circulation *increases*. Imagine that you are working in a cupcake factory, putting the icing on cupcakes as they go by on a conveyor belt. If they go by relatively quickly, inevitably you will miss a few. Now imagine there is an increased demand for cupcakes, so the conveyor belt goes by at a doubled rate....you are likely to miss a lot more cupcakes, and they will be released into the world without

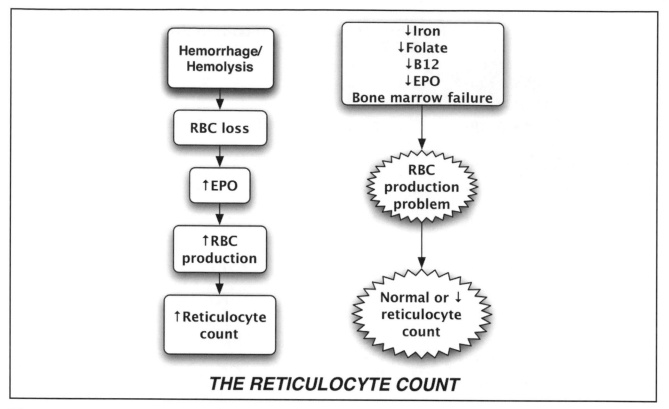

Figure 6-6

icing. Similarly in anemia, the body seeks to churn out RBCs more quickly to respond to the increased demand, and in so doing, more immature cells than usual make it out into the circulation unfinished.

The reticulocyte count is useful for evaluating anemia. Some of the anemias are caused by *blood loss* (hemorrhage, hemolytic anemia), whereas some are due to difficulties in *synthesizing RBCs* (iron, B12, or folate deficiency, loss of EPO, or bone marrow failure). If RBC count is *low*, the appropriate response is to increase RBC production, which will *increase reticulocyte count*. Thus, a *normal or low* reticulocyte count in the presence of anemia *signifies that there is a problem with RBC **production*** (e.g., a bone marrow problem or iron, B12, or folate deficiency). A high reticulocyte count can only occur if the anemia is *not* a problem of *production*. So the combination of anemia and an elevated reticulocyte count suggests RBC *loss* is causing the anemia, either from hemorrhage or hemolytic anemia.

Anemia of Chronic Disease

Fig. 6-7. Ferritin and transferrin (TIBC) in anemia of chronic disease. Chronic systemic diseases (autoimmune diseases, cancer, chronic infections) can cause anemia for various reasons, one of which is dysfunc-

tional iron *utilization*. That is, in anemia of chronic disease, iron is inappropriately stored instead of being released to tissues that need it. If there is impaired *release* of iron, what will happen to ferritin and TIBC? Since iron is stored in excess (inappropriately) and ferritin is used for storage, *ferritin is elevated*. The *TIBC decreases* in anemia of chronic disease: because the iron is already mostly (inappropriately) bound, there is very little capacity left to bind more. So in *anemia of chronic disease, ferritin increases and TIBC decreases*. (Note: This is the *opposite* of what is seen in iron deficiency, where ferritin decreases and TIBC increases.)

Blood Smear

We can broadly classify the anemias discussed above based on the appearance of RBCs on blood smear as microcytic (smaller-than-normal cells), macrocytic (larger-than-normal cells), or "funny shaped." *Microcytic* anemia occurs in iron deficiency (mnemonic: without iron, the red cells are little and pale). Thalassemia also leads to microcytic anemia (mnemonic: thalassemia leads to decreased amounts of hemoglobin and thus smaller cells). Thalassemia can also cause target-shaped RBCs to appear. *Macrocytosis* occurs when RBCs are released too early from the bone marrow. This can occur when there is B12 or folate de-

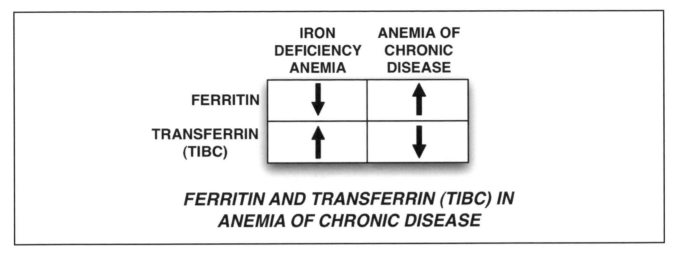

FERRITIN AND TRANSFERRIN (TIBC) IN ANEMIA OF CHRONIC DISEASE

Figure 6-7

ficiency, since maturation of the red cells is disturbed by lack of the materials fundamental for proper DNA synthesis. In B12 and folate deficiency, WBC nuclei are also affected, resulting in hypersegmented PMNs. As for *funny shaped* RBCs, there are many of them, but the ones we referred to in this section are sickled cells, spherocytes, schistocytes, helmet cells, and target cells.

Treatment of Anemia

Treatment of anemia depends on the underlying etiology and severity. Iron, folate, and B12 supplementation can be used to remedy deficiencies of these nutrients. Blood transfusion may be necessary in severe cases. If the anemia is a result of an underlying disease process (e.g., autoimmune disease), the primary disease must be treated.

Review of Anemia

Anemia is a decrease in red cell number or function. Anemia can be classified by *mechanism*: *decreased production* vs. *blood loss* vs. *production of defective RBCs*. Causes of decreased production include iron, B12, or folate deficiency; bone marrow problems; and loss of EPO in renal failure. Causes of blood loss can be internal or external hemorrhage or hemolysis. Hemolysis can be further subcategorized as secondary to defects that are *intracorpuscular* (membrane, hemoglobin, or metabolic enzyme problem) vs. *extracorpuscular* (autoimmune, drug, infection).

Anemia can also be classified by **blood smear findings**: microcytic vs. macrocytic vs. funny shaped (see previous section).

The reticulocyte count *should* increase in response to anemia, because in an effort to replenish the RBC count, the bone marrow starts churning out immature RBCs (reticulocytes) before they are finished. How-

ever, if anemia is due to a problem with RBC *production* (EPO problem; bone marrow problem; iron, B12, or folate deficiency), the reticulocyte count will be inappropriately *normal or even decreased* since it is the production that is impaired. Alternatively, in hemolysis or hemorrhage, the anemia is due to a *loss* of RBCs. In hemolysis or hemorrhage, reticulocyte production is unimpaired, and is thus *increased* in an effort to counter the anemia.

Too Many RBCs: Polycythemia

Polycythemia is an *increase* in the number of RBCs. An increase in the number of red cells makes the blood more viscous, which can lead to headache, or worse, thrombosis and/or stroke.

Causes of Polycythemia

RBC production occurs in the bone marrow under the stimulation of erythropoietin (EPO). So a *hyperproliferative state of the bone marrow* or *excess EPO secretion* could lead to polycythemia.

Hyperproliferative State of the Bone Marrow: Polycythemia Vera. *Polycythemia vera* is a myeloproliferative disease that increases production of RBCs (and usually other hematologic lineages). The cause is not fully understood. What would you expect to happen to EPO levels in polycythemia vera? If the RBC count is inappropriately high, this should cause negative feedback on EPO, and thus *EPO level is low in polycythemia vera*.

Elevated EPO. Elevated EPO could occur either as a normal response to needing more RBCs, or from an anomalous over-production (i.e., by a tumor). Why would we need more RBCs? The job of the RBC is oxygen transport. In any condition in which oxygen supply to the tissues is inadequate, EPO will increase in an attempt to raise RBC count to increase oxygen delivery to the tissues. Chronic lung disease, living at a high altitude, chronic carbon monoxide exposure, sleep apnea, and right-to-left cardiac shunts can all cause chronic hypoxia. This hypoxia leads to an elevation of EPO in an attempt to raise the oxygen-carrying capacity of the blood. Although initially this is an appropriate response, if the hypoxia is *chronic*, the EPO elevation will be chronic, and this can cause excessive RBC production (polycythemia).

A tumor can also be a source of elevated EPO. The most common tumor sources of elevated EPO are renal cell carcinoma (which makes sense, since the kidneys produce EPO), hepatocellular carcinoma, hemangioblastoma, and uterine fibroids.

Lab Findings in Polycythemia

Hematocrit and hemoglobin rise in polycythemia. EPO will be decreased in polycythemia vera, but increased if there is an ectopic source of EPO or if the polycythemia is secondary to hypoxia.

Treatment of Polycythemia

If the polycythemia is secondary to hypoxia, one must remedy the cause of the hypoxia. If the cause of polycythemia is a myeloproliferative disorder, chemotherapy is usually necessary. In the meantime, to reduce hematocrit to a safer level and make the blood less viscous, phlebotomy is used to remove some of the excess blood.

WHITE BLOOD CELLS AND IMMUNOLOGY

The white blood cells (WBCs) are responsible for immunity against infection. As with red blood cells, there can either be too few or too many WBCs. Since WBCs fight infection, an elevated number of WBCs is expected to occur in infection. Increased WBC count also occurs in inflammatory conditions. An extremely high number of one specific WBC lineage can indicate hematologic malignancy. Over-activity of WBCs (*hypersensitivity*) can cause autoimmunity and allergy. Too few WBCs or decreased activity of WBCs can lead to *immunodeficiency*.

WBCs are a diverse group specialized for various aspects of immunity. Neutrophils, monocytes, and macrophages ingest and destroy foreign material. Lymphocytes produce antibodies (which are for immune memory as well as for opsonization).[1] Basophils, eosinophils, and mast cells are important in the allergic response. The complement proteins are another component of the immune system. Any of these cell types (or complement) can be present in extremely low levels or in excess, for a variety of reasons.

Hypersensitivity

Fig. 6-8. Hypersensitivity. Sometimes the host response to antigens is excessive, causing this response to be destructive while trying to be protective. Overactivity of the immune system is at the root of hypersensitivity, which underlies allergy, anaphylaxis, and autoimmune disease.

Immunodeficiency

If any type of WBC (or complement) decreases in *quantity* or in its *ability to function*, the result is *immunodeficiency*: a predisposition to infections. Immunodeficiency can lead to *opportunistic infections*, i.e., infections that do not usually occur in normal hosts. Examples include *Pneumocystis carinii, Cryptosporidium, Toxoplasmosis, Cryptococcus, Histoplasmosis, M. tuberculosis, Mycobacterium avium intracellulare* (MAI), and cytomegalovirus (CMV). Causes of immunodeficiency are *decreased number* or *decreased function* of any element of this system (WBCs, complement, or antibodies).

Decreased Number of WBCs

Decreased WBCs can occur secondary to *decreased production* (bone marrow problem or congenital deficiency) or *loss* (e.g., *infection of WBCs*).

Since WBCs form in the bone marrow, anything that adversely affects the bone marrow can lead to a de-

---

[1] Opsonization is the attachment of antibody and complement to foreign material, targeting this foreign material for phagocytosis and destruction.

Figure 6-8 Hypersensitivity

TYPE	MECHANISM	MEDIATED BY:	EXAMPLES
Type I	Anaphylaxis	IgE → mast cells basophils	Allergy (food, dust, insect bite)
Type II	Cytotoxic	IgG, IgM antibodies	Incompatible blood transfusion, some drug reactions, autoimmune hemolytic anemia, Goodpasture's Disease, rheumatic fever, antiphospholipid antibodies, pernicious anemia, myasthenia gravis, Graves' Disease
Type III	Immune Complex	Antigen-Antibody complexes → tissue damage	Post-infectious glomerulonephritis, rheumatoid arthritis, systemic lupus erythematosis, polyarteritis nodosa
Type IV	Cell mediated/delayed	Previously sensitized T-lymphocytes release cytokines and/or attack targets	Response to tuberculosis test, rejection of transplanted organs

crease in WBCs. Examples include radiation, drugs (e.g., chemotherapeutic agents), infection (e.g., HIV, Epstein-Barr virus), and infiltration by primary or metastatic tumor. A decrease in *all* WBC lineages (along with RBCs and platelets) most likely indicates a problem with the bone marrow. A decrease in one specific lineage most likely indicates either a congenital deficiency in the production of that lineage (e.g., DiGeorge syndrome: T cell deficiency secondary to impaired thymus development) or an infection specific to that lineage (e.g., HIV for lymphocytes).

Decreased Function of WBCs

Fig. 6-9. Overview of the immune system and its pathology. First, foreign material is *opsonized* (by complement and antibodies). This opsonization chemically attracts WBCs (*chemotaxis*). Via *adhesion* to blood vessel walls and *locomotion* through tissue, WBCs arrive at the foreign material and *phagocytize* it, and *destroy it with toxins* (namely oxidative radicals).

Pathology can occur at any of these levels. As numbered in the figure: (1) *complement deficiency* or *antibody deficiency* can lead to failure of *opsonization*, (2) *leukocyte adhesion deficiency* causes *adhesion* problems, (3-4) *Chediak-Higashi disease* causes problems with *locomotion* and *phagocytosis*, and (5) failure of *toxin production* occurs in *chronic granulomatous disease* and *myeloperoxidase deficiency*.

What follows are brief specifics related to each specific cell of the WBC family.

Neutrophils

Increased Neutrophils

Infection, inflammatory diseases, and malignancy can all lead to elevated levels of neutrophils. The neutrophils are part of the myelogenous lineage, so acute myelogenous leukemia (*AML*) and chronic myelogenous

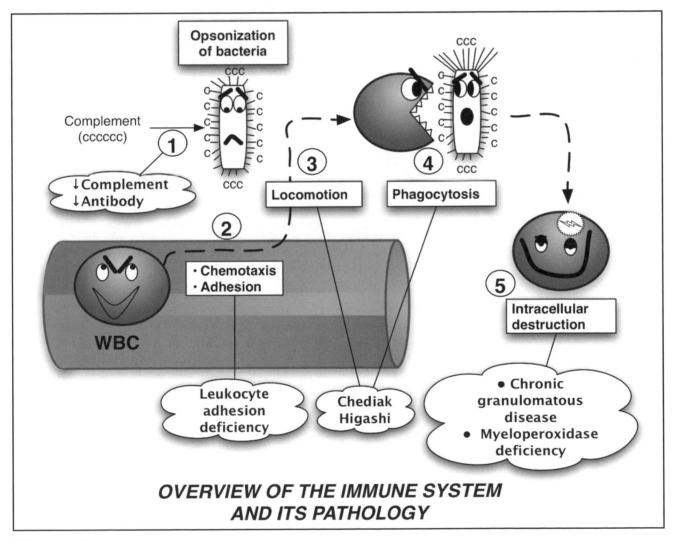

OVERVIEW OF THE IMMUNE SYSTEM AND ITS PATHOLOGY

Figure 6-9

leukemia (*CML*) are the two hematologic malignancies involving this lineage.

Decreased Neutrophils (or Decreased Function of Neutrophils)

A decrease in neutrophil number can occur from drug toxicity, chemotherapy, infections, rare congenital deficiencies, or in the setting of pancytopenia (e.g., secondary to bone marrow failure). A decrease in neutrophil function can occur at any of the points discussed in Fig. 6-9.

Lymphocytes

Increased Lymphocytes

Neutrophils generally arrive first at the site of inflammation, while lymphocytes typically arrive later. Lymphocytes can thus be elevated in chronic inflammatory diseases. Lymphocyte count is also preferentially elevated in some viral and fungal infections, whereas neutrophil count is generally elevated in bacterial infections. Acute lymphoblastic leukemia (*ALL*) and chronic lymphocytic leukemia (*CLL*) are the lymphocyte lineage's analogues of AML and CML. (ALL can also be called acute lymphocytic leukemia.)

Decreased Lymphocytes (or Decreased Function of Lymphocytes)

A decrease in lymphocyte number can occur from drug toxicity, chemotherapy, infections (e.g., HIV), congenital deficiencies, or in pancytopenia (since all blood cell lineages decrease in pancytopenia, e.g., secondary to bone marrow failure). In *severe combined immunodeficiency* (SCID), a genetic defect leads to premature death of B and T cells (e.g., a lack of adenosine deaminase, which leads to inability to catabolize toxins produced in purine metabolism). One of the chief functions of lymphocytes is *antibody production*. Problems with antibody production include genetic diseases such as *X-linked agammaglobulinemia*, *common variable immune deficiency*, and *selective IgA deficiency*.

Basophils, Mast Cells, and Eosinophils

Basophils, mast cells, and **IgE** are involved in allergy. (Mnemonic: **IgE** is involved in aller**gE**).

Eosinophils can be elevated in neoplasia, allergy, asthma, collagen vascular disease, and parasitic infections.

The Hematologic Malignancies of WBC Lineage

In any malignancy, some cell line escapes normal regulation and reproduces itself in an out-of-control fashion. In the hematologic system, this falls into two broad classes: leukemia and lymphoma. ***Leukemias*** *are pro-* *liferations of white cells in the* **bone marrow,** whereas ***lymphomas*** *are proliferations of white cells in* **lymphatic tissue** (e.g., lymph nodes, spleen). Symptoms/signs of leukemia and lymphoma are quite non-specific and can include fever, weight loss, fatigue, malaise, lymph node enlargement, and night sweats.

Leukemias

If one cell line in the bone marrow escapes normal regulation and begins hyperproliferating, production of other hematologic cell lineages decreases since their space and resources in the bone marrow become inadequate. So leukemia can lead to a high number of cells in one white cell lineage and a decrease in others, as well as decreases in RBCs (causing anemia) and platelets (causing spontaneous mucosal bleeding, easy bruising). Myelogenous leukemias (AML and CML) arise from the lineage that gives rise to granulocytes (neutrophils, eosinophils, basophils, and monocytes), erythrocytes, and platelets. Lymphocytic leukemias (ALL and CLL) involve the lymphocyte lineage (that gives rise to T and B lymphocytes). Acute leukemias in either lineage are due to a proliferation of precursor cells, whereas chronic leukemias result from proliferation of mature cells. ALL is more common in children, whereas the others are all more common in adults.

Lymphomas

Lymphomas are divided into Hodgkin's and non-Hodgkin's lymphomas. Remember that lymphomas are proliferations of white cells in lymphoid tissue (nodes, spleen, etc.), whereas leukemias are proliferations in the marrow. Non-Hodgkin's lymphoma is a proliferation of B or T cells, whereas the precursor that proliferates in Hodgkin's disease is unknown. A pathological hallmark of Hodgkin's disease is the *Reed-Sternberg cell*, whose classic appearance resembles "owl eyes" under the microscope.

Multiple Myeloma

Multiple myeloma is a proliferation of plasma cells (terminally differentiated B cells) that occurs most commonly in bone. Multiple myeloma can thus cause bony destruction, which can result in hypercalcemia, bone pain, spinal cord compression, and/or pathological fractures. The malignant cells over-produce non-functional antibodies, resulting in immunodeficiency, elevated serum protein, and elevated urine protein (*Bence Jones proteinuria*). This elevated protein can lead to kidney damage.

Radiation and chemotherapy are used to treat hematologic malignancies.

Review of WBCs

The WBCs are components of the immune system and fight infection. Thus, a decrease in WBCs (or their function) will result in immunodeficiency. An increase can occur in response to infection or inflammation (including autoimmune disease), or as a result of hematologic malignancy. If there is a decrease in a certain WBC type with all others remaining normal, think "What could be affecting this cell type?" The answer could be drugs, an infection, or a rare genetic disease. If there is immunodeficiency with normal cell counts, this could be due to decreased function of a certain cell type (i.e., there is a normal number but the cells themselves are nonfunctional) or a deficit in some other immune component (e.g., complement or antibody). If the cell number is decreased while another cell type is markedly increased, this should raise suspicion for a hematologic malignancy. If there is a decrease in several WBC lineages, there may be bone marrow disease (e.g., secondary to infection, primary or metastatic malignancy, radiation). If there is a modest increase in one type of WBC, this could be due to infection or inflammation. Typically, neutrophil number increases in acute processes and lymphocyte number increases in chronic processes, although some types of infections do not follow this pattern: viruses can have elevated lymphocytes in the acute phase, while parasites can have elevated eosinophils. An extremely high WBC count is more consistent with a malignant process.

PLATELETS AND COAGULATION FACTORS

The coagulation system has two components: *platelets* and *coagulation factors*. Platelets and coagulation factors interact to plug sites of bleeding. Deficiencies in either platelets (or their function) or any of the coagulation proteins can lead to excessive bleeding, i.e., a hyp*o*coagulable state. An excess of platelets or a deficiency of anti-thrombotic proteins (e.g., protein C, S, antithrombin III) can lead to hyp*er*coagulability.

Hypocoagulable States: Tendency to Bleed

If platelets or coagulation factors are low, the ability to effectively form a clot diminishes. This can lead to excessive bleeding/bruising from minor trauma, nosebleeds, blood in the urine (*hematuria*), bleeding into the joints (*hemarthrosis*), excessive bleeding during a menstrual period (*menorrhagia*), and/or bleeding *between* periods (*metrorrhagia*). Mnemonic: Metro is *between* periods and a *metro goes between* two places. **P**etechiae, pinpoint red dots on the skin, are more common in **p**latelet dysfunction or when the number of **p**latelets is low, whereas deep bleeding is more common when there is a disorder of coagulation factors.

Hypocoagulable states arise from either *decreased coagulation factors, decreased platelet function,* or *decreased platelet number* (thrombocytopenia*)*.

Decreased Coagulation Factors

The clotting factors are proteins, many of which are synthesized in the liver, and some of which (II, VII, IX, and X) need vitamin K for their synthesis. Deficiency in clotting factors can thus occur from *liver failure*, from *vitamin K deficiency*, or as with any protein, from a genetic mutation leading to a dysfunctional protein or inadequate amount of it. *Hemophilia* is an example of a genetic disease (X-linked) that leads to clotting factor deficiency. Hemophilia A (Classic hemophilia) is a deficiency of factor VIII. Hemophilia B (Christmas disease) is a deficiency of factor IX. von Willebrand's disease leads to a decrease in von Willebrand's factor (vWF), a protein that stabilizes factor VIII. Decrease in vWF can thus result in a decrease in factor VIII.

Fig. 6-10. PT, PTT, heparin, and coumadin. There are two clotting pathways: intrinsic and extrinsic. The *intrinsic* pathway is initiated when there is damage on the *in*side of a blood vessel and the extrinsic pathway is initiated when there is tissue injury (extrinsic to the blood vessel, which exposes tissue factor to the circulation). Both feed into the common pathway: factors X, V, and II. When there is a problem with the clotting cascade, it takes *longer* for coagulation to occur. Prothrombin time (PT) and partial thromboplastin time (PTT) are laboratory measurements used to examine how long clotting takes, thus assessing the integrity of the clotting cascade. *Prothrombin time (PT) assesses the extrinsic pathway* (VII). *Partial thromboplastin time (PTT) assesses the intrinsic pathway* (XII, XI, IX, VIII). Mnemonic: PTT is a *longer* name than PT and the intrinsic pathway has more factors. Also, PTT has an extra T *"in*side" it and it measures the *in*trinsic pathway. Of course, PT and PTT also assess the final common pathway. Thus, an abnormal (i.e., prolonged) PT could mean a problem with the extrinsic pathway *or* the final common pathway. Abnormal PTT could mean a problem with the intrinsic pathway *or* the final common pathway. This is why PT and PTT are tested together. For example, a normal PTT with an abnormal PT tells you that XII-XI-IX-VIII-X-V-II must be working (since PTT is normal), so the problem must be with factor VII. A normal PT with an abnormal PTT tells you that VII-X-V-II is working, so the problem must be with XII, XI, IX, or VIII.

Coumadin, an anticoagulant, interferes with coagulation by affecting the vitamin K-dependent factors: II, VII, IX, X. *PT is used to monitor the effect of coumadin therapy.* Heparin, another anticoagulant, works by increasing antithrombin III activity. *PTT is followed in heparin therapy.* Remember Extrinsic = VII = PT = Coumadin. Intrinsic= PTT = XII, XI, IX, VIII = Heparin. Mnemonic: "**Hint**" **H**eparin = **Int**rinsic pathway.

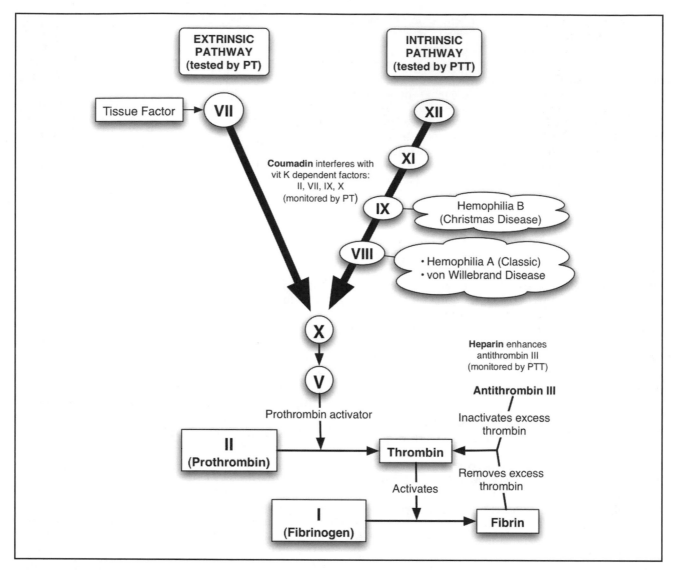

Figure 6-10

Decreased Platelet Function or Number

Platelet dysfunction

Fig. 6-11. Platelet function and pathology. To make a clot, platelets need to adhere to the vessel wall, secrete substances to call more platelets to the site, and then stick to each other to form an aggregate clot. Adhesion to the vessel wall requires von Willebrand's factor, which serves as a bridge from the vessel wall to the platelet, specifically to glycoprotein Ib-IX on the platelet membrane. The platelet is then activated to secrete molecules that signal other platelets to come to the site (e.g., thromboxane, serotonin, ADP). Upon arrival, platelets are linked together by forming fibrin bridges between GPIIb/GPIIIa receptors on the platelets' surfaces. The big picture: Platelets stick to vessel wall, call more platelets, and then stick to each other.

Pathology can occur at any of these steps. In *von Willebrand's disease* there is a decrease in, or absence of, von Willebrand's factor (vWF), which results in a decrease in the ability of platelets to bind to the vessel wall.[2] In *Bernard-Soulier syndrome*, there is a defect in GP Ib-IX (the link to vWF), which also leads to decreased ability of the platelet to bind to the blood vessel wall. In *storage pool diseases*, there is a decrease in the storage pool of signaling molecules normally

---

[2] vWF also stabilizes factor VIII of the coagulation cascade, so von Willebrand's disease detrimentally affects both the platelet clotting mechanism *and* the coagulation cascade.

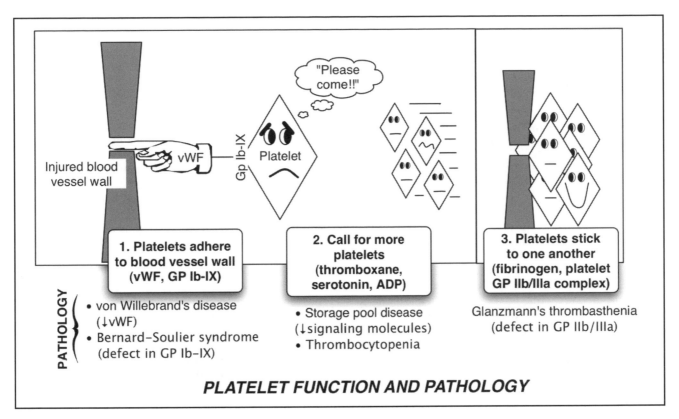

PLATELET FUNCTION AND PATHOLOGY

Figure 6-11

released by the platelet. In *Glanzmann's thrombasthenia*, a defect in the GP IIb/IIIa complex causes inability to bind with other platelets via fibrinogen.

Decreased Platelet Number: Thrombocytopenia.
Why would platelet count decrease? As with the other blood elements, either there is decreased production of platelets, or platelets are somehow getting destroyed:

Decreased Production, i.e., *marrow failure* due to:
• Malignancy (some other cell proliferating and crowding bone marrow space)
• Radiation
• Drugs (e.g., chemotherapy agents)
• Infection

Platelet loss / destruction due to:
• Infection
• Drugs (e.g., heparin, alcohol, quinidine)
• Autoimmunity (e.g., idiopathic thrombocytopenic purpura (ITP))
• Consumption/inappropriate platelet aggregation
  – Thrombotic thrombocytopenic purpura/hemolytic uremic syndrome (TTP/HUS).
  – Disseminated intravascular coagulation

In *thrombotic thrombocytopenic purpura / hemolytic uremic syndrome (TTP/HUS)*, damage to microvasculature (microangiopathy) and/or genetic predisposition[3] can lead to platelet aggregation and thrombus formation. The platelet aggregation causes thrombocytopenia. The microvascular occlusion results in widespread ischemia, classically presenting as fever, purpura, altered mental status, neurological signs, renal dysfunction, thrombocytopenia, and/or hemolytic anemia (secondary to damage to RBCs as they pass through thrombus-occluded microvasculature). Causes of initial microvascular injury include autoimmune processes, pregnancy, infection (e.g., HIV, *E. coli*), cancer, and drugs.

HUS and TTP are thought to have the same underlying pathophysiology, but HUS is generally the name given to the syndrome when it occurs following a diarrheal illness (e.g., caused by *E. coli, Shigella*), which occurs more commonly in children. Laboratory signs include thrombocytopenia and hemolytic anemia (manifesting as decreased red cells, increased reticulocytes, schistocytes on smear, elevated LDH). In contrast to disseminated intravascular coagulation (see below), coagulation factors are not affected, and PT and PTT are thus normal. TTP can be fatal if plasmapheresis (plasma exchange) is not

---

[3] Deficiency in a von Willebrand factor-cleaving metalloproteinase (gene: ADAMTS13) can lead to platelet aggregation and TTP. In patients without this genetic defect, the inhibition of this enzyme (e.g., by an autoantibody) plays a role in the pathophysiology of the disease.

initiated immediately and continued until symptoms and signs improve. Plasmapheresis is thought to remove offending toxins and also replace deficient serum factors.

Disseminated intravascular coagulation (DIC) can lead to both thrombosis *and* bleeding. DIC can be caused by:

- Infections (e.g., gram negative sepsis, Rocky Mountain spotted fever, malaria)

- Massive trauma or surgery

- Any neoplastic, chronic infectious, or chronic inflammatory disease

- Complications of child birth (amniotic fluid embolus, retained dead fetus, abruptio placentae)

These conditions can activate the clotting cascade directly (by release of pro-coagulants or inhibition of anti-coagulant proteins) or indirectly due to endothelial injury in the blood vessels. The resultant diffuse clotting can lead to thrombosis, and the diffuse thrombosis can consume so many platelets and coagulation factors so as to lead to bleeding. Thus, bleeding, bruising, and ischemia of any organ can occur along with features of the underlying disease; respiratory, renal, hepatic, and/or neurological dysfunction may be present. In acute DIC, PT and PTT can be elevated (because of consumption of clotting factors in clots), platelets can be decreased, and fibrin split products such as D dimer (evidence of clotting) can be elevated. Schistocytes (damaged RBCs) may be observed on smear because RBCs are damaged when passing through the sites of thrombus. There is some variability in possible lab findings, and not all of these features are always present. Chronic DIC can occur over a more subacute time course with more variability in lab findings. In addition to treating the underlying cause, management of the manifestations is complex because one must balance anticoagulation (e.g., heparin) and pro-coagulation (i.e., fresh frozen plasma and/or platelet transfusion).

Summary of Hypocoagulable States

The clotting system consists of the platelets and the coagulation cascade. Deficits or dysfunction of platelets or coagulation factors can thus lead to decreased ability to form clots, which can cause bleeding problems. Why would platelets be low? Since they are produced in the bone marrow, any problem with the bone marrow can lead to thrombocytopenia (hematologic malignancy or metastasis to bone marrow, radiation,

infection, or drugs). Thrombocytopenia can also occur from *loss of platelets in the periphery*, e.g., in ITP or TTP/HUS. Platelet dysfunction can occur at various levels due to the platelets' inability to bind with the vessel wall, with other platelets, or lack of secretory compounds necessary to facilitate this process.

Alternatively, clotting factor decrease or defects can lead to bleeding problems despite normally functioning platelets. Vitamin K is necessary for the synthesis of certain clotting factors, and some coagulation factors are formed in the liver. Thus, vitamin K deficiency or liver dysfunction can lead to decreases in clotting factors and bleeding. Additionally, genetic defects leading to decreased or defective clotting proteins (e.g., hemophilia) can lead to decreased clotting ability and hence bleeding.

Hypercoagulable States: Tendency to Clot

Hypercoagulability can lead to clot formation. Depending on where the clot lodges, this can have various consequences. Examples include pulmonary embolism if the clot goes to the pulmonary artery, stroke if the clot ends up in the cerebral vasculature, and mesenteric ischemia if the clot lodges in the mesenteric vasculature.

Protein C, S, and antithrombin III serve as checks and balances in the clotting system to prevent venous thrombosis. Mutation can lead to deficiency of one of these proteins. Without this control on the system, there can be a tendency toward hypercoagulability. Factor V Leiden, a mutation of factor V, causes factor V to be unable to be inactivated by protein C, leading to hypercoagulability.

Other predisposing factors to hypercoagulability include anti-phospholipid antibodies (which can be associated with lupus or occur independently), pregnancy, malignancy, oral contraceptives, turbulent flow (e.g., in atrial fibrillation), heart failure, and stasis. Stasis occurs when people are immobile, for example in a hospitable bed or on an airplane. Stasis can lead to deep venous thrombosis (DVT): clot formation in a deep vein (most commonly a deep leg vein). Parts of the clot can break off and embolize, for example, to the lung (*pulmonary embolus*). That is why prophylactic measures (e.g., subcutaneous heparin, support stockings, etc.) are often used in hospitalized patients who are not moving around very much.

CHAPTER 7. THE NERVOUS SYSTEM

ANATOMICAL OVERVIEW

Clinical reasoning in neurology proceeds in two steps:

1. Localizing the lesion within the nervous system
2. Determining a differential diagnosis for what could cause a lesion at this location

The nervous system may be divided most simply into the *central nervous system* (brain and spinal cord) and the *peripheral nervous system* (peripheral nerves). When localizing a lesion, one attempts to determine whether the lesion is in the *brain*, the *spinal cord*, the *peripheral nerve(s)* (motor, sensory, or both?), at the *neuromuscular junction*, or in the *muscle* itself. The brain is further divided into the *cerebral hemispheres* (frontal lobes, temporal lobes, parietal lobes, occipital lobes), *subcortical structures* (e.g., thalamus, basal ganglia), *cerebellum*, and *brainstem* (midbrain, pons, and medulla). Each area performs specific functions, and changes in these functions can be clues to the site of pathology.

In addition to the anatomical regions at the macro level, the nervous system is divided into gray and white matter on the micro level. *Gray matter* is clusters of neuron cell bodies, and *white matter* is their myelinated axon pathways. *Schwann cells* provide the myelin in the periphery while *oligodendrocytes* myelinate the central nervous system. Disease processes can affect the neurons themselves (e.g., neurodegeneration), the myelin (e.g., multiple sclerosis, Guillain-Barré), or both (e.g., stroke).

The brain is a control center for everything from higher cognitive functions (reasoning, attention, language, etc.) to initiating, planning, and coordinating movement, to perceiving and interpreting sensory stimuli from the outside world and the viscera. The cranial nerves transmit sensory information from the head (e.g., sight, smell, taste, hearing, facial sensation) to the brain, while the peripheral nerves transmit sensory information from the rest of the body to the brain by way of the spinal cord. The motor output of the brain occurs via some of these same nerves: cranial nerves innervate various parts of the head (for moving the facial muscles, the eyes, the tongue, etc.), while peripheral nerves innervate the rest of the body. The vagus nerve (cranial nerve X) is an exception: although it is a cranial nerve, one of its roles is communication between the brain and the thoracic and abdominal viscera.

Although this chapter is organized by region, not all diseases fit neatly into a regional category. Multiple sclerosis (MS) can affect the entire central nervous system (spinal cord and brain) and amyotrophic lateral sclerosis (ALS) affects the motor pathway in both the central nervous system and in the peripheral nervous system.

NEUROANATOMY AND LOCALIZATION

Motor and Sensory Pathways

Motor Pathway: Upper Motor Neurons vs. Lower Motor Neurons

Fig. 7-1. Motor (corticospinal) pathway. The primary motor pathway is comprised of two main components: *upper motor neurons* (projecting from cortex to spinal cord) and *lower motor neurons* (projecting from spinal cord to muscle). The cell bodies in the motor cortex project their axons (through the internal capsule) in the *corticospinal tract*, the main motor pathway. These fibers descend in the brainstem, cross (*decussate*) in the lower medulla (in the medullary pyramids), and then descend as the lateral corticospinal tracts in the spinal cord. These corticospinal tract fibers, from the cortex through the spinal cord, are called *upper motor neurons* (UMN). The upper motor neurons synapse on anterior horn cells in the anterior spinal cord. These anterior horn cells and their axonal projections in

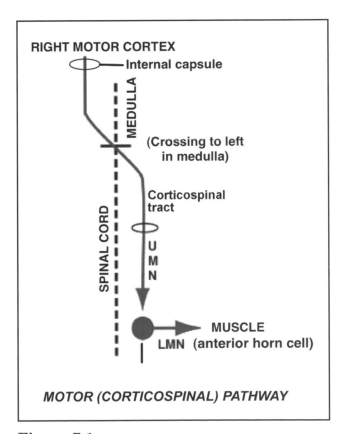

RIGHT MOTOR CORTEX — **Internal capsule**

MEDULLA

(Crossing to left in medulla)

Corticospinal tract

SPINAL CORD

U M N

MUSCLE
LMN (anterior horn cell)

MOTOR (CORTICOSPINAL) PATHWAY

Figure 7-1

peripheral nerves are called *lower motor neurons* (LMN). These lower motor neurons synapse on the muscles. Because of the crossing (*decussation*) of the corticospinal tract in the medulla, the right motor cortex controls the left side of the body, and the left motor cortex controls the right side of the body.

If there is a lesion anywhere in the motor pathway, the result will be *weakness* of the affected muscle(s). However, depending on whether this lesion affects the upper or lower motor neurons, there will be different signs accompanying this weakness.

Fig. 7-2. Upper and lower motor neuron lesions. Imagine a *lower motor neuron* lesion (i.e., injury of anterior horn cells and/or the peripheral nerve(s) in which their axons travel). What do you think would happen to the affected muscle(s)? You could try to tell the muscle(s) to move, but the signal would never arrive. The muscle(s) would be paralyzed and would be floppy (*flaccid*). Reflexes would be diminished or lost. The muscle would no longer be under any control, and left to its own devices it would twitch (*fasciculate*). The classic symptoms of a lower motor neuron lesion are *flaccid paralysis, diminished or absent reflexes, fasciculations,* and, over time, *muscle atrophy*.

Now consider a lesion of an *upper motor neuron,* anywhere from the motor cortex through the corti-

cospinal tract in which its axons run (i.e., in the internal capsule, brainstem, or spinal cord). The affected muscles become paralyzed. In addition, because of the loss of higher control, the lower motor neuron fires spontaneously, causing *spasm* in the affected muscles, a state of tonic contraction. With this loss of inhibition from above, reflexes eventually become exaggerated or hyperactive. Also, primitive reflexes can resurface because of the loss of upper motor neuron inhibition. One example is Babinski's sign. If you stroke the bottom of the foot, the toes should *normally* curl down. If the big toe goes *up*, this is *Babinski's sign,* and is *abnormal* in adults.[1] Babinski's sign indicates an upper motor neuron lesion anywhere from the motor cortex through the corticospinal tract's path in the brainstem and spinal cord. Babinski's sign is not found with lower motor neuron lesions.[2]

Clonus is repetitive, rhythmic contraction of a muscle when it is stretched, commonly seen in the ankle. Clonus is another example of disinhibition. Although a bit of clonus (or other hyperreflexia) can be normal, especially if it is present symmetrically bilaterally, *unilateral* clonus

---

[1] In newborns, since myelination is not yet complete, the big toe will go up. Babinski's sign is *normal* in newborns.
[2] *Acute* upper motor neuron lesions (e.g., spinal shock from an infarct) can present with flaccid paralysis and loss of reflexes, *without* classic "upper motor neuron signs."

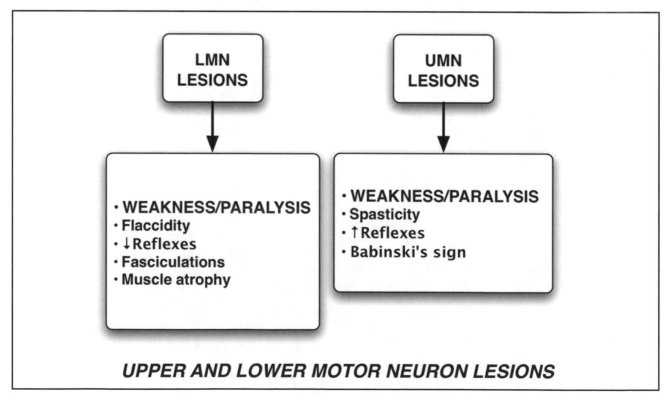

Figure 7-2

(or other hyperreflexia) should raise suspicion for an underlying upper motor neuron lesion. Thus, the classic symptoms of an upper motor neuron lesion are *spastic paralysis* and *increased reflexes*, including *disinhibition* of primitive reflexes (e.g., Babinski's sign) and *clonus*.

If the lesion is *above the decussation of the corticospinal tract* in the medullary pyramids, the motor deficit will be on the *opposite (contralateral)* side of the body from the lesion. If the lesion is *below the decussation* (e.g., in the spinal cord or a peripheral nerve), the motor deficit will be on the *same (ipsilateral)* side of the body as the lesion.

Sensory Pathways

Fig. 7-3. Sensory pathways. The two main sensory pathways are the *posterior columns* (also known as the dorsal columns) and the *spinothalamic tracts* (also

known as the anterolateral tracts). The posterior columns transmit discriminative touch, vibration, and position sense *(proprioception)*. The spinothalamic tract carries pain and temperature sensation. Both pathways also transmit some light touch sensation. All of this sensory input comes from the periphery (skin, muscle spindle, etc.) via peripheral nerves that enter the spinal cord posteriorly. Important anatomy: The *spinothalamic pathways cross **immediately** in the cord, forming the spinothalamic tracts. The posterior columns stay ipsilateral (same side) until the brainstem, and then cross in the **medulla**, continuing as the medial lemnisci (which project to the thalamus).* Why is this significant? Imagine a lesion of the posterior column on the left side at about the level of the belly button. Since the sensory information has come from that *same* side of the body (and stays on that side until the brainstem), one would lose discriminative touch/vibra-

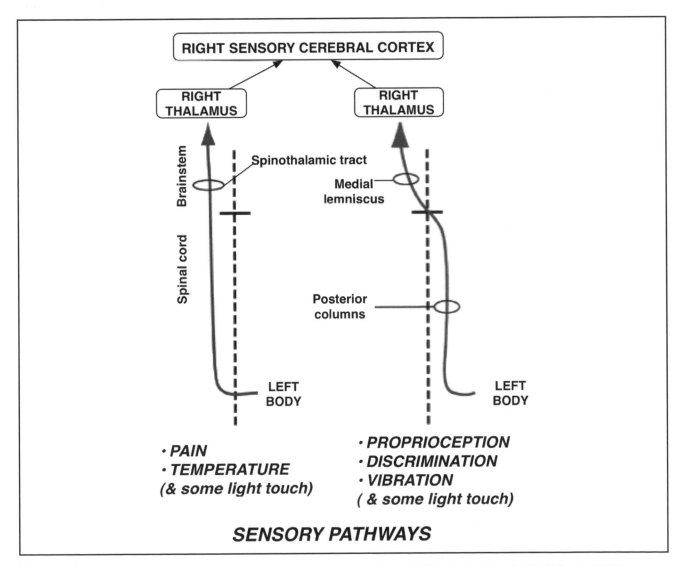

Figure 7-3. Modified from Goldberg: *Clinical Neuroanatomy Made Ridiculously Simple*, MedMaster 2005

tion/position sense on the *same side, distal* to the lesion (i.e., from there down). What about a lesion of the spinothalamic tract on the *left* side? Since the fibers in that tract came from the *right* side, a lesion of the spinothalamic tract on the *left* would lead to loss of pain and temperature sensation below the lesion *on the contralateral side, in this case on the **right** side.*

More precisely, in the *spinothalamic tract*, first order sensory neurons synapse immediately upon arrival in the cord, and the second-order neurons cross and ascend as the spinothalamic tract. In the *posterior columns*, most of the axons of the first order sensory neurons travel all the way to the medulla, where they synapse onto neurons that cross there and ascend to the thalamus as the medial lemniscus. *However, some fibers carrying light touch actually cross right away in the spinal cord.* As a result, ipsilateral lesions of the spinal cord often do not result in much loss of light touch, since some light touch sensation is preserved in fibers that cross.

Fig. 7-4. Brown-Séquard syndrome. What if a lesion destroyed the entire left half of the cord? Remember, *only the spinothalamic tract (pain and temperature fibers) crosses **in the spinal cord.*** So *paralysis* and *discrimination / vibration sense / proprioception* loss will occur *on the **same** side of the body* below the level of the lesion, whereas loss of *pain / temperature* will occur on the **contralateral** side of the body below the level of the lesion. *If one entire half of the spinal cord is damaged, all the deficits will be on the ipsilateral side of the*

*body **except** pain and temperature loss, which will occur on the contralateral side of the body.* Note that *light touch* can be relatively spared because it runs in both the spinothalamic tract and the posterior (dorsal) columns.

If *everything* (strength, light touch, pain, temperature sensation, etc.) is all lost on *only one* side of the body (with the other side entirely normal), could this possibly be due to spinal cord pathology? It could *not*, because a spinal cord lesion would typically have some *contralateral* effect because of the crossing of the spinothalamic tract. Loss of *everything* on *only one side* must localize to somewhere outside of the spinal cord. For example, a middle cerebral artery stroke can cause ischemia/infarction of both the motor cortex and the sensory cortex on one side, leading to contralateral hemiparesis and sensory loss. A peripheral nerve lesion could also lead to loss of motor and sensory function together on one side, but this would be in a region limited to the distribution of the nerve. Compression of *sensory* (posterior/dorsal) nerve roots as they enter the spinal cord leads to symptoms confined to specific *dermatomes*, stripes in a zebra-like sensory map (Fig. 7-5). Dermatomal sensory deficits only occur with focal spinal cord lesions or nerve root compression. The difference between symptomatic patterns resulting from lesions of roots, peripheral nerves, etc., is discussed in more detail later in this chapter.

Fig. 7-5. Dermatomes.

Summary of Motor and Sensory Systems

The cortex is the starting point of the motor system and the end of the sensory systems (i.e., where ascending sensory input from the body finally arrives). The internal capsule contains the subcortical white matter from the motor system traveling toward the brainstem as well as sensory projections from the thalamus to the sensory cortex. The motor and sensory pathways run very close to each other but separately through the brainstem and spinal cord, and exit as separate anterior (ventral) motor and posterior (dorsal) sensory roots. The fibers in these roots then join to form mixed motor/sensory peripheral nerves.

Relatively large lesions commonly affect both motor and sensory pathways where these pathways run close to each other. Examples include large cerebral strokes (e.g., middle cerebral artery), brainstem lesions, and peripheral nerve lesions.[3]

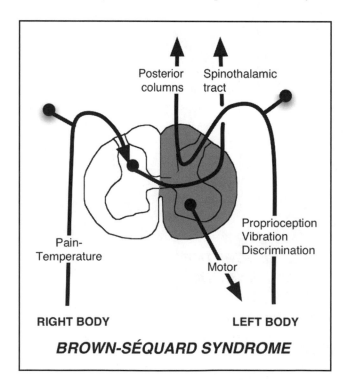

Figure 7-4

---

[3] As discussed later in this chapter, the story with peripheral neuropathy is not quite so simple. There are disease processes that affect specific fiber types and can thus lead to a purely sensory or purely motor peripheral neuropathy. Also, some distal branches of peripheral nerves carry only sensory or only motor fibers.

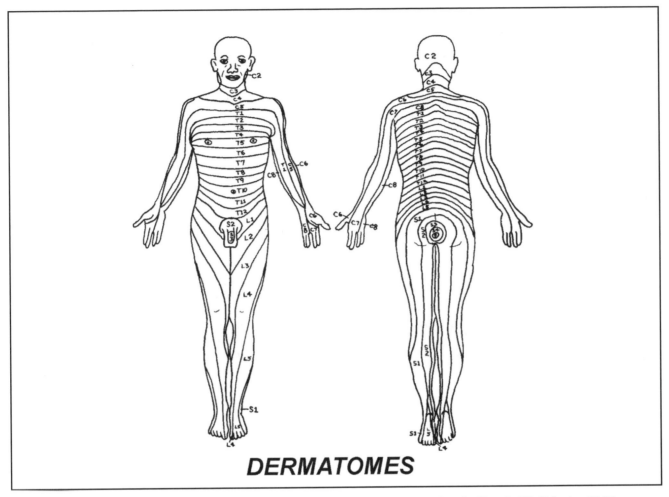

DERMATOMES

Figure 7-5. Modified from Goldberg: *Clinical Neuroanatomy Made Ridiculously Simple*, MedMaster 2005

In the **CNS**, *isolated* motor or sensory deficits typically occur with small isolated lesions in *very specific* places. An example is a lacunar infarct, which is an occlusion of a small penetrating vessel in the brain. These small lesions can lead to stroke with only motor deficits or only sensory deficits. "Pure motor" strokes, for instance, can occur from small lacunar infarcts of the motor fibers of the internal capsule or the motor pathway in the brainstem. "Pure sensory" strokes can result from infarction of the thalamus or sensory pathways in the brainstem.

In the **PNS**, causes of *isolated* motor or sensory deficits include root lesions or diseases affecting the motor or sensory systems specifically. Prolapsed discs or tumors that compress *only* the anterior (ventral) or posterior (dorsal) roots can also lead to isolated motor or sensory findings, respectively. This is because the motor and sensory fibers are relatively separate in the spinal cord and spinal roots (whereas they tend to be mixed in peripheral

nerves). Recall that sensory (posterior/dorsal) root compression leads to symptoms in a dermatomal distribution (Fig. 7-5). Some disease processes selectively affect only motor or only sensory neurons/nerves. For example, amyotrophic lateral sclerosis affects only motor neurons, and certain types of peripheral neuropathy selectively impair sensory fibers.

Brainstem and Cranial Nerves

Brainstem

Fig. 7-6. Cranial nerve nuclei of the brainstem. The brainstem contains most of the cranial nerve nuclei, connections with the cerebellum, and the descending motor and ascending sensory pathways just discussed. From top to bottom, the brainstem is divided into *midbrain, pons,* and *medulla.* A mnemonic to remember where the cranial nerves exit/enter is: 1-4 are in the midbrain, 5-8 are in the pons, and 9-12 are in the medulla. This is not

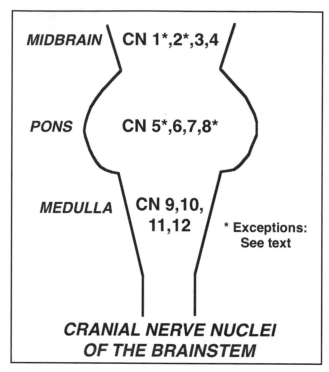

MIDBRAIN CN 1*,2*,3,4

PONS CN 5*,6,7,8*

MEDULLA CN 9,10, 11,12   * Exceptions: See text

CRANIAL NERVE NUCLEI OF THE BRAINSTEM

Figure 7-6

perfectly true, but the general scheme is a helpful one. There are four main exceptions:

1. Cranial nerve I (olfactory nerve) does not project to the brainstem at all but to olfactory cortex.

2. Cranial nerve II (optic nerve) does contain fibers that project to the midbrain (pretectal nucleus) for the afferent limb for the pupillary light reflex, but the visual pathway carried in cranial nerve II does *not* project to the brainstem. The visual pathway fibers in cranial nerve II project to the lateral geniculate nucleus of the thalamus.

3. The spinal trigeminal nucleus, which receives facial sensation information from cranial nerve V (trigeminal nerve), spans much of the brainstem and extends into the upper spinal cord.

4. The vestibular nuclei of cranial nerve VIII (vestibulocochlear nerve) straddle the ponto-medullary junction.

The cranial nerves generally exit the brainstem anteriorly and project ipsilaterally. The primary exception is cranial nerve IV (the trochlear nerve), which exits the brainstem posteriorly and projects to the contralateral superior oblique muscle.

It is not until the medullary pyramids (at the bottom of the medulla) that motor fibers in the corti-

cospinal tract cross to the other side. Sensory fibers (from the posterior columns) also cross nearby in the medulla (becoming the medial lemnisci as they ascend). So a brainstem lesion *above* this decussation in the medulla will impair motor and sensory function on the *opposite* side of the *body* but impair *cranial nerve* function on the *same* side (since the cranial nerves project ipsilaterally). These **crossed signs** *are characteristic of brainstem lesions*. For example, if cranial nerve function is diminished on the *left* with paralysis and/or sensory loss on the *right side of the body* below the head, this would indicate a brainstem lesion on the left. If cranial nerve function and paralysis and/or sensory loss below the head are on the *same side*, this generally implies a lesion *above* the brainstem (e.g., cerebral cortex, internal capsule, thalamus).[4]

Cranial Nerves

Cranial Nerve I, the *olfactory nerve*, transmits smell information from the nose to the brain. So a lesion of cranial nerve I leads to *anosmia*, loss of smell. If a patient has lost his/her sense of smell, the most common cause is nasal obstruction (e.g., from a cold or sinusitis). Other causes of anosmia include aging, trauma (skull fracture impinging on the olfactory nerve), Kallmann's syndrome (loss of olfactory neurons and GnRH-secreting cells, leading to hypogonadism), or a tumor (e.g., a meningioma) impinging on the olfactory nerve. Do you think a tumor is more likely to cause unilateral or bilateral anosmia? A tumor (e.g., meningioma, frontal lobe mass) would probably lead to unilateral loss of smell as it would generally impinge on CN I on only one side.

*Cranial nerve I is the only cranial nerve that does **not** connect **at all** to the brainstem. CN I projects to the temporal lobe olfactory area.*

Cranial Nerve II, the *optic nerve*, conveys visual information from the eyes to the brain for visual processing (Fig. 7-7). So a lesion of CN II or its pathway leads to a visual defect (i.e., blindness in part or all of the visual field in one or both eyes). CN II is also the afferent (sensory) limb of the pupillary light reflex (Fig. 7-9).[5] The visual pathway (Fig. 7-7) does *not* connect to the brainstem like most other cranial nerve pathways. However, the afferent limb of pupillary light reflex that is carried in CN II travels to the midbrain, fitting

---

[4] In some cases of small midbrain or upper pons lesions, deficits may not be crossed. That is, these lesions can produce patterns similar to cerebral lesions: all signs in the face and body occurring on the *same* side. This is because some of the fibers from the cortex can incur lesions on their way down before arriving at their brainstem nuclei. Thus, although crossed signs can **only** occur with brainstem lesions, crossed signs do *not* occur with *all* brainstem lesions.

[5] Cranial nerve II also sends minor projections to the suprachiasmatic nucleus of the hypothalamus (involved in circadian rhythms) and the superior colliculus (function in humans poorly understood; may be involved in eye-head orienting reflexes).

into the **1-4 (midbrain)**, 5-8 (pons), 9-12 (medulla) schematic.

Fig. 7-7. Visual pathways and lesions. Light hits the retina, which converts the light information into electrical impulses. These electrical impulses travel in the optic nerves, half of whose axons cross at the *optic chiasm*, after which they are known as the *optic tracts*. The optic tracts synapse in the lateral geniculate nuclei (LGN) of the thalamus. From there, there are two projections (on each side), one going superiorly, and one going inferiorly (Meyer's loop). These pathways synapse in the occipital cortex, which is the posterior-most portion of the cerebral cortex. The lesions and associated visual deficits in this figure will be discussed below.

The easiest way to remember where information from the visual fields travels in this system is to start with *how light comes into the eye*. For example, if you look straight ahead and imagine a beam of light coming from the extreme right, that beam will hit the *left* portions of both retinas, whereas a beam of light coming from the extreme left will hit the *right* portions of both retinas. A beam from the top will hit the bottom of the retinas, whereas one from the bottom will hit the top. *This pattern is maintained in the brain:* the left brain contains information about the right visual field and the right brain contains information about the left visual field. Light coming from the left zaps into the right brain, light from the right zaps into the left brain. Similarly, light coming from the top zaps into the bottom of the brain and light coming from the bottom zaps into the top of the brain.

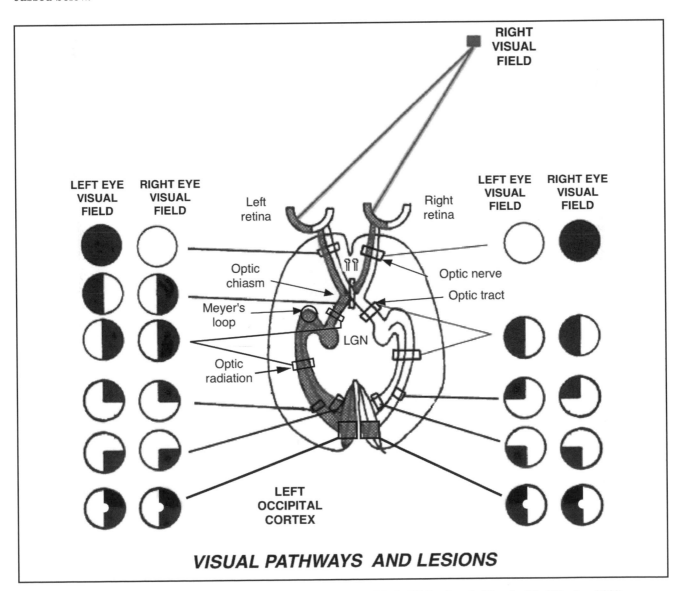

VISUAL PATHWAYS AND LESIONS

Figure 7-7. Modified from Goldberg: *Clinical Neuroanatomy Made Ridiculously Simple*, MedMaster 2005

Fig. 7-8. Schematic of visual pathway. Following the steps below, draw a diagram that will help you remember how this system works.

1. Draw the eyes seen from above.

2. Draw two lines coming straight off the *outer* portions of them.

3. Draw two lines coming off the *inner* portions that cross to join the outer lines.

4. Draw two parallel light beams coming from the right. This is the right visual field, and these beams hit the *left portions* of both retinas.

Note: The information from the right *visual field* is carried in the *outermost* line from the left eye and the *innermost* line from the right eye. Notice that all information from the right visual field ends up *on the left* side of the brain.

Another observation from this diagram is that the *lateral* (also called *temporal*) visual fields end up on the *medial surface* of each retina, and the *medial* (also called *nasal*) visual fields end up on the *lateral surface* of each retina. Information from the medial retinas crosses at the chiasm, while information from lateral retinas stays ipsilateral.

Just as information from the visual fields ends up on the contralateral side of the brain, the upper portion of the visual field ends up in the inferior portion of the brain (temporal lobe and inferior occipital cortex), and the lower visual field ends up in the superior portion of the brain (parietal lobe and superior occipital cortex). If you follow logically how the light hits the retinas, this should make sense.

The following discussion refers to Fig. 7-7.

Lesion of the optic nerve. Since no information is going from this eye to the brain, this eye is blind and the other eye is fine.

Lesion of the optic chiasm at the midline. Information from the *lateral parts* of both retinas still makes it to the brain. What information is this? From the right eye this is the left (nasal) visual field, and from the left eye this is the right (nasal) visual field. What's *lost* is the information that crosses, which comes from the *medial* parts of the retinas: the left (temporal) visual field of the left eye and the right (temporal) visual field of the right eye. So the result is loss of the *lateral (temporal) visual fields on both sides* (because the outer visual fields hit the inner retinas). This is *bitemporal hemianopsia*. What could cause this? Think anatomically. The pituitary lies right beneath the optic chiasm, and

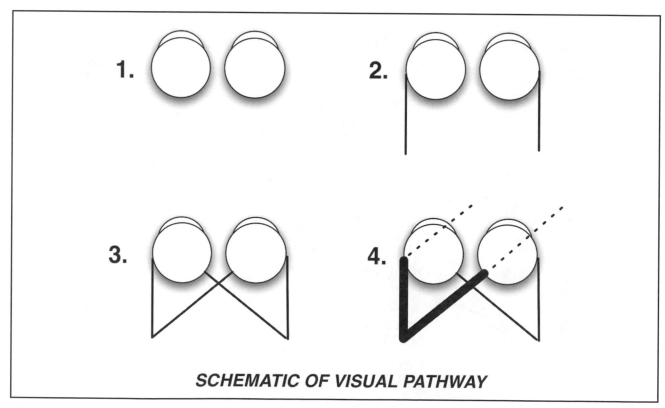

SCHEMATIC OF VISUAL PATHWAY

Figure 7-8

thus a midline pituitary tumor could press on the chiasm at the midline, causing bitemporal hemianopsia. When you test the outer visual fields in a patient, you are assessing the integrity of the fibers that cross in the chiasm. Mnemonic: ***coyote*** = chi—outy. The crossing fibers in the **chi**asm carry the **out**er visual fields, so a chiasmatic lesion causes loss of the outer (temporal) visual fields (bitemporal hemianopsia).

Lesion of the optic tract. The optic tracts carry all of the information from the *contralateral* visual field (the lateral retinal fibers from the ipsilateral eye and the crossed medial retinal fibers from the contralateral eye). A postchiasmatic lesion of one optic tract thus leads to loss of the entire *contralateral* visual field.

Lesion of the visual pathway in the optic radiations (parietal and temporal lobe). Visual information from the lateral geniculate nucleus of the thalamus on each side travels toward the visual cortex in an upper loop in the parietal cortex and a lower loop in the temporal lobe (*Meyer's loop*). Maintaining the "opposites" pattern, lower visual field information travels in the upper loop, and upper visual field information travels in the lower loop. Of course, the left-sided loops carry information about the right visual field, and the right-sided loops carry information about the left visual field. So what kind of visual deficit would a *left Meyer's loop* lesion cause? A loss of the *right upper* visual field, also called a right upper quadrantanopsia, or a "pie in the sky" lesion. An upper loop lesion leads to a contralateral lower quadrantanopsia.

Lesion of the occipital cortex. A lesion of the entire occipital cortex on one side leads to complete loss of the *contralateral* visual field (*homonymous hemianopsia*). A strictly superior lesion leads to contralateral lower quadrant field loss, and a strictly inferior lesion leads to contralateral upper quadrant field loss. Since the center of the visual field (corresponding to the macula or the retina) is arguably the most important, it is extensively represented, and receives dual blood supply from both middle and posterior cerebral arteries. Thus, lesions involving only one of these vascular territories can lead to homonymous hemianopsia with *macular sparing*: loss of the entire (contralateral) visual field with a small half-circle of vision preserved at the center.

Visual loss can also be caused by non-neurological diseases of the eye, including retinal disease, cataract formation, or age-related changes to the eye. How can one distinguish visual loss caused by a visual pathway lesion from visual loss caused by a problem with the eye itself? *Any type of visual **field** deficit (e.g., hemianopsia, quadrantanopsia) indicates a lesion of the visual pathway (i.e., optic nerve, tract, radiations, or occipital cortex).* To assess the eye itself, ophthalmologic examination can be performed to look for retinal disease and cataracts.

Refractive errors such as near-sightedness (*myopia*), far-sightedness (*hyperopia*), age-related accommodation/focusing difficulty (*presbyopia*), will *improve* if the patient reads through a pinhole or with appropriate corrective lenses. Such refractive errors can be corrected with glasses or contact lenses: concave lenses for myopia, convex lenses for hyperopia and presbyopia.

Cranial Nerve III, the *oculomotor nerve*, innervates four extraocular muscles: the inferior oblique and the superior, inferior, and medial rectus muscles. In other words, it innervates all extraocular muscles that are *not* innervated by cranial nerve IV (which innervates superior oblique) and cranial nerve VI (which innervates lateral rectus). Cranial nerve III also innervates the levator palpebrae muscle (which raises the eyelid) and provides *parasympathetic* innervation to the pupil. Do you expect parasympathetic input to constrict or dilate the pupil? Well, when would the pupils dilate? When someone is "wide eyed with fear," wanting to fight or flee...so pupillary dilation is sympathetic and *constriction is parasympathetic*. Parasympathetic constriction is *mediated by fibers traveling in CN III*. So a lesion of III weakens all eye muscles on that side *except* superior oblique (which intorts and depresses the eye, innervated by cranial nerve IV) and lateral rectus (which abducts [laterally moves] the eye, innervated by cranial nerve VI). Since the inferior oblique, superior, inferior, and medial rectus muscles stop working in a complete cranial nerve III lesion, the superior oblique and lateral rectus muscles are unopposed and pull the eye *down and out*. Since the levator palpebrae muscles and pupillary constrictors are also lost, we are left with a dilated pupil and a drooping eyelid (ptosis). So a complete lesion of cranial nerve III causes an ipsilateral eye that is "down and out" with a fixed, dilated ("blown") pupil and drooping eyelid.

Cranial nerve III can be compressed by aneurysm, tumor, infectious or inflammatory processes, or damaged by vascular or inflammatory disease.

Fig. 7-9. Pupillary light reflex. When light shines into the eye, the pupil normally constricts in response. This reflex is accomplished by the optic nerve (afferent) and the oculomotor nerve (efferent).[6] If this pathway is intact bilaterally, shining light into either eye causes constriction of both pupils, because the efferent signal is sent via both oculomotor nerves to both pupils so as to cause a symmetrical pupillary response (7-10A).

---

[6] The CN II projections for the pupillary reflex exit CN II prior to the lateral geniculate nucleus of the thalamus (where visual information is sent) and synapse instead in the pretectal nucleus of the midbrain. This nucleus then sends bilateral projections to the ipsilateral and contralateral nuclei of Edinger-Westphal in the midbrain (EW nuc in Fig. 7-9). The Edinger-Westphal nuclei send parasympathetic fibers via the oculomotor nerve (III) to the ciliary ganglion, which sends fibers to the muscles of pupillary constric-

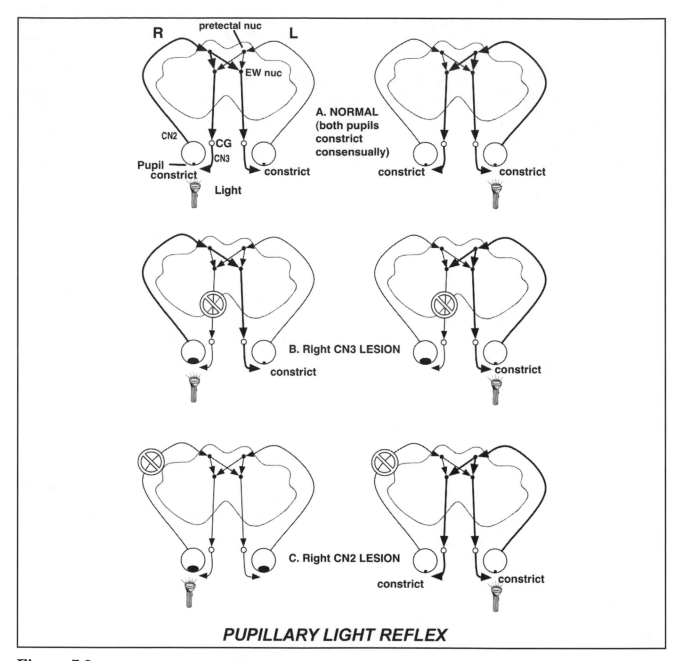

PUPILLARY LIGHT REFLEX

Figure 7-9

Pupillary constriction in response to light in the ipsilateral eye (into which light is shined) is called the *direct response*, and constriction in the contralateral eye is called the *consensual response*. A *right CN **III*** lesion would prevent the right eye from constricting in response to light in either eye; *however*, if CN II is still intact on the right, light shined in the right eye can still be transmitted through this afferent pathway and cause constriction of the left pupil (7-10B). A *right CN **II*** lesion would lead to *no* pupillary constriction of either eye if light is shined in the *right* eye (since the right

CN II does not transmit the afferent information); however, *both* eyes would constrict if light is shined in the *left* eye since the afferent signal arrives in the brainstem and the efferent pathway (both CN IIIs) is intact (7-10C). The situation in 7-10C (CN II lesion) is called a *relative afferent pupillary defect*, and the affected pupil can be called a *Marcus Gunn pupil*. A relative afferent pupillary defect can be demonstrated by the swinging flashlight test. In this test, when one moves a light back and forth between the two eyes, one notes *dilation* of the pupil on the side of the CN II (afferent) defect. This is because that pupil is re-equilibrating after constricting consensually from light shined in the contralateral eye, and it does not respond to light shined directly on it.

The pupils not only constrict in response to light, but also as part of accommodation for focusing on near objects. Although the light and near responses are usually lost together, *Argyll-Robertson pupils*, classically caused by syphilis, constrict in accommodation but do *not* react to light. Mnemonic: An **A**rgyll-**R**obertson pupil **A**ccommodates but does *not* **R**eact. Argyll-Robertson pupils also tend to be small and unequal.

Adie's pupil is a dilated pupil that constricts only very gradually when exposed to light, often responding more normally during accommodation. Mnemonic: **Adi**e = **A di**lated pupil. Adie's pupil can be caused by damage to the ciliary ganglion (which contains the parasympathetic input from CN III that constricts the pupil). Holmes-Adie syndrome is the association of Adie's pupil with absent deep tendon reflexes (usually in the leg and ankle) and orthostatic hypotension (and/or other autonomic dysfunction). The syndrome is most common in younger women (i.e., average onset in 30s).

Horner's syndrome is the triad of *ptosis* (drooping eyelid), *miosis* (constricted pupil) and *anhidrosis* (loss of sweating) due to lesion of the sympathetic pathway somewhere along its path from its origin in the hypothalamus down to the cervical spinal cord to the superior cervical ganglion back up to the face and eyes. Lateral brainstem infarcts, spinal cord lesions, and apical pulmonary tumors can all cause Horner's syndrome. The constricted pupil in Horner's syndrome still responds normally to light and near stimuli (accommodation response) since parasympathetic (i.e., constricting) input is still intact. The ptosis results from loss of sympathetic input to the tarsal muscles, which retract the eyelids.

Many drugs, legal and illegal, can have a variety of effects on the pupils. Most commonly, systemically administered drugs will cause symmetrical effects in both eyes, but administration of a drug into only one eye can cause a unilateral effect. Pupillary asymmetry is referred to as *anisocoria*.

***Cranial Nerve IV**, the *trochlear nerve*, has one job: it innervates the superior oblique muscle. Because of the way this muscle attaches to the eye, the superior oblique *intorts* and depresses the eye.[7] So a lesion of cranial nerve IV would reduce the ability to intort and depress the eye, leading to extortion and weakness of

downward gaze, especially when the eye is adducted (turned medially). This is because the superior oblique's depressor function is strongest when the eye is adducted. Whenever there is a loss of one of these rotatory functions (intortion/extortion), there may be a head tilt to compensate. Cranial nerve IV is the only cranial nerve that projects contralaterally. So deficits are ipsilateral to a peripheral CN IV lesion, but contralateral to a lesion in the brainstem nucleus.

***Cranial Nerve V**, the *trigeminal nerve*, has several functions:

- *Sensory*:
  - *Facial sensation*: including skin, sinuses, tongue (*not* taste, just sensation) and cornea
  - Other sensation: part of the tympanic membrane and part of the meninges
- *Motor*
  - Innervation of the *chewing muscles*
  - Innervation of the *tensor veli palitini* muscle (a muscle of the soft palate)

There are three branches of CN V that bring sensory information to the brain from the face: *ophthalmic, maxillary,* and *mandibular*. Thus, sensory loss localized to only *one* of these facial regions would imply a lesion *between the face and the trigeminal ganglion* from which the branches emerge. Sensory loss on one *entire* side of the face would imply a lesion *between the brain and the trigeminal ganglion*. Remember that part of cranial nerve V follows 1-4= midbrain, **5**-8 = **pons,** 9-12 = medulla, and part does not: Facial light touch, proprioception, and motor (to chewing muscles) are found in the pons, while the spinal nucleus of V spans much of the brainstem and extends into the upper spinal cord (Fig. 7-6).

CN V is the afferent (sensory) limb of the *corneal reflex,* a blink of the eyelid in response to stimulation of the cornea. CN VII (facial nerve) is the efferent (motor) limb. So this blink reflex can be absent in either a CN V or a CN VII lesion.

***Cranial Nerve VI,** the **abducens** nerve,* innervates the lateral rectus, which **abducts** the eye (turns it laterally). *Thus, a lesion of cranial nerve VI leads to ipsilateral inability to abduct the eye.*

Fig. 7-10. Conjugate gaze pathway. When you want to look to the left, both eyes must move left in a synchronized fashion. To accomplish this, your left eye ab**ducts** (turns laterally) and your right eye ad**ducts** (turns medially). What muscles are responsible for these actions, and what nerves innervate these muscles? To look to the left, the left lateral rectus, innervated by the left abducens nerve (VI), abducts the eye (turns it laterally). The right medial rectus, innervated by the right oculomotor nerve (III) ad**ducts** the right eye (turns it

---

[7] Note: *Superior **oblique** depresses* the eye; *superior **rectus** elevates* it. *Inferior **oblique** elevates* the eye; *inferior **rectus** depresses* it. ***Superior** oblique intorts* the eye; ***inferior** oblique extorts* it.

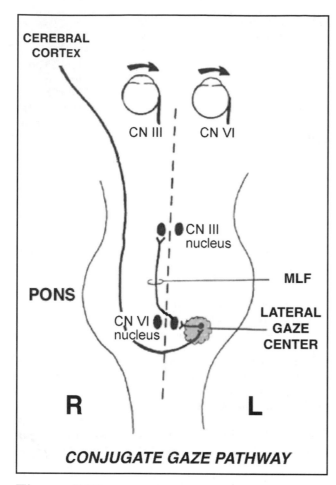

Figure 7-10. Modified from Goldberg: *Clinical Neuroanatomy Made Ridiculously Simple*, MedMaster 2005

medially). To accomplish these conjugate eye movements, the *medial longitudinal fasciculus* (MLF) in the brainstem allows for communication between the nucleus of VI (in the pons) and the *contralateral* nucleus of III (in the midbrain). The communication is *contralateral* because the MLF coordinates abduction in one eye with adduction in the contralateral eye.

A lesion of the MLF results in *internuclear ophthalmoplegia* (INO), in which the eye ipsilateral to the lesion cannot adduct (turn medially) during attempted conjugate gaze. The side of the lesion is named for the side of medial rectus dysfunction, which is the same side as the MLF *after* it has crossed to the side of the affected CN III nucleus. For example, a lesion of the *right* MLF means that the left abducens (VI) nucleus in the pons cannot communicate with the right oculomotor (III) nucleus in the midbrain. So when the patient looks to the left, the left eye abducts (turns left) but the right eye cannot adduct (turn left). How can you prove that this is an INO and not some problem with the right medial rectus or the right cranial nerve

III? Since *convergence* uses a different pathway, the right eye will still adduct on convergence. Adduction on convergence proves that the right medial rectus and right CN III are intact and that the lesion must thus be in the right MLF. The most common causes of INO are brainstem strokes and multiple sclerosis. It is possible to have bilateral INOs (from bilateral MLF lesions): on leftward gaze the right eye does not adduct (turn left) and on rightward gaze the left eye does not adduct (turn right).

Cranial Nerve VII is the *facial* nerve, whose functions include:

- Innervation of the *facial musculature* and the *stapedius* muscle of the inner ear

- *Taste* sensation from the anterior 2/3 of the tongue (CN IX does the rest of the tongue)

- *Salivary gland* stimulation (submaxillary and submandibular; CN IX does the parotid)

- *Lacrimal gland* stimulation

- *Sensation* from *parts of the inner and exterior ear*

Fig. 7-11. Upper and lower motor neurons of CN VII. Each motor cortex *forehead* area projects to *both* the contralateral VII nucleus *and* the ipsilateral one. The motor cortex *lower face* area projects *only* to the *contralateral* VII nuclei. The facial nerve (CN VII) carries *all* of this information from *both* sides of the cortex. Thus, the facial nerve on each side receives contralateral cortical input for the forehead *and* lower face in addition to ipsilateral cortical input for the forehead. Since innervation to the forehead comes to the facial nerve from both sides of the brain, unilateral *cortical* lesions can affect the muscles of the lower face, while sparing the forehead.

A lesion of the *facial nerve* (CN VII) will cause weakness of the muscles of the *whole* face, *forehead included*, on that same side (middle panel of Fig. 7-11). Causes of facial nerve palsy include infectious diseases (e.g., Lyme Disease, Herpes-Zoster, HIV), trauma, multiple sclerosis, sarcoidosis, and tumor impinging on the seventh nerve (e.g., acoustic neuroma). Bell's palsy is an idiopathic palsy of CN VII.

A patient with an *upper motor neuron lesion* (e.g., a cortical stroke) will have *loss of contralateral **lower face*** movements, *but* normal forehead movements, since the facial nerve is still carrying input to the forehead from ipsilateral cortex (right-most panel of Fig. 7-11).

Note: For simplicity, the figure shows the input to the *left* CN VII. Though the left motor cortex says "to forehead," it of course also projects to both right forehead and lower face. Similarly, in addition to the contralat-

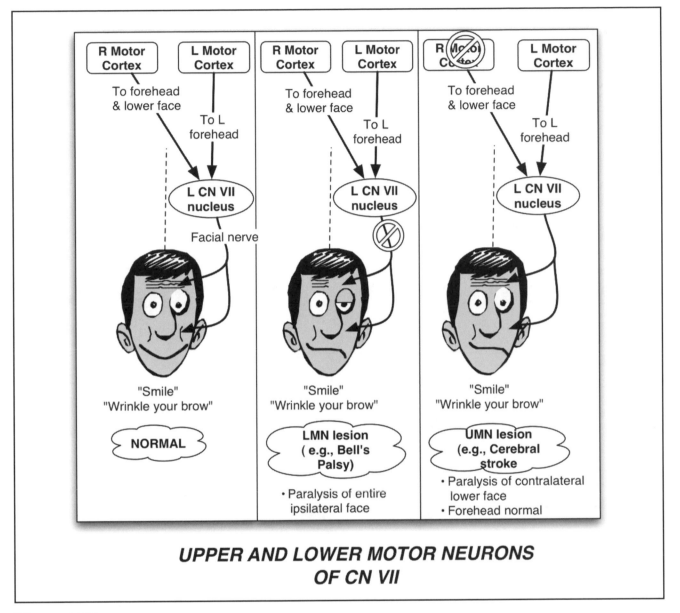

Figure 7-11

eral projections of the right motor cortex, it projects to the ipsilateral forehead via the right facial nerve.

Cranial Nerve VIII, the *vestibulocochlear nerve,* conveys sound and head movement/position information to the brainstem from the cochlea and semicircular canals. Auditory information arrives in the brainstem in the pons as expected (given "5-8 = pons"), but most vestibular information arrives lower, straddling the pons and medulla. An example of a lesion that affects the eighth nerve is an *acoustic neuroma,* also called *vestibular schwannoma.* These slow-growing tumors of CN VIII can lead to unilateral hearing and/or vestibular deficits. *Non*-neurological causes of hearing loss in-

clude middle ear infection/congestion and damage to the tympanic membrane, ossicles, or cochlea. *Non*-neurological causes of dizziness and balance problems include various systemic diseases (e.g., cardiovascular disease, anemia), and inner ear diseases (e.g., benign paroxysmal positional vertigo, Meniere's disease).

The *vestibulo-ocular reflex* keeps vision steady while the head moves by causing the eyes to move in the opposite direction from the head as the head turns (assuming the eyes are not trying to follow a moving object). Try it. Turn your head back and forth as if saying "no" while continuing to read, and you will notice that your eyes try to maintain straight-ahead position by turning in the *opposite* direction from that of your head. This is a complex reflex; the brainstem gets information from CN VIII and transmits it to the relevant eye movement nuclei (CN III, CN IV, and/or CN VI), generating the appropriate eye movements. When you do a "doll's eye" test in a comatose patient, you test the integrity of this system. If when the head is turned in one direction, the eyes move in the opposite direction, the brainstem is intact. If the eyes move in the same direction as the head, this implies that the vestibulo-ocular reflex is not working, and thus a brainstem lesion may be the cause of the coma. A doll's eye maneuver should not be performed if cervical spine injury is suspected.

Nystagmus is oscillation of the eyes, e.g., what the eyes do when observing passing telephone poles out the window of a moving train - repetitively moving slowly to one side and then flicking back rapidly. The direction of nystagmus is named for the *fast phase* (i.e., the direction of the flicking back). Nystagmus can occur normally at the extremes of gaze, but can also

occur pathologically. Pathological causes include lesions of the peripheral vestibular system, brainstem, or cerebellum, or certain drugs.

Fig. 7-12. Cold calorics. Putting cold water into one ear (*cold caloric testing*) mimics a temporary lesion of the vestibular system on that side. In normal, conscious patients, this causes the eyes to move slowly *toward* the cold side, followed by a quick return in the *opposite* direction (i.e., toward the side *without* cold water). Cold calorics assess the integrity of the vestibular/VIII/VI/ MLF/III system. If the eyes do not deviate in response to the cold water, there may be a lesion anywhere along this pathway (or there may be too much wax in the ear to perform the test adequately). Lack of response to cold calorics can also occur secondary to some types of drug intoxication. In comatose or unconscious patients with an *intact* brainstem, slow deviation toward the cold water side will occur *without* the subsequent quick return. Before performing cold calorics, the tympanic membrane should be examined to assure that it is intact.

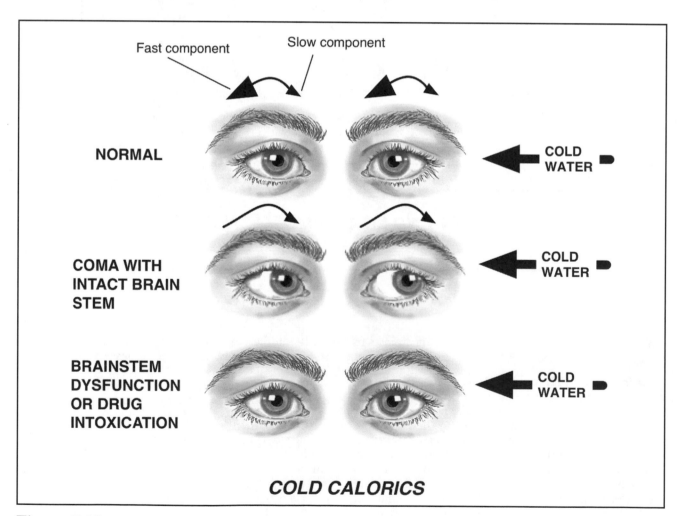

Figure 7-12

Cranial Nerve IX, the *glossopharyngeal nerve*, has several functions:

• *Sensation and taste from the posterior third of the tongue* and *sensory input from the palate*

• *Motor input to the stylopharyngeus muscle of the pharynx*

• Stimulation of the *parotid gland*

• Transmitting *visceral sensory information* from the *carotid body* (oxygen tension) and *carotid sinus* (volume) receptors to the nucleus solitarius of the medulla

• *Sensation* from *part of the external ear* and *tympanic membrane*

Note the complementary relationship between CN VII and CN IX with regard to taste (anterior 2/3 of tongue = CN VII; posterior 1/3 = CN IX) and salivation (submandibular and submaxillary glands= CN VII; parotid gland = CN IX).

CN IX is the afferent component of the gag reflex (CN X is the efferent component), so CN IX lesion can lead to absent gag reflex.

Cranial Nerve X is the *vagus nerve*.   When you think vagus, think *parasympathetic*. The vagus supplies the parasympathetic input to the heart, lungs, and most of the GI system. (The bladder, descending colon, rectum, and genitals receive their parasympathetic input from sacral spinal cord.) The vagus nerve has a variety of other functions as well:

• Carries *sensory* information to the brainstem from the *viscera* and the *aortic arch* (oxygen tension and blood volume information)

• Provides *motor* input to one muscle of the tongue (*palatoglossus*) and all muscles of the *larynx* and *pharynx except* the stylopharyngeus muscle (CN IX) and tensor veli palatini muscle (CN V)

• *Sensation* from the *pharynx, ear,* and *tympanic membrane* (note sharing of function in these regions by CNs V, VII, IX, and X)

Fig. 7-13. Palate deviation. When you ask a patient to "Open wide and say 'Ahhh,'" you are assessing the vagus nerve. If the uvula elevates symmetrically in the midline, both sides of the pharynx are tugging symmetrically. If the uvula deviates to the *left*, where is

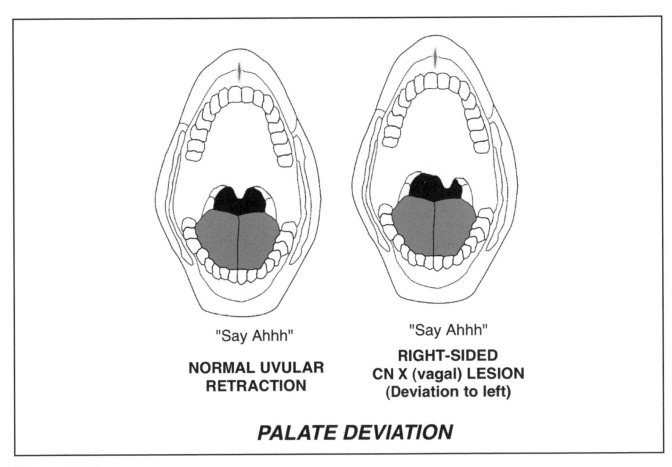

"Say Ahhh"

NORMAL UVULAR RETRACTION

"Say Ahhh"

RIGHT-SIDED CN X (vagal) LESION (Deviation to left)

PALATE DEVIATION

Figure 7-13

the lesion? If the uvula is pulled more to the left, this must mean that the *right* is weak. Thus, a lesion of the right vagus nerve allows the left side to win the tug-of-war, and the uvula deviates to the *normal* side.

Symptoms of vagus nerve damage include hoarseness (from the loss of laryngeal muscle innervation), trouble swallowing, and absent gag reflex. The recurrent laryngeal nerve, a branch of the vagus, can be compressed by tumor or damaged in neck surgery (e.g., thyroid surgery). Recurrent laryngeal nerve lesions result in hoarseness.

Cranial Nerve XI, the *spinal accessory* nerve, innervates the sternocleidomastoid and the trapezius muscles. When you ask a patient to shrug against resistance and to turn his/her head against your hand, testing strength and symmetry, you are assessing CN XI. A lower motor neuron lesion on one side would lead to ipsilateral shoulder drop and weakened shrugging, as well as weakness turning the head against resistance toward the *opposite* side (because the sternocleidomastoid muscle normally rotates the head to the contralateral side).

CN XII, the *hypoglossal* nerve, innervates the musculature of the tongue (except palatoglossus, which is innervated by CN X).

Fig. 7-14. Tongue protrusion. The tongue muscles on each side push the tongue to the opposite side. If they both work perfectly together, the tongue will go straight out. If one side is lesioned, the other side will push the tongue *toward the weak side*. If the lesion affects the lower motor neurons, the weak side is ipsilateral to the lesion. If the lesion affects the upper motor

neurons (i.e., from cortex down to but not including the nucleus in the medulla), the weak side is contralateral to the lesion.

Fig. 7-15. Summary of cranial nerve functions.

Cerebellum and Basal Ganglia

The cerebellum and basal ganglia are both involved in coordinating movements.

Cerebellum

The cerebellum uses feedback from the spinocerebellar tracts (which travel uncrossed from the spinal cord) to monitor movements while they are taking place, and sends output to the cerebral cortex (by way of the thalamus) to adjust these movements. The cerebellum is also involved in balance and posture. Thus, cerebellar lesions can result in *ataxia* (uncoordinated movement, as demonstrated in finger-to-nose and heel-to-shin tasks), *dysdiadochokinesia* (inability to perform rapid alternating movements), *intention tremor* (normal at rest, tremor when intending to move, e.g., to touch a target or to pick up a glass), *imbalance*, *nystagmus*, and/or *vertigo*. Cerebellar deficits occur *ipsilateral* to the side in which the lesion occurs. Cerebellar dysfunction can be caused by toxins (e.g., alcohol), stroke, multiple sclerosis, tumor, and/or paraneoplastic syndromes.

Basal Ganglia

The basal ganglia (caudate, putamen, subthalamic nucleus, nucleus accumbens, globus pallidus, and substantia nigra) are part of a loop circuit that begins and ends in the cortex. In contrast to cerebellar lesions,

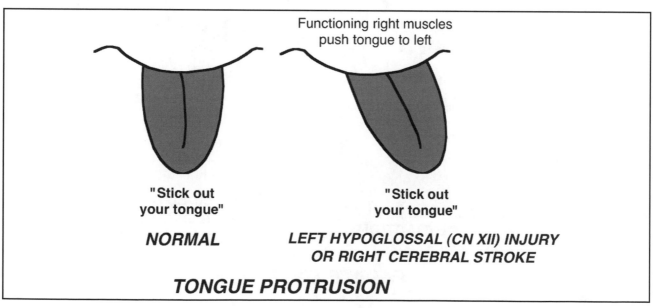

Figure 7-14

Figure 7-15 Summary of cranial nerve functions

Nerve	Name	Function	Projects to/from:	Lesion can lead to:
CN I	Olfactory	Smells	Olfactory cortex in temporal lobe	• Anosmia (loss of smell)
CNII	Optic	Sees	• Lateral geniculate nucleus of thalamus (vision) • Pre-tectal nucleus of midbrain (pupillary light reflex) • Hypothalamus (circadian reflexes) • Superior colliculus (eye-head reflexes)	• Visual defect • Impaired pupillary response to light
CN III	Oculomotor	• Moves eyes : all muscles except lateral rectus (done by VI) and superior oblique (done by IV) • Constricts pupils • Accommodates lens • Elevates upper eyelids	Midbrain	• Eye down and out • Pupil dilated
CN IV	Trochlear	Superior oblique (depresses and intorts eye)	Midbrain	Weakness of downward gaze, Extortion (can cause head tilt)
CN V	Trigeminal	• Facial sensation (including face itself, tongue, meninges, cornea, and part of tympanic membrane) • Chewing muscles • Tensor veli palitini muscle	Pons (except spinal nucleus, which spans brain stem and extends into upper spinal cord)	• Decreased facial sensation • Absent corneal reflex • Weakness of chewing
CN VI	Abducens	Lateral rectus (Abducts eye)	Pons	Inability to abduct eye
CN VII	Facial	• Innervates facial musculature • Taste (anterior 2/3 of tongue) • Submandibular and submaxillary glands • Lacrimal glands • Sensory from parts of inner ear	Pons	• Facial weakness • Decreased taste • Dry eye
CN VIII	Vestibulocochlear	• Hearing • Balance	Pons (some vestibular nuclei extend into the medulla)	• Hearing loss • Tinnitus • Balance difficulties • Vertigo • Nystagmus
CN IX	Glossopharyngeal	• Sensory to palate • Swallowing • Taste (posterior third of tongue) • Parotid gland • Carotid body and carotid sinus	Medulla	Impaired gag reflex
CN X	Vagus	• Parasympathetic input to and sensory from viscera • Larynx • Swallowing/Palatal elevation	Medulla	• Hoarseness (recurrent laryngeal nerve) • Difficulty swallowing • Impaired palatal elevation
CN XI	Spinal accessory	• Sternocleidomastoid (turns head to opposite side • Trapezius (elevates shoulders)	Medulla	• Weakness turning head to opposite side • Shoulder drop/weakness
CN XII	Hypoglossal	Innervates tongue musculature for tongue protrusion (to opposite side)	Medulla	• Tongue deviation to weak (affected) side

which tend to cause problems during *intended movement*, lesions of the basal ganglia tend to cause unwanted movements *at rest*. Examples include the *resting tremor* of Parkinson's (see below), *dystonia* (painful muscular contraction leading to undesired and often unusual postures), *hemiballismus* (violent, unilateral, involuntary movements resulting from contralateral lesion of the subthalamic nucleus), and *chorea* (involuntary choreiform (dance-like) movements). Chorea can also occur secondary to Wilson's disease (see Chapter 5), drugs, Huntington's disease (autosomal dominant-inherited degeneration of the caudate/putamen), and Sydenham's chorea (chorea in rheumatic fever).

Parkinson's Disease

Parkinson's disease is a degeneration of the substantia nigra, an area of the midbrain that sends dopaminergic projections to the striatum (caudate and putamen). The loss of dopamine input to the striatum commonly results in the symptomatic triad of *bradykinesia* (slow movement), *resting tremor,* and *cogwheel rigidity*. Additionally, patients may have a shuffling, hunched-over gait, and have difficulty starting, stopping, and making turns when walking.

Fig. 7-16. Parkinson's disease. The substantia nigra projects to the striatum (caudate and putamen), which sends projections to the cerebral cortex via a few intermediate structures. Dopaminergic projections to the striatum synapse on two pathways, a *direct pathway* (internal segment of the globus pallidus (GPi) → ventrolateral nucleus of the thalamus (VL) → motor areas of the cerebral cortex) and an *indirect pathway* (external segment of the globus pallidus (GPe) à subthalamic nucleus (STN) → GPi → VL → motor areas of the cerebral cortex). The direct pathway excites the cortex and the **in**direct pathway **in**hibits it (7-16A). Dopamine input from the substantia nigra to the striatum excites the direct pathway and **in**hibits the **in**direct pathway. *Thus, the overall result of normal dopaminergic input to the striatum is increased cortical excitation.* This is because the direct pathway is stimulated to excite cortex, while the indirect pathway, which normally inhibits the cortex, has been inhibited (i.e., prevented from inhibiting) (7-16B). Loss of dopamine from substantia nigra degeneration in Parkinson's leads to decreased activity of the direct pathway and **in**creased activity of the **in**direct pathway. Thus, in Parkinson's disease there is *decreased excitation* of the cortex and *increased inhibition* of the cortex (7-16C). This causes an *overall decrease* in motor cortical activity, resulting in bradykinesia and rigidity. Notice that the indirect pathway is *always* associated with inhibition: It inhibits the cortex, and the substantia nigra normally inhibits it. Parkinson's disease disinhibits the indirect pathway, allowing it to inhibit the cortex.

Since Parkinson's disease involves a shortage of dopamine, treatment attempts to restore dopamine, either directly (L-dopa) or indirectly. Indirect strategies include agonists of the dopamine receptors (*bromocriptine, ropinirole, pergolide, pramipexole*) and drugs that decrease dopamine breakdown (e.g., monoamine oxidase inhibitors such as *selegiline*). Refractory cases can sometimes benefit from surgical lesion of the GpI (part of the over-active inhibitory indirect pathway) or deep brain stimulation of the subthalamic nucleus.

What would you expect side effects of dopamine agonists to be? Well, what disease is caused by *too much dopamine*? Schizophrenia. So dopamine therapy can lead to hallucinations. The corollary is that dopamine *ant*agonists used to treat schizophrenia can lead to *dyskinesias* (abnormal movements). Finally, remember that dopamine *inhibits* prolactin, so some of these very same dopamine agonists used in the treatment of Parkinson's disease can also be used to shrink prolactinomas (see Chapter 5).

DISEASES OF THE BRAIN

As with any organ, the brain can be affected by *infection* (viral encephalitis, abscess, meningitis[7]), *tumors* (primary or metastatic), *metabolic disorders, endocrine diseases, inflammatory diseases, drugs, congenital diseases, trauma, vascular disease* (e.g., stroke, hemorrhage), etc. Any of these can result in *headache, mental status changes, seizures, coma, focal neurological deficits, and/or elevated intracranial pressure.*

Mental Status Changes: Dementia and Delirium

Dementia is a *progressive* change in cognitive function. Cognitive decline can include changes in memory, personality, and speech as well as delusions and disinhibition. Before considering a diagnosis of a dementia syndrome such as Alzheimer's disease, frontotemporal dementia, or Lewy body disease, *it is important to rule out other causes of cognitive decline, some of which are treatable*. Such causes include infections (e.g., HIV, Lyme disease), cerebrovascular disease (e.g., multi-infarct dementia), hypothyroidism, medications, hydrocephalus, and depression.

Dementia differs from *delirium* in its time course. *Delirium* is an *acute* change in mental status. Otherwise, like dementia, delirium can be caused by infections, vascular disease, endocrine disease, drugs, or psychological disorders.

---

[7] Meningitis is actually an infection of the meninges, not the brain.

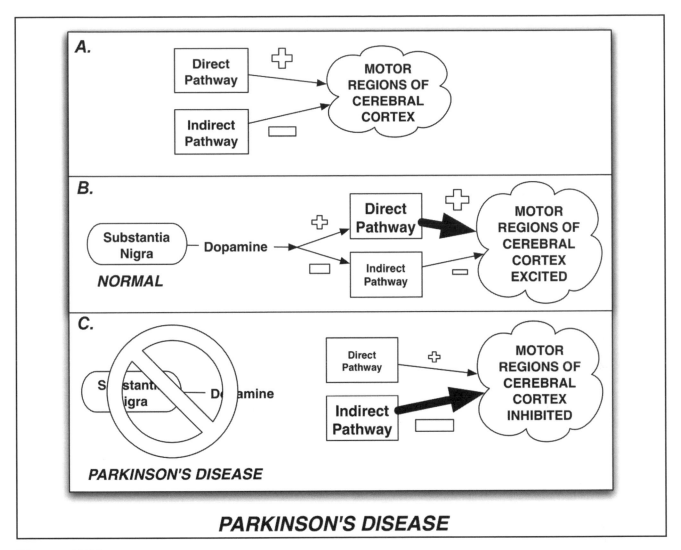

Figure 7-16

Seizures

Isolated seizures arise from abnormal electrical activity in the brain and can be caused by electrolyte or glucose abnormalities, medications, drug withdrawal, head trauma, infections, fever, stroke, and structural abnormalities of the brain (e.g., tumor), to name a few of countless causes. Additionally, disorders of decreased inhibition/increased excitation in the brain can cause *epilepsy*, or recurrent seizures. Some of these disorders may be caused by ion channel malfunction (*channelopathy*). In children, seizure disorders can also be due to congenital structural abnormalities of the brain. In adults, a first seizure warrants a search for some structural lesion (e.g., tumor, vascular malformation, stroke).

It is important to distinguish a seizure from *syncope* (fainting). The presence of an aura (visual, olfactory, or auditory), tongue biting, loss of bowel/bladder control, and/or repetitive stereotyped motions can all be characteristic of seizure, though aura can also occur in migraine, and some people convulse a bit after syncope. When in doubt, an EEG (electroencephalogram) can pick up abnormal firing patterns in the brain that could indicate underlying seizure foci.

Single isolated seizures usually do not require antiepileptic treatment, though they do require a search for an underlying cause. Recurrent seizures (e.g., in epilepsy, post-surgery) require ongoing treatment with antiepileptics.

Antiepileptics

Antiepileptics either ***inhibit*** *excitation* of neurons or ***increase*** *inhibition* of them. Glutamate is the main excitatory neurotransmitter in the brain, while GABA is the main inhibitory one. So antiepileptic drugs either *inhibit* glutamate activity or *increase* GABA activity.

Glutamate can be inhibited by decreasing its release from the presynaptic neuron or preventing the postsynaptic neuron from responding. As for inhibiting release of glutamate, one could inhibit calcium channels of the presynaptic neuron that allow the calcium influx that leads to synaptic vesicle fusion/release of neurotransmitter (e.g., *ethosuximide*). Or, one could inhibit sodium channels that stimulate the action potential in the presynaptic neuron (e.g., *phenytoin, carbamezapine, valproic acid*) and/or postsynaptic neurons (e.g., *topiramate*, which blocks the AMPA glutamate receptor).

To increase GABA or its effectiveness, one can decrease synaptic degradation of GABA (*vigabatrin*) or block GABA reuptake in the presynaptic neuron (*tiagabine*). Note that both of these drugs have "gab" in their names for GABA. Benzodiazepines and barbiturates act at the post-synaptic chloride channel where GABA acts; they enhance chloride influx, thus increasing inhibition (hence decreasing firing) of these neurons.

Elevated Intracranial Pressure

The intracranial space is limited, so tumors, edema (from infection, post-stroke, inflammatory disease, etc.), and bleeding can elevate intracranial pressure. Symptoms of increased intracranial pressure (ICP) include nausea, headache, visual changes, seizures, behavioral changes, and neurological deficits. One sign of increased ICP is *papilledema* (swelling of the optic nerve as seen on retinoscopy). Extreme ICP elevation can cause *herniation* of the brain through the foramen magnum, which can result in the rapid onset of neurological symptoms and signs (e.g., fixed, dilated pupil, hemiparesis) and/or coma or death. IV mannitol can be administered to decrease ICP: mannitol increases the osmolarity of the blood so as to draw water *from* the edema *into* the blood. If a patient has elevated ICP, a lumbar puncture can be dangerous since it can create a negative pressure in the spinal canal that can precipitate herniation. This is why many patients receive a CT scan before undergoing lumbar puncture: to look for signs of intracranial pressure (e.g., ventricular dilatation) or any pathology that could raise intracranial pressure.

Hydrocephalus

Cerebrospinal fluid (CSF), produced by the choroid plexus, circulates through the ventricles and bathes the brain. Its production is in equilibrium with its reabsorption back into the venous system via the arachnoid granulations. A disturbance in this equilibrium causes hydrocephalus and elevates ICP. Hydrocephalus can be caused by *increased CSF production* (e.g., choroid plexus tumor), *decreased CSF*

reabsorption (from blockage of arachnoid villi, e.g., in subarachnoid hemorrhage, infection), or *ventricular obstruction* (e.g., by tumor or congenital malformation, e.g., Arnold-Chiari, Dandy-Walker). Nonobstructive causes are examples of *communicating* hydrocephalus, since there is no obstruction to prevent CSF from communicating within the ventricular system or between the ventricles and the subarachnoid space. Obstructive causes of hydrocephalus are also referred to as non-communicating hydrocephalus, since ventricular obstruction prevents communication within the ventricular system or between the ventricles and the subarachnoid space.

Symptoms and signs of hydrocephalus include visual disturbances, papilledema, headache, urinary incontinence, unsteady gait, mental status changes, hypertension, bradycardia, and/or irregular respiratory patterns. The last three (hypertension, bradycardia, and irregular respirations) are known as *Cushing's triad* or *Cushing's response*. The increased CSF causes the ventricles to enlarge, which can be seen on MRI or CT. Treatment includes removing CSF via lumbar puncture (in communicating hydrocephalus) or placing a shunt from the ventricular system that drains either into the abdomen or the atrium of the heart (in obstructive hydrocephalus).

Pseudotumor Cerebri

In *pseudotumor cerebri* (also known as *idiopathic/benign intracranial hypertension*), symptoms and signs of elevated ICP are present, but the brain appears *normal* when scanned (i.e., there is *no* ventricular enlargement as in hydrocephalus). Pseudotumor cerebri is most common in women, particularly obese women. Although it can be seen as a reaction to medication, during pregnancy, and during systemic illness, it can also occur idiopathically. Symptoms/signs include headache, visual changes (e.g., blurred vision, blackouts, double vision), nausea, vomiting, papilledema, and elevated ICP on lumbar puncture. Acetazolamide, a carbonic anyhdrase inhibitor, is often used for treatment. This is thought to decrease CSF production, leading to a decrease in ICP.

Intracranial Infection and Bleeding

Fig. 7-17. Sites of intracranial bleeding and infection. The dura mater adheres tightly to the inner surface of the skull, but there is some space between it and the posterior aspect of the vertebrae in the spine. The *subdural* space lies between the dura mater and the arachnoid. The *subarachnoid* space is the space between the arachnoid and the pia mater, which directly adheres to the brain. The subarachnoid space contains the CSF. Infection or bleeding can occur in any of these places or in the brain itself.

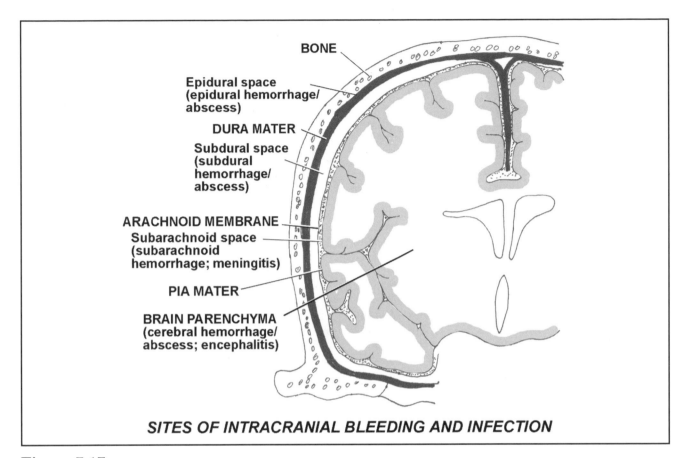

BONE

Epidural space
(epidural hemorrhage/
abscess)

DURA MATER

Subdural space
(subdural
hemorrhage/
abscess)

ARACHNOID MEMBRANE

Subarachnoid space
(subarachnoid
hemorrhage; meningitis)

PIA MATER

BRAIN PARENCHYMA
(cerebral hemorrhage/
abscess; encephalitis)

SITES OF INTRACRANIAL BLEEDING AND INFECTION

Figure 7-17

Infectious agents can arrive at the brain or meninges via hematogenous spread from other sites (endocarditis, pneumonia), spread from nearby infections (sinusitis, orbital cellulitis, or otitis in the case of intracranial infection; osteomyelitis, paraspinous abscess, or psoas abscess in the case of spinal infections), or from infection during trauma or neurosurgery.

Any bleeding or infection in or around the brain can cause headache, nausea/vomiting, seizure, mental status changes, elevated ICP (and its associated signs/symptoms), and/or papilledema. Fever is often present in infection. Subarachnoid hemorrhage and meningitis irritate the meninges, resulting in *meningeal signs*.

Meningeal Signs

Irritation of the meninges (e.g., in subarachnoid hemorrhage or meningitis) can lead to pain during any maneuver that puts traction on them. This is why meningeal irritation causes a *stiff neck*: to avoid such traction, the neck stiffens (like guarding in peritonitis). On physical exam, if one attempts to flex the patient's neck, this will cause involuntary flexing of the

hip and knees (*Brudzinski's sign*). If one flexes the thigh at the hip, and attempts to straighten the patient's leg at the knee, this will be met with resistance (*Kernig's sign*).

Epidural Bleeding and Infection

Epidural Hematomas are caused by trauma to the skull that ruptures the middle meningeal artery, leading to bleeding between the dura mater and the skull. Symptoms and signs include headache, nausea and vomiting, seizure, and symptoms/signs of elevated ICP. Sometimes patients with epidural hematoma maintain (or regain) consciousness for a period after the trauma, called a *lucid interval*. Blood is drained surgically by drilling burr holes in the skull.

Epidural Abscesses can be caused by hematogenous spread of infectious agents or spread from nearby infection. Such infections include osteomyelitis, paraspinous abscess, or psoas abscess in the spine; sinusitis, orbital cellulitis, or otitis in the skull; or infection during a neurosurgical procedure. In the skull, epidural abscess can cause the symptoms of elevated ICP (headache, nausea/vomiting), focal neurological signs, and/or seizures. In the spinal cord, epidural abscess can cause back pain, radicular pain (pain radiating along a dermatomal distribution), and/or bowel/bladder incontinence. Spinal epidural abscesses are more likely to occur than intracranial ones because there is more space between the dura mater and overlying bone in the spine than in the cranium (where the dura is tightly adherent to the skull). *Staph. aureus* and *Streptococcus* are common pathogens. Treatment involves antibiotics and surgical drainage.

Subdural Bleeding and Infection

Subdural Hematomas are caused by head trauma that tears bridging veins between the brain and the dura. Clotting disorders, thrombocytopenia, and alcoholism (because of both head trauma and thrombocytopenia from liver dysfunction) can increase the risk of subdural hematoma. Symptoms are those of increased intracranial pressure and/or focal neurological deficits. These symptoms can arise acutely following trauma or more insidiously over weeks/months (*chronic subdural hematoma*). Chronic subdural hematoma in the elderly can be caused by brain atrophy, which stretches the bridging veins, predisposing them to spontaneous rupture with even minor trauma (e.g., a fall). If extensive, blood from subdural hematoma must be drained surgically.

Subdural Abscesses (empyema) can arise via spread of infectious material from intracerebral abscess, meningitis, sinusitis, trauma/surgery, intracerebral infections, otitis, or hematogenous spread from a distant site. Symptoms and signs are those of increased ICP. *Staph. aureus, Streptococcus*, and gram negative bacteria are the most common pathogens. Abscesses are treated by antibiotics and surgical drainage.

Subarachnoid Bleeding and Infection

Subarachnoid Hemorrhage is most commonly secondary to rupture of an aneurysm or less commonly to rupture of an arteriovenous malformation (AVM). The sudden-onset headache of subarachnoid hemorrhage is classically described by the patient as the "worst headache of my life." Meningeal signs and signs of elevated ICP may also be present. Diagnosis is made by seeing blood in the CSF on lumbar puncture and evidence of bleeding on CT or MRI. Patients should be stabilized and prepared for surgical clipping of the aneurysm or intravascular coiling, an interventional radiologic procedure that blocks off the aneurysm with micro-coils.

Meningitis is infection of the meninges and CSF from hematogenous spread (e.g., *Strep. pneumoniae* from pneumonia), entry via the upper respiratory tract (*N. meningitidis*) or ear infection (*Hemophilus influenza*), or post-surgery or trauma (*Staph.*, gram negatives). Fever, headache, meningeal signs, stiff neck, photophobia (increased sensitivity to seeing light), seizures, and/or mental status changes may occur.

The most common offending organisms are:

- In neonates: group B *Streptococcus*

- In children: *H. influenza, Strep. pneumoniae, N. meningitidis*

- In adults: *Strep. pneumoniae* and *N. meningitidis*.

- Tuberculosis and *Listeria monocytogenes* can also cause meningitis.

Viral meningitis (enterovirus, varicella zoster virus, herpes simplex virus, HIV) and fungal meningitis (e.g., cryptococcus, candida, histoplasmosis—more common in immunocompromised patients) can cause similar symptoms, but usually have a more subacute presentation than bacterial meningitis.

Diagnosis is made by CSF examination (see below). Treatment involves antibiotics targeted to the infectious organism.

Bleeding and Infection in the Brain

Intraparenchymal Hemorrhage can be caused by hypertension, trauma, aneurysm/arteriovenous malformation (AVM) rupture, intracranial tumor bleeding, and post-stroke hemorrhage. Symptoms/signs can include headache, seizure, focal neurological deficits, or mental status changes. Meningeal signs can also occur if the bleeding extends into the subarachnoid space. Surgical treatment is often necessary unless the amount of hemorrhage is small, in which case the patient can be stabilized and observed.

Brain Abscess. A cerebral abscess can arise when infection spreads to the brain from nearby infections (meningitis, sinusitis, otitis), distant infections (via hematogenous spread), or during surgery. Symptoms/signs may include fever, headache, nausea/vomiting, seizure, focal neurological deficits, and mental status changes. *Staph. aureus, Streptococcus*, anaerobes, *H. influenza*, tuberculosis, fungi, and protozoans can all cause cerebral abscesses. Treatment involves appropriate antibiotic therapy and surgical drainage.

Encephalitis is usually viral (e.g., herpes simplex virus, enterovirus, mumps, rabies, mosquito borne viruses such as West Nile Virus and St. Louis Encephalitis), but it can also be caused by parasites (e.g., toxoplasmosis) or some atypical bacteria (e.g., *Listeria, Bartonella, Rickettsia, Mycoplasma*). Fever, headache, nausea/vomiting, seizures, focal neurologic deficits, and/or altered mental status may be present. Diagnosis is made by identifying evidence of the infectious agent in the CSF, or in some cases by brain biopsy. Treatment is directed against the offending organism (e.g., acyclovir for herpes simplex virus) if available. When treatment does not exist for a particular organism, patients' systemic manifestations are treated as necessary for stabilization.

Cerebrospinal Fluid (CSF) Examination

Examining the CSF by lumbar puncture (spinal tap) is key in the diagnosis of suspected meningitis/encephalitis. In any infection, WBC count and protein will be elevated. In bacterial meningitis, there will be a predominance of polymorphonuclear cells (PMNs), while mononuclear cells typically predominate in fungal and viral meningitis and encephalitis. Gram stain can be used to identify bacterial pathogens and PCR can be used to identify viral ones. Tuberculosis and bacteria also cause a decrease in CSF glucose to less than 2/3 the amount of serum glucose.

Blood in the CSF can indicate intracranial bleeding (e.g., subarachnoid hemorrhage). How can this be distinguished from blood simply from the trauma of the tap? In a lumbar puncture, multiple tubes of CSF are taken. If the tap is traumatic, the amount of blood in the CSF samples will decrease with each successive tube. If there is intracranial bleeding, the amount of blood in each tube will be relatively constant. Additionally, blood that has been in the CSF for more time (6-12 hours) will be broken down, giving the CSF a yellowish color (*xanthochromia*). Blood arising from the trauma of the tap will not have time to break down, and thus will not produce xanthochromia.

Central Nervous System Tumors

Tumors of the brain or meninges can cause headache, seizure, nausea/vomiting, focal neurological deficits, mental status changes, and/or elevated ICP (and its associated symptoms/signs). Spinal cord tumors can cause symptoms of nerve compression, Brown-Séquard syndrome (Fig. 7-4), or syrinx (discussed below in the Spinal Cord section). Primary tumors or metastases from other sites can cause any of these signs/symptoms.

Meningiomas are typically benign tumors that can occur on any portion of the meninges, thus causing practically any neurological symptom or sign depending on the brain region(s) or cranial nerve(s) that are impinged upon by the tumor. Surgical removal is standard treatment, though radiation is used if the tumor is inoperable.

Acoustic neuroma/vestibular schwannoma is a benign tumor of cranial nerve VIII (vestibulocochlear) that can cause unilateral hearing loss, vertigo, and/or other cranial nerve deficits if the tumor impinges on the brainstem.

Gliomas include astrocytoma (including glioblastoma multiforme), oligodendroglioma, and ependymoma. *Ependymomas* arise from cells of ventricular lining and can thus lead to obstruction/hydrocephalus. *CNS lymphoma* can be primary (most common in immunocompromised patients, e.g., AIDS) or secondary (metastasis from another site of lymphoma). All of these tumors develop more commonly in the cerebral hemispheres though they can occur elsewhere in the brain. *Medulloblastoma* is a childhood tumor that, in contrast, is most common in the cerebellum.

Treatment of all CNS tumors is by some combination of surgery, radiation, and/or chemotherapy.

Stroke

Occlusion of cerebral vasculature from plaque formation, emboli, or thrombosis can lead to acute cerebral ischemia (*stroke*). Ischemia can be caused by:

- *Emboli* that lodge in the cerebral vasculature (e.g., from a fibrillating atrium, vegetations on an infected valve, or from a hypercoagulable state)

- *Atherosclerotic plaque*, which can occlude the carotid arteries, the vertebro-basilar system, or their branches in the brain

- *Venous occlusion* (e.g., secondary to thrombosis)

- *Arterial dissection* in the carotid or vertebro-basilar system following trauma or chiropractic manipulation

- *Severe hypotension,* which can be caused by cardiac dysfunction (e.g., arrhythmia, cardiac arrest, post-surgery) and severe hypovolemia. This can lead to infarction of cerebral areas at the boundaries of the major vascular territories (*watershed infarcts*).

A *transient ischemic attack* (TIA) is a harbinger of stroke to come. Critical narrowing of the carotid or vertebrobasilar system or small pieces of plaque that embolize can cause stroke-like symptoms that only last for a few seconds, minutes, or hours. *Amaurosis fugax* is one classic TIA symptom: transient ischemia in the ophthalmic artery (a branch of the internal carotid) causes temporary blindness. Patients often describe this as appearing "like a curtain coming down." (Patients may also describe retinal detachment in a similar way.)

Treatment of an acute event (e.g., with thrombolysis) and prevention (e.g., lowering blood pressure, quitting smoking, decreasing cholesterol, taking aspirin to inhibit platelets) are similar to such measures in myocardial ischemia/infarction.

Cerebral Vasculature

Fig. 7-18. Cerebral Circulation.

Anterior Circulation. The common carotid arteries branch to form the external and internal carotid arteries. The internal carotids give rise to the *middle* and *anterior cerebral arteries*. The middle cerebral arteries supply much of the lateral surfaces of the hemispheres while the anterior cerebrals supply much of the medial surfaces.

Posterior Circulation. The *vertebral arteries* arise from the subclavian arteries. The vertebral arteries feed the medial medulla and give off the *posterior inferior cerebellar arteries* (PICAs), which supply the lateral brainstem and inferior cerebellum. The vertebral arteries then fuse over the medulla to form the *basilar artery*. The basilar artery feeds the medial pons and gives off the AICAs (*anterior inferior cerebellar ar-*

teries), which supply the lateral portions of the pons and the anterior cerebellum. The basilar artery also gives rise to the *superior cerebellar arteries* (which supply the brainstem and cerebellum) before splitting into the *posterior cerebral arteries* (which supply the occipital lobes). *Posterior communicating arteries* link the anterior and posterior circulation, creating what is known as the Circle of Willis.

Based on the neurological symptoms/signs during the stroke, one can determine the part of the brain and vascular supply that are affected.

Fig. 7-19. Homunculus and vascular territories of ACA and MCA. Imagine the homunculus as sunbathing on the brain, legs dangling between the hemispheres, leaning back over the external surface. Based on the vascular anatomy, a stroke of the middle cerebral artery will affect the face, as well as the arm, and to a

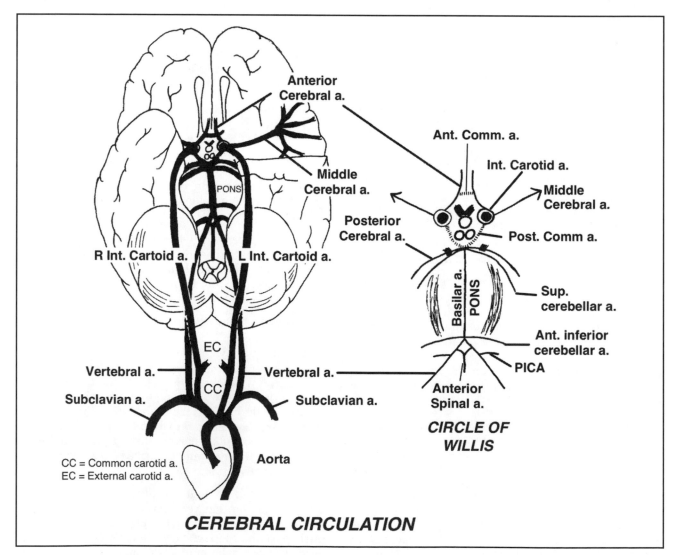

CEREBRAL CIRCULATION

Figure 7-18. Modified from Goldberg: *Clinical Neuroanatomy Made Ridiculously Simple*, MedMaster 2005

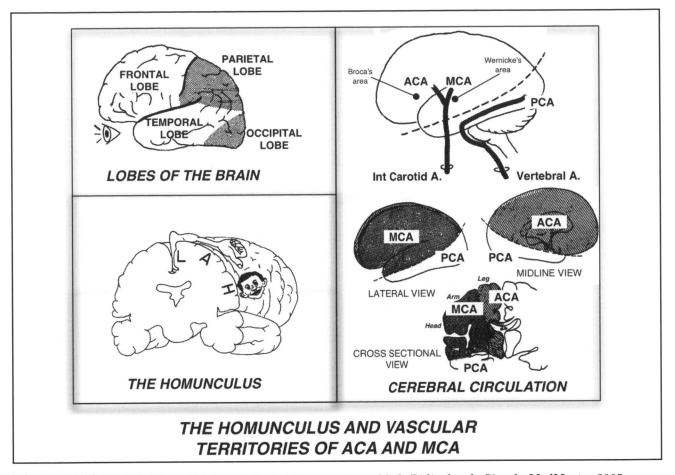

Figure 7-19. Modified from Goldberg: *Clinical Neuroanatomy Made Ridiculously Simple*, MedMaster 2005

lesser extent, the leg (all on the *contralateral side* since we are far above the decussation in the medulla). Alternatively, a stroke of the anterior cerebral artery will cause sensory and motor dysfunction that is greater in the leg than in the arm (again, all on the *contralateral* side). Anterior cerebral artery strokes can also lead to *abulia*, a lack of motivation due to ischemia/infarction of part of the frontal lobe.

The left hemisphere houses the areas responsible for language production (Broca's area) and comprehension (Wernicke's area). Broca's area receives its blood supply from the anterior branch of the middle cerebral artery, whereas Wernicke's area receives its blood supply from the posterior branch of the middle cerebral artery. Broca's aphasia is an *expressive* aphasia: there is difficulty producing spoken and written language, but *preserved comprehension*, and thus preserved ability to follow commands. Wernicke's aphasia is a *receptive* aphasia: difficulty understanding language (both spoken and written), leading to flowing yet senseless speech and inability to follow commands. Thus, a middle cerebral stroke can be further localized to the anterior branch of the middle cerebral artery (which can cause Broca's aphasia) or the posterior branch (which can cause Wernicke's aphasia) by the patient's pattern of language deficits. A more proximal occlusion of the middle cerebral artery can lead to combined aphasia: loss of both language production and comprehension.

Note that certain lesions at any variety of locations may cause *dysarthria*, a problem producing the mouth/tongue movements necessary for speech. In such lesions, speech will be affected, but patients will still be able to understand spoken and written language.

The posterior cerebral artery supplies the posterior part of the brain, namely the occipital lobe. What visual defect would you expect from damage to one occipital lobe? Homonymous hemianopsia on the contralateral side (Fig. 7-7).

Lacunar infarcts involve the small penetrating branches that feed deeper brain structures. These strokes can cause isolated motor or isolated sensory deficits. For example, pure motor deficits can occur from lacunar infarct of the motor fibers of the internal capsule or the corticospinal tract in the brainstem. A pure sensory deficit can occur from infarct of the thalamus.

Strokes of the brainstem are more complicated since there is a lot of anatomy/function packed into a tiny space. Keep in mind the main basic principle of brainstem anatomy: midbrain = cranial nerve nuclei 1-4, pons = cranial nerve nuclei 5-8, and medulla = cranial nerve nuclei 9-12. (Also review the exceptions, Fig. 7-6). Recall that brainstem lesions are the only lesions that can cause *crossed signs*: symptoms/signs involving the face ipsilateral to the lesion and the body contralateral to it.

The midbrain is supplied by the top of the basilar artery, the superior cerebellar arteries, and the posterior cerebral arteries.

The pons is supplied by the middle of the basilar artery and anterior inferior cerebellar arteries.

The medulla is supplied by the vertebral arteries and the posterior inferior cerebellar arteries. Different patterns of clinical findings depend on which vascular territory is affected.

Midbrain stroke (posterior cerebral artery ischemia) can cause:

- *Ipsilateral* **cranial nerve III** palsy (the affected eye appears down and out, with a fixed and dilated pupil)

- *Contralateral* **hemiplegia** (body/limb weakness) from effect on the corticospinal tract

(Remember, despite the 1-4 mnemonic for the midbrain, cranial nerve I does *not* project to the brainstem, and though the afferent pathway for the pupillary reflex travels in CN II to the brainstem, the visual pathway of CN II does *not*.)

Pontine stroke (basilar and/or anterior inferior cerebellar artery ischemia) can cause any or all of the following:

- *Ipsilateral* **CN V** deficit (facial numbness)

- *Ipsilateral* **CN VI** deficit (loss of eye abduction)

- *Ipsilateral* **CN VII** deficit (facial weakness)

- *Contralateral* **hemiplegia** (body/limb weakness) from effect on the corticospinal tract

Medullary stroke (PICA, vertebral, and/or basilar artery ischemia) can cause any or all of the following:

- Deficit of the *lower portion* of *ipsilateral* **CN V** (ipsilateral loss of facial sensation)

- Deficit of the *vestibular portion* of **CN VIII** (vertigo, vomiting)

- Deficits of **CN IX** and **CN X** (dysarthria/dysphagia and/or deviation of uvula *away* from the lesioned side)

- Deficit of **CN XII** (ipsilateral tongue weakness—tongue deviates toward side of lesion)

- *Ipsilateral* **Horner's syndrome** (loss of descending sympathetic fibers, leading to ipsilateral ptosis, miosis, anhidrosis)

- *Contralateral* **hemiplegia** (body/limb weakness) from effect on the corticospinal tract

- *Contralateral* **sensory changes** in the body/limbs from effect on the medial lemniscus and spinothalamic tract

- *Ipsilateral* **ataxia** and **dysdiadochokinesia** from effect on the cerebellum

Multiple Sclerosis

If one thinks of nerve axons as electrical wire, it is myelin that provides their insulation. In multiple sclerosis, the "insulation" gets damaged in the *central nervous system (brain and spinal cord)*. The pathophysiology is not yet fully elucidated but is postulated to involve autoimmunity, infection, genetics, and/or a combination of these factors. The term "multiple" in the name refers to the characteristic multiple lesions in multiple sites in the CNS, which can arise at multiple points in time. Multiple sclerosis has various types of clinical courses, but the most common is the relapsing-remitting course, which evolves in a series of normal periods punctuated by flares.

The loss of myelin in the CNS leads to a slowing of nerve conduction. Symptoms vary depending on the site of the lesion: subcortical white matter lesions can result in cognitive dysfunction; brainstem lesions can cause dysfunction of any cranial nerve; cerebellar lesions can lead to ataxia, dysdiadochokinesia, etc.; spinal cord tract lesions can cause pain/temperature/vibration sense loss and/or motor dysfunction. What type of motor deficits would you expect, upper or lower motor neuron-type lesions? Multiple sclerosis is limited to the *central* nervous system; the peripheral nervous system is unaffected. Thus, it is *upper* motor neurons that are affected in multiple sclerosis, which can cause spasticity, increased reflexes, Babinski's sign, etc.

The bladder also has upper motor neurons (in the spinal cord) and lower motor neurons arising from sacral levels 2-4 (S 2,3,4), which travel in peripheral nerves. Just as upper motor neuron lesions of skeletal muscles cause spasticity, upper motor neuron lesions of the bladder cause *spasticity* of the bladder, which can present as urinary frequency and urgency.

*Any **CNS** deficit can occur in multiple sclerosis.*

Some classic multiple sclerosis signs: *Uthoff's phenomenon* is a worsening of symptoms in the heat (classically weakness or sensory changes after a hot bath or vigorous exercise). *L'Hermitte's sign* is when electrical sensations run down the spine when the patient bends his/her head forward. Multiple sclerosis is also a common underlying cause of internuclear ophthalmoplegia (INO) (Fig. 7-11). Where is the demyelinating lesion in this case? For INO, the lesion must be in the MLF *ipsilateral* to the eye that cannot adduct when the other eye abducts (though it should still adduct on convergence).

Treatment for multiple sclerosis is immunomodulatory, including *interferon* and/or *glatiramer acetate* (*Copaxone*). Glatiramer acetate is a mixture of small peptides related to proteins in myelin. Glatiramer acetate's mechanism of action is thought to occur by modifying the immune processes involved in the pathogenesis of multiple sclerosis. Multiple sclerosis can present in a wide variety of severities and courses, and treatments have various side effects. This makes its management complex, determined by many factors in each individual case.

DISEASES OF THE SPINAL CORD

Fig. 7-20. The spinal cord. The spinal cord's organization is "inside out" compared with the brain: in the spinal cord, the white matter runs on the outside and the gray matter is on the inside. Within the tracts of the spinal cord, the fibers from different regions of the body are aligned in a specific way (*lamination*). Mnemonic: Imagine two people lying comfortably on top of the cord. Also imagine people lying on either side of the cord, falling perilously toward its center. The people falling towards the center are falling with their *arms out in front of them*. The people relaxing on top

are oriented in the *opposite* way, with feet toward the center. The people relaxing on the top represent the *posterior columns* (arm fibers lateral, leg fibers medial). The people falling perilously toward the center represent the *corticospinal* and *spinothalamic tracts* (arm fibers medial, leg fibers lateral). Note that although this mnemonic puts heads on the figures, the nerves to and from the head are *not carried* in the spinal cord, but in cranial nerves.

Let's take the example of a *syrinx* to review the anatomical layout. In *syringomyelia*, the central canal expands. The first fibers to be affected are the pain/temperature fibers crossing to become the spinothalamic tract (Fig. 7-3). Since only the *crossing* fibers are affected, there is bilateral loss of pain/temperature sensation in one ring around the body at that level with normal function above and below (*suspended sensory level*). Expansion of the syrinx can affect the lateral corticospinal and spinothalamic tracts in a *cervical to sacral progression*, since the bulging presses first against the more centrally located fibers of these tracts. An expanding syrinx causes sensory and motor deficits *below* it (since sensory and motor fibers entering and exiting *above* the syrinx will be unaffected).

NERVE ROOT COMPRESSION

Notice in Fig. 7-20 that the dorsal/posterior (sensory) fibers enter and ventral/anterior (motor) fibers exit via roots that join to form *peripheral nerves*. Discs that prolapse and impinge on either a sensory or motor root can thus cause isolated sensory or motor symptoms in a dermatomal distribution, i.e., along a "zebra stripe" of a dermatomal diagram (*radiculopathy*). See Fig. 7-5 for review of dermatomes.

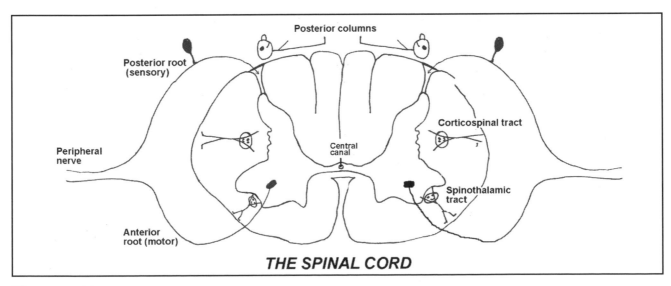

THE SPINAL CORD

Figure 7-20

Nerve roots can be compressed by prolapsed/herniated disc(s), tumor(s), or spinal stenosis. A prolapsed disc usually affects the root *below* it, so the L4 disc hits the L5 root, the L5 disc hits the S1 root, etc. Lateral herniation (L4 disc to L4 root, L5 disc to L5 root, etc.) can also occur, but it is much less common. In nerve root compression, sensory findings tend to occur *only in the dermatome of the affected root*. This is in contrast to distributions of symptoms such as the complete loss of sensation that occurs below a certain point in spinal cord compression; a "stocking/glove" pattern of sensory deficits in peripheral polyneuropathy; a specifically affected area in mononeuropathy (e.g., palmar surface of the hand and the first two fingers in median nerve compression); or the involvement of a large area that is *not* restricted to a single dermatome in cortical or brainstem lesions.

Fig. 7-21. Commonly tested reflexes. In nerve root compression, motor findings are localizable to the specific spinal root. Mnemonic: Touch your ankles and say 1-2, knees and say 3-4, palmar surface of arm and say 5-6, elbow (dorsal surface) and say 7-8. The ankle reflex uses S1-2 (gastrocnemius), patellar uses L3-4 (quadriceps), biceps/brachioradialis is innervated by C5-6, and triceps is innervated by C7-8.

S 2, 3, and 4 control bowel, bladder, and erectile function, so compression at this level can lead to incontinence and impotence.

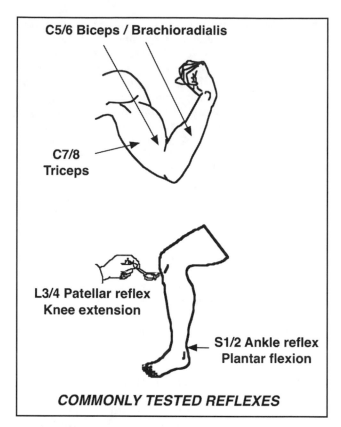

COMMONLY TESTED REFLEXES

Figure 7-21

DISEASES OF LOWER MOTOR NEURONS, NEUROMUSCULAR JUNCTION, AND MUSCLE

Review figure 7-20. The axons of anterior horn cells (lower motor neurons) exit the spinal cord anteriorly (ventrally) as the anterior (or ventral) roots. These roots join with the posterior (or dorsal) roots (sensory fibers) to form the peripheral nerves. Thus, the peripheral nerves generally carry *both* motor fibers traveling to the muscles and sensory fibers from the skin, joints, and muscles. The sensory fibers bring back information about light touch, pain, temperature, and proprioception. Additionally, there are visceral motor fibers to sweat glands, sympathetic fibers to the various organs, etc. (By the way, where do the parasympathetic neurons come from? The vagus nerve and sacral spinal cord.) Motor neuron axons traveling in peripheral nerves eventually synapse with muscle cells at the neuromuscular junction (NMJ). Only excitation is possible at the NMJ, and the neurotransmitter is acetylcholine.

There are diseases that affect the anterior horn cells, those that affect the peripheral nerves, those that affect the NMJ, and those that affect the muscles themselves. These are grouped together because their clinical presentations often share a common feature: *weakness*. If lesions affecting any component of the motor system will lead to weakness, what other signs/symptoms can help localize the site of the lesion? If the weakness involves damage to lower motor neurons (i.e., anterior horn cell, nerve root, or peripheral nerve), we would expect other lower motor neuron signs, such as fasciculations, decreased/absent reflexes, and muscle atrophy. Peripheral neuropathy typically leads to *distal* muscle weakness, while myopathy typically leads to *proximal* muscle weakness.

What if there were weakness and also sensory changes (loss of feeling, numbness, pain/temperature sensation loss)? Weakness and sensory changes together can only occur with lesions of peripheral nerve(s), the cerebral hemispheres (e.g., contralateral middle cerebral artery stroke), the brainstem (e.g., stroke), or with a spinal cord lesion affecting both motor and sensory pathways (e.g., transverse myelitis in multiple sclerosis). If there is loss of motor function and light touch/proprioception on one side and pain/temperature sensation loss on the opposite side, this indicates a spinal cord lesion (Fig. 7-4). Weakness *alone* with no sensory changes implies a problem specifically affecting motor pathways (e.g., pure motor stroke, amyotrophic lateral sclerosis), the neuromuscular junction, or the actual muscle(s).

Diseases of Anterior Horn Cells

The *juvenile spinal muscular atrophy syndromes* affect the anterior horn cells. The details of classification are beyond the scope of this text, but the symptoms are what you would expect from a disease process that exclusively affects the anterior horn cells: weakness/flaccid paralysis, fasciculations, muscle atrophy, decreased/absent reflexes. *Poliomyelitis* can also selectively affect the anterior horn cells.

Amyotrophic lateral sclerosis (ALS) affects the anterior horn cells *and* the corticospinal tract. This leads to a mixture of *both* upper and lower motor neuron findings: weakness, spastic paralysis, some increased reflexes, some decreased.

In disease processes that affect anterior horn cells *without affecting the peripheral nerves*, sensory function will be normal.

Diseases of Peripheral Nerves

Many types of pathology can cause peripheral neuropathies: *infection* (e.g., AIDS, leprosy), *systemic diseases* (e.g., diabetes, polyarteritis nodosa), *toxins* (e.g., lead, chemotherapy agents, alcohol), *genetic diseases* (e.g., hereditary motor and sensory neuropathies such as Charcot-Marie-Tooth syndrome), *paraneoplastic syndromes, autoimmune diseases* (e.g., Guillain-Barré), and *metabolic deficiencies* (B12 deficiency). Peripheral neuropathy can be caused by damage to either the axons themselves or the myelin (Guillain-Barré is an example of a demyelinating peripheral neuropathy). Nerve conduction studies can help distinguish between axonal and demyelinating causes of neuropathy. One type of disease process *slows nerve conduction*; the other *decreases the amplitude of nerve conduction*. Which do you think is which? Myelin insulates the axon so as to allow for *faster* nerve conduction. So *myelin loss decreases velocity* of nerve conduction. *Axonal damage decreases the amplitude* of nerve conduction.

Peripheral neuropathy can cause sensory deficits, motor deficits, or both, depending on whether the pathology is specific for a given fiber type. The motor deficits in peripheral neuropathy are of the lower motor neuron variety: flaccid paralysis/weakness, decreased or absent reflexes. The sensory deficits in peripheral neuropathy can include loss of light touch, loss of pain/temperature sensation, loss of proprioception, and/or symptoms such as neuropathic pain, numbness, and/or tingling.

The extent of deficits is useful in classifying peripheral neuropathies. Is only one nerve involved, or are there multiple sites of pathology? A *mononeuropathy* (problem limited to one nerve) could indicate entrapment (e.g. the median nerve in carpal tunnel), trauma, or ischemia/infarct. *Mononeuropathy multiplex* (multiple individual mononeuropathies) indicates a systemic underlying pathology such as diabetes, vasculitis, infection, or toxicity (e.g., lead). *Peripheral neuropathy* (multiple distal portions of nerves affected, e.g., "stocking/glove" distribution) also typically results from systemic pathology (e.g., diabetes, drug toxicity).

Diseases of the Neuromuscular Junction
Myasthenia Gravis

In myasthenia gravis, autoantibodies are produced against the acetylcholine receptors on muscle cells at the neuromuscular junction. These antibodies block the receptor so that acetylcholine cannot bind and stimulate muscular contraction. While many cases are idiopathic, myasthenia can also occur secondary to a *thymoma* (a tumor of the thymus). Myasthenia produces weakness, and its clinical hallmark is that muscles are more likely to *fatigue*. The muscles of the face are often profoundly affected, which can manifest as *ptosis* (drooping eyelids) and quick fatigue of eyelids during prolonged upward gaze (*ptosis time*), trouble swallowing (*dysphagia*), and/or trouble speaking (*dysarthria*). Relatively rapid fatigue can also be demonstrated by the patient's inability to maintain arm abduction for more than a brief period.

Myasthenia gravis must be distinguished from weakness caused by disease of peripheral nerve or disease of the muscle. In myasthenia gravis, one would *not* expect sensory deficits (as can be present in peripheral neuropathy) or pain (as can be present in inflammatory muscle disease). The diagnosis of myasthenia gravis can be confirmed by detecting the acetylcholine receptor antibody in the blood or by EMG (electromyelography) study, which demonstrates fatigue during repetitive stimulation. This EMG finding confirms what is seen clinically: sustained firing that leads to fatigue.

At the neuromuscular junction the motor neurons release the neurotransmitter acetycholine, which stimulates post-synaptic receptors on the muscle cells. Since we do not want our muscles to stay contracted permanently, there must be a mechanism for getting rid of that acetylcholine. This is accomplished by acetylcholinesterase, an enzyme that cleaves acetylcholine into its component parts for reuptake by the presynaptic neuron. So blocking acetylcholinesterase decreases acetylcholine breakdown, increasing the amount of acetylcholine in the synapse that can compete with antibodies for postsynaptic binding. This fact can be used for diagnosis (Tensilon test) and treatment (pyridostigmine) of myasthenia gravis.

Tensilon is the trade name of edrophonium, a competitive inhibitor for binding sites on acetylcholinesterase, which thus increases the life of acetylcholine in the synapse. Tensilon acts quite quickly, so a patient with myasthenia gravis will feel a fast (but temporary) improvement of weakness. This *Tensilon test* is not a sure-fire proof of myasthenia gravis; any patient with muscle weakness might feel slightly better from increased stimulation of their muscles by acetylcholine. However, dramatic improvement following the Tensilon test generally indicates myasthenia gravis.

One treatment for myasthenia is *pyridostigmine*, which blocks acetylcholinesterase. Although pyridostigmine can improve symptoms of weakness, it does not correct the underlying cause of the weakness: the immune system's production of autoantibodies. Thus immunosuppression is used if myasthenia gravis is severe. In some cases, removal of the thymus can lead to improvement of symptoms.

Lambert-Eaton Syndrome

A myasthenia-like syndrome, *Lambert-Eaton syndrome*, can occur as a *paraneoplastic* syndrome. Lambert-Eaton syndrome is most commonly seen with small cell lung cancer, though it can also arise with other cancers. The pathophysiology is slightly different from myasthenia gravis: autoantibodies form against the pre-synaptic calcium channels, leading to decreased synaptic activity at the NMJ. As in myasthenia, this results in weakness, though muscles of the face are affected to a lesser extent than in myasthenia. In Lambert-Eaton syndrome, because the problem is failure of calcium influx to trigger acetylcholine release, repetitive stimulation (clinically or by EMG) actually produces transient *improvement*; this is the exact *opposite* effect of what occurs in myasthenia gravis.

Diseases of the Muscle

Weakness can also be due to a problem with the muscles themselves, independent of a perfectly functioning nervous system. This too would present as weakness but should *not* have sensory changes or changes in reflexes. Additionally, muscular problems (unless they are from injury) tend to be fairly symmetrical, since there is usually some underlying systemic process affecting the muscles. Muscle problems also tend to present with *proximal weakness* as opposed to the distal weakness typically noted in neuropathies.

Diseases of the muscle can essentially be divided into the *dystrophies, inflammatory myopathies*, and the *metabolic myopathies*. The dystrophies are genetic diseases with specific patterns of involvement (e.g., Duchenne's muscular dystrophy, myotonic dystrophy, facioscapulohumeral dystrophy). Inflammatory diseases include dermatomyositis and polymyositis (see Fig. 8-1). Metabolic myopathies include mitochondrial myopathies and glycogen storage diseases, as well as steroid-induced myopathy and myopathies from underlying endocrine dysfunction (e.g., hyper- or hypothyroidism). Inflammatory diseases of the muscles typically cause *muscle pain and tenderness*. Muscle pain and tenderness can help to distinguish myopathy from neuropathy or myasthenia as causes of weakness.

CHAPTER 8. RHEUMATOLOGY

Rheumatology deals with diseases involving joints, autoimmunity, or both. In autoimmune diseases, the normal self-tolerance of the immune system breaks down, and the immune system attacks the body. Infectious triggers and genetics may play a role in susceptibility to autoimmunity, but the pathophysiology of these diseases has not yet been fully elucidated.

Autoimmune diseases are a diverse group. Some autoimmune diseases affect only individual organs (e.g., diabetes type I affects the pancreas; primary biliary cirrhosis affects the bile ducts; Hashimoto's thyroiditis affects the thyroid), and some can affect nearly all organ systems. Many autoimmune diseases have serum auto-antibodies associated with them, though such autoantibodies are neither 100% specific nor 100% sensitive for the diseases. In some autoimmune diseases, it is uncertain whether these autoantibodies are part of the cause of the disease or a result of the underlying disease process.

Fig. 8-1. Features of selected rheumatologic diseases. The primary features of several diseases and their associated autoantibodies are listed in this table. In addition to the features characteristic of any given autoimmune disease, constitutional symptoms (fever, malaise) are often present as a result of the inflammatory process. Also, inflammatory markers such as ESR (erythrocyte sedimentation rate) and CRP (C-reactive protein) may be elevated in the serum in any of these diseases.

TREATMENT OF AUTOIMMUNE DISEASES

Since the underlying cause of the loss of self-tolerance and/or over-activity of the immune system is not fully understood, treatment is directed against the inflammatory response itself, which can be blocked at various levels. Of course, due to the inhibition of the immune system that some of these drugs produce, bone marrow suppression and subsequent immunosuppression can result, predisposing to infection.

Immunosuppressive and Anti-Inflammatory Drugs

Drugs inhibit the immune system at various levels by:

- *Causing death of inflammatory cells (cytotoxic agents).* Methotrexate, cyclophosphamide, azathioprine, leflunomide, and mycophenolic acid alter DNA synthesis, causing death of rapidly dividing cells, among them lymphocytes involved in the inflammatory response.

- *Preventing the secretion of inflammatory cytokines.* Cyclosporine specifically inhibits T-lymphocytes, preventing them from secreting interleukins. Corticosteroids, among the most commonly used immunosuppressive agents, alter gene expression, leading to a decrease in the inflammatory response. Corticosteroid treatment can cause Cushing's syndrome (See Fig. 5-4).

- *Inhibiting cytokine synthesis* (e.g., NSAIDs, COX-2 inhibitors)

- *Blocking cytokines, preventing them from acting* (e.g., anti-TNF antibodies, soluble TNF receptors)

In joint disease, first-line anti-inflammatory therapy often involves NSAIDs (non-steroidal anti-inflammatory drugs), which block cytokine synthesis (specifically prostaglandins). Older NSAIDs (e.g., ibuprofen, naproxen) inhibit both COX (cyclooxygenase)-1 and COX-2 enzymes. Though blocking COX-2 leads to the desired anti-inflammatory effect, one side effect of COX-1 inhibition is decreased prostaglandin synthesis in the gut, which can predispose to ulcer. COX-2 inhibitors (drugs whose names end in "–coxcib") selectively block the COX-2 enzyme, thus inhibiting inflammation with fewer gastrointestinal side effects. Soluble TNF (tumor necrosis factor) receptors and anti-TNF antibodies block TNF, an inflammatory cytokine.

JOINT DISEASE: ARTHRITIS

Arthritis is inflammation of a joint or several joints, and can be caused by infection, autoimmune disease, or joint trauma. Symptoms can include joint pain, stiffness, warmth, and/or swelling.

Causes of arthritis are classified as *inflammatory* (e.g., rheumatoid arthritis, spondyloarthritis, infection, crystal-induced) or *non-inflammatory* (e.g., osteoarthritis, trauma, hemarthrosis). Any type of arthritis can cause pain, limitation of motion, swelling, and/or tenderness of the joint. *Inflammatory* causes will also tend to have systemic features (constitutional systems or effects on other organ systems), aggravation with rest (e.g., prolonged morning stiffness), relief with use, and warmth and redness of joints. *Non-inflammatory* arthritis tends to be aggravated by motion and relieved by rest. Arthritis can affect a single joint (*monoarticular*), several (2-4) joints (*oligoarticular*) or many joints (*polyarticular*). Any cause of polyarticular arthritis can also present first in a single joint.

Figure 8-1   Features of Selected Rheumatologic Diseases

DISEASE	CLASSIC FEATURES	ADDITIONAL FEATURES	SEROLOGICAL MARKERS	TREATMENT
Behçet's Disease	Oral and genital aphthous ulcers, uveitis	GI ulceration, CNS lesions, glomerulonephropathy, peripheral neuropathy, arthritis, vasculitis, skin lesions	(none)	Steroids
Dermatomyositis	Proximal muscle weakness, often painless, though myalgia sometimes occurs. Dermatologic manifestations: heliotrope rash (around eyes), "mechanic's hands" (hyperkeratosis of hands), Gottron's papules over joints	Interstitial fibrosis of lungs, cardiomyopathy, arthritis, dysphagia, increased risk of malignancy	Anti-Jo-1, anti-Mi-2, elevated creatine kinase (from muscle breakdown); diagnosis confirmed by muscle biopsy	Steroids ± other immunosuppressives
Polymyositis	Proximal muscle weakness, often painless, though myalgia sometimes occurs	Interstitial fibrosis of lungs, cardiomyopathy, arthritis, dysphagia	ANA, Anti-SRP, anti-Jo-1, elevated creatine kinase (from muscle breakdown); diagnosis confirmed by muscle biopsy	Steroids ± other immunosuppressives
Sarcoid	Pulmonary (cough, dyspnea), arthritis, lymphadenopathy	Any organ system can be affected: e.g., CNS, cardiac, renal	Elevated serum ACE; granulomas on biopsy	Steroids
Scleroderma	Thickened skin, Raynaud's phenomenon (cold or stress-induced closure of peripheral arteries leading to pallor and cyanosis, e.g., in fingertips)	Pulmonary fibrosis, esophageal dilatation and GERD, myocardial fibrosis, pericardial effusion, renal involvement; CREST variant: **c**alcinosis, **R**aynaud's, **e**sophageal dysmotility, **s**clerodactyly, **t**elangectasia	Anti-Scl-70; Anti-centromere in CREST	Anti-inflammatories for arthritis, ACE-I for renal involvement/hypertension, calcium channel blockers for Raynaud's; Penicillamine (mechanism uncertain) in some cases
Sjögren's Syndrome	Dry eyes, dry mouth	Pulmonary fibrosis, peripheral neuropathy, increased risk of other autoimmune diseases (e.g., rheumatoid arthritis) and B cell lymphoma, parotid gland enlargement	Anti SS-A (Ro) and Anti SS-B (La)	Symptomatic: eyedrops
Systemic Lupus Erythematosus (SLE)	Malar rash (butterfly rash on cheeks), photosensitivity, fever	Can affect ANY organ system: arthritis, pleuritis, pericarditis, seizures, psychosis, immunodeficiency, thrombocytopenia, nephrotic or nephritic syndrome...	ANA, anti-DNA, anti-SM, anti-Ro, anti-La; anti-histone in drug induced lupus	Steroids, azathioprine, cyclophosphamide, methotrexate, cyclosporine

ANA stands for anti-nuclear antibodies. Autoimmune diseases not on this table but discussed elsewhere in this book: rheumatoid arthritis (Fig. 8-2); autoimmune hepatitis, primary biliary cirrhosis, and primary sclerosing cholangitis (Chapter 4); and Hashimoto's thyroiditis and Graves' disease (Chapter 5).

Synovial Fluid Analysis

In monoarticular arthritis, since the disease process is specifically localized, synovial fluid analysis from the involved joint is used for diagnosis. Synovial fluid analysis can detect infectious agents, crystals, blood, and WBCs. Crystals may indicate gout or pseudogout; blood (*hemarthrosis*) could result from trauma, hemophilia, or anticoagulant treatment. Synovial fluid is classified as noninflammatory, inflammatory, or septic (infectious) based on the number of white blood cells (WBCs). Non-inflammatory < 2000 WBCs; inflammatory > 2000 WBCs; septic > 100,000 WBCs.

Fig. 8-2. Arthritis. The features of the different types of arthritis are summarized in this table.

Rheumatoid Arthritis (RA)

Rheumatoid arthritis is an autoimmune disease, though the cause(s) of this disorder have not yet been fully elucidated. In rheumatoid arthritis, inflammation of the synovium (the inner lining of the joint capsule) and the resultant cascade of inflammatory molecules lead to joint damage. Like many autoimmune diseases, RA is more common in women. *Any joint(s) can be affected*, but symmetrical involvement of the hands and/or feet is a common presentation.

Fig. 8-3. Joints of the hand. In the fingers, the MCP (metacarpal phalangeal) and PIP (proximal interphalangeal) joints are often affected in rheumatoid arthritis. The DIP (distal interphalangeal) joint is the only joint in the hand *not* usually affected in RA (though it is commonly affected in osteoarthritis).

Although a short period of stiffness in the morning and/or after any period of inactivity can occur in any joint disease, *prolonged* morning stiffness (e.g., greater than 30 minutes) is more typical of RA and other types of inflammatory arthritis (i.e., *not* in osteoarthritis). As with any autoimmune disease, constitutional symptoms can be present in rheumatoid arthritis (malaise, weakness, fatigue). Any organ system can be affected by the underlying inflammatory disease process in RA, leading to any or all of the following: vasculitis, anemia, lymphadenopathy, splenomegaly, pulmonary nodules, pleural effusions, pericarditis, and/or scleritis. Serum rheumatoid factor (RF) is present in the majority of cases. Over the long term, joint inflammation/destruction can lead to nodule formation and deformities in the joints.

Osteoarthritis (OA)

Osteoarthritis is the most common cause of arthritis in adults. Aging, excess weight, joint trauma, and/or genetic predisposition can lead to damage of articular cartilage. Gradual onset of pain in one or several joints is the primary feature of osteoarthritis. This pain tends to occur with activity of the joint. Although morning stiffness may occur, it is typically brief as opposed to the prolonged stiffness in rheumatoid arthritis. Knee, hip, spine, and hand joints are the most commonly affected in OA. PIP *and* DIP joints can *both* be affected (vs. RA, which usually does *not* affect the DIP, see Fig. 8-3). The MCP joints are typically *unaffected* in osteoarthritis (vs. RA, which usually *does* affect the MCP, see Fig. 8-3). Osteophytes (bone spurs) can form, which can lead to spinal stenosis, nerve compression, esophageal compression (if the osteophyte is on the anterior spine and compresses the esophagus), Heberden's nodes (DIP spurs), and/or Bouchard's nodes (PIP spurs).

Spondyloarthritis

Spondyloarthritis is characterized by *spinal arthritis* (which can cause back pain/stiffness), *enthesopathy* (inflammation of insertions of tendons and ligaments to bone, which can lead to *dactylitis,* also called "sausage digits"), *peripheral arthritis, extra-articular features* (including eye, skin, and GI pathology), *no* rheumatoid factor (RF) in the serum, and a genetic association with *HLA-B27.* The spondyloarthropathies include anklyosing spondylitis, reactive (Reiter's) arthritis, inflammatory bowel disease-associated arthritis, and psoriatic arthritis. The features of these diseases are listed in Fig. 8-2.

Infectious Arthritis

Infectious arthritis can arise from hematogenous spread from another site of infection, contiguous spread (e.g., from osteomyelitis), trauma, or surgery. Predisposing factors include diseased joints, prosthetic joints, IV drug use, immune deficiency, and trauma. Infection most commonly affects one single joint (commonly the knee), and concurrent fever is usually present in addition to the signs/symptoms of joint inflammation. Diagnosis is made by synovial fluid analysis (> 100,000 WBCs). Because infectious arthritis typically presents acutely, gout must be ruled out due to its similar acute presentation. Common pathogens include *Gonorrhea*, *Staph. aureus* and gram negatives. *Salmonella* arthritis can occur in sickle cell disease. More rarely, mycobacteria, a variety of viruses (parvovirus B19, HIV, rubella, hepatitis), and fungi (blastomycosis, candida, coccioidomycosis, cryptococcosis, histoplasmosis, sporotrichosis) can also cause arthritis.

Lyme disease is another infection that can cause arthritis. The infectious organism, *Borrelia burgdorferi,* is typically transmitted by tick bite. The tick bite often (but not always) causes a target-shaped rash (*erythema migrans*). Symptoms can include fever, malaise, lymphadenopathy, and arthritis. If untreated, Lyme disease can progress to chronic arthritis,

Figure 8-2 Arthritis

DISEASE	EPIDEMIOLOGY	JOINTS INVOLVED	FEATURES OF ARTHRITIS	OTHER FEATURES	SERUM	SYNOVIAL FLUID	TREATMENT
Rheumatoid arthritis	More common in women	Symmetrical; any joint, but hands and feet common (especially MCP and PIP of hand)	Prolonged morning stiffness; long term: deformation of joints and nodule formation	Constitutional symptoms; vasculitis, anemia, pulmonary nodules, pericarditis, scleritis	RF	Inflam.	NSAIDS, sulfasalazine, anti-malarials, steroids, methotrexate, TNF alpha antagonists
Osteoarthritis	Most common in older adults	Knee, hip, spine, hand (DIP and PIP)	Gradual onset, pain with activity, much shorter period of morning stiffness than RA	Osteophyte formation can cause spinal stenosis, esophageal compression		NON- inflam.	Weight loss, physical therapy, NSAIDS, COX 2 inhibitors, steroid injections, surgery
Ankylosing spondylitis	More common in men, often emerges in young adulthood	Spine, sacroiliac joint, peripheral joints	Gradual onset of back pain, stiffness	Peripheral enthesopathy, dactylitis, conjunctivitis, uveitis; spinal changes can cause restrictive lung disease; cardiac involvement*	HLA-B27	Inflam.	NSAIDS, TNF alpha antagonists
Psoriatic arthritis	Any age, men and women equally affected	Hands, wrists, ankles, feet, DIP	Can be acute onset (mimicking gout) or more RA-like presentation; arthritis mutilans (bone resorption) can occur	Psoriasis is a silver scale that appears most commonly on the elbows, knees, and scalp; ocular involvement; cardiac involvement*	HLA-B27	Inflam.	NSAIDS, steroids, TNF alpha antagonists
Reactive arthritis (Reiter's syndrome)	Several weeks after GU or GI infection	Feet/legs, hands/arms most common	Inflamed joint(s) 2-4 weeks after infection	Skin/eye	HLA-B27	Inflam.	NSAIDS, steroids, antibiotics
IBD-associated arthritis	Associated w/Crohn's or ulcerative colitis (UC)	Spine, sacroiliac, peripheral joints	Gradual onset of pain and stiffness	UC, Crohn's and associated features	HLA-B27	Inflam.	Steroids, sulfasalazine
Infectious arthritis	Predisposition: IV drug use, trauma, prosthetic joints, immunocompromise	Commonly single joint (knee) but multiple joints possible	Acute onset of joint pain, swelling, redness		Hyperuricemia may be present	Infectious, organisms	Antibiotics
Gout	More common in men	Most common: big toe, but other joints possible	Acute onset of joint pain, swelling, redness	Tophi in chronic gout		Inflam., monosodium urate crystals	• Acute: Anti-inflammatories (NSAIDS, colchicine) • Chronic:
Pseudogout	More common in men	Can have monoarticular presentation (knee common) or polyarticular presentation	Acute (mimicking gout) or indolent (mimicking RA)			Inflam., calcium pyrophos-phate crystals	NSAIDS, colchicine

*Cardiac involvement (in psoriatic arthritis and ankylosing spondylitis) can include valvular disease, arrhythmia, and/or myocarditis.

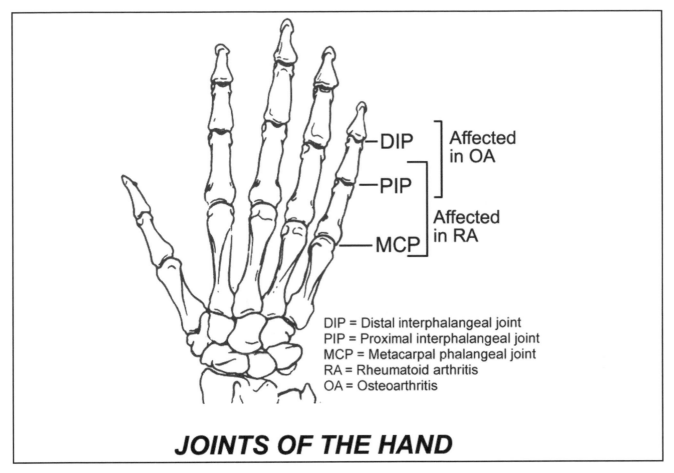

JOINTS OF THE HAND

Figure 8-3

neurological disease (CN VII lesion is common, see Fig. 7-11), and heart block. Diagnosis is made by identification of antibodies to *B. burgdorferi* in the serum.

In all cases of infectious arthritis, antibiotic treatment is directed against the offending organism.

Gout and Pseudogout

In these two diseases, joint inflammation is caused by crystals that form in the synovial fluid. In gout, these are uric acid crystals; in pseudogout, they are calcium pyrophosphate crystals. Both diseases are more common in men.

Gout

Gout is joint inflammation caused by uric acid crystals. Uric acid crystals only form in the setting of hyperuricemia (uric acid excess). Uric acid is a normal breakdown product of purines, which may come from the body itself (e.g., nucleic acid metabolism) or from diet (e.g., meats).

Uric acid excess can occur if there is:

- *Decreased excretion* of uric acid (e.g., renal failure, diuretics)

- *Overproduction* of uric acid
  - Overconsumption of purines in meats and alcoholic beverages (note: alcohol can also increase urate production)
  - Increased cellular turnover, e.g., hematologic malignancy
  - Obesity
  - HGPRT (hypoxanthine-guanine phosphoribosyltransferase) deficiency, e.g., Lesch-Nyan syndrome: an X-linked syndrome with severe HGPRT deficiency, causing hyperuricemia, mental retardation, self-mutilation, and spasticity

A classic acute gout attack is pain/warmth/swelling in a single joint, most commonly the big toe (called *podagra*), but other sites of first presentation are possible. A gout attack can be provoked by trauma, alcohol, or drugs (e.g., diuretics). Chronic hyperuricemia can lead to renal insufficiency, kidney stones, and the formation of *tophi*. Tophi are clumps of uric acid crystals in soft tissues that can be palpated on exam.

Diagnosis of gout is confirmed by seeing needle-shaped monosodium urate (MSU) crystals in synovial fluid. Uric acid crystals are strongly negatively birefringent, meaning that they are yellow when parallel to polarized light and blue when perpendicular to this light (the opposite is true of calcium pyrophosphate crystals in pseudogout). Synovial fluid will be *inflammatory* in gout (i.e., it will have > 2000 WBCs).

Treatment of an acute attack of gout is aimed at decreasing the inflammatory response, while the goal of chronic therapy is to lower serum uric acid. Anti-inflammatories commonly used for acute gout attacks are NSAIDs, colchicine, and steroids. Weight loss and decreased consumption of alcohol and purine-rich foods (meat, alcohol) are important components of long-term prevention of gout attacks. In addition, urate-lowering agents can be used. These agents function by *decreasing uric acid production* (e.g., *allopurinol*, which inhibits xanthine oxidase, an enzyme at a late step in purine metabolism) or *decreasing renal uric acid reabsorption* (e.g., *probenecid*).

Pseudogout

Pseudogout is joint inflammation caused by calcium pyrophosophate crystals. Unlike gout, pseudogout is not caused by elevated plasma level of a crystal-forming substance, but by increased accumulation of such substances in the synovial fluid. The cause of this accumulation is unknown but is thought to be secondary to production of calcium pyrophosphate in the joint by chondrocytes. There may be an association with hyperparathyroidism, hypothryoidism, and/or hemochromatosis, but these are debated. Pseudogout can present acutely in one joint like gout (though more commonly in the knee, as opposed to the big toe in gout), or it can sometimes have a more indolent onset, mimicking rheumatoid arthritis. Diagnosis: Synovial fluid demonstrates inflammation (>2000 WBCs) and rhomboid-shaped crystals that are weakly positively birefringent, meaning that on polarized light, they are blue when parallel and yellow when perpendicular (note, all opposites of MSU crystals). As with gout, treatment involves anti-inflammatories such as NSAIDs and colchicine.

CHAPTER 9. MALE AND FEMALE REPRODUCTIVE SYSTEMS

MALE REPRODUCTIVE ORGAN PATHOPHYSIOLOGY

Prostate

The prostate gland surrounds the urethra and secretes some of the seminal fluid. Because of its location, pathology of the prostate can cause symptoms of urethral obstruction: incomplete emptying of the bladder, poor urinary stream strength, frequency (frequent need to urinate), urgency (sudden need to urinate), hesitancy (starting and stopping of urinary stream), and nocturia (increased urination at night). Infection (*prostatitis*) or enlargement (*benign prostatic hypertrophy*) of the prostate can cause any or all of these symptoms

Prostatitis

Prostatitis (inflammation of the prostate) can be acute or chronic. Bacterial causes include *E. coli* and other gram negative rods, *N. gonorrhoeae,* and *Chlamydia trachomatis*. These bacteria can enter the prostate via the urethra, hematogenously, or during urologic procedures. Symptoms can include fever, chills, dysuria (pain during urination), other urinary symptoms (frequency, urgency, etc.), and/or pain in the low back, pelvis, and/or on ejaculation. The inflamed prostate is tender and soft ("boggy") on exam. Urinalysis demonstrates WBCs and can be used to culture causative organisms. Chronic prostatitis can lead to recurrent UTIs.

So-called "non-bacterial" prostatitis can cause any/all of the above symptoms and signs, including WBCs on urinalysis, but no organism can be cultured from urinalysis. Some suspect difficult-to-culture organisms as causes, e.g., *Chlamydia, Mycobacteria, Mycoplasma,* or fungi.

Antibiotics are used for treatment; fluoroquinolones and trimethoprim-sulfamethoxazole (TMP-SMZ) have the best prostate penetration. NSAIDs and sitz baths (sitting in warm water) can be used to relieve pain.

Benign Prostatic Hypertrophy

With age, the prostate enlarges. Enlargement can compress the urethra, leading to a variety of urinary symptoms, such as incomplete bladder emptying, poor urinary stream strength, urinary frequency, urgency, hesitancy, and/or nocturia. Obstruction can weaken the bladder over time, leading to retention of urine, which predisposes to urinary tract infection. Treatment is either pharmacologic or surgical. Inhibition of 5-alpha reductase (e.g., *finasteride*) decreases testos-terone formation, decreasing testosterone stimulation of prostate growth. Alpha blockade (e.g., *prazosin, terazosin*) relaxes smooth muscle, easing urinary flow through the urethra. If pharmacologic therapy fails, the prostate can be removed by transurethral resection of the prostate (TURP) or open surgery if it is too large to be removed by TURP.

Prostate Cancer

Prostate cancer is one of the most common cancers in men, with a high incidence in older men. Prostate cancer arises most often in the peripheral part of the prostate, so the urethra often remains unaffected, and thus the patient may be asymptomatic. Screening via digital rectal exam (DRE) and serum prostate-specific antigen (PSA) are therefore extremely important in men over 50. Diagnosis is made by transrectal ultrasound-guided biopsy. Bone metastases are common, and back pain resulting from spine metastases can be a presenting symptom. Treatment can include surgery, radiation, chemotherapy, and/or hormonal therapy. Hormonal therapy seeks to remove hormonal stimulation (mainly testosterone stimulation) of the prostate. This can be accomplished by orchiectomy (removing the testicles removes the main source of testosterone), anti-androgen therapy (blocking testosterone), or LHRH (LH releasing hormone) agonists. LHRH agonists initially increase LH secretion (and testosterone secretion) but the over-stimulation of LHRH receptors eventually leads to their down-regulation, causing a decrease in LH secretion and a subsequent decrease in testosterone secretion.

Testicles

During development, the testicles descend from the abdomen to their place outside the body in the scrotum. Their function is to produce sperm and seminal fluid. The testicles can become inflamed (*orchitis*), "tangled" (*torsion*), and they can develop testicular cancer.

Orchitis

Orchitis is testicular inflammation. Mumps is the most common cause of orchitis, though *Gonorrhea* and *Chlamydia* are also potential culprits. In immunocompromised patients, orchitis can be caused by fungi and mycobacteria. *Gonorrhea* and *Chlamydia* can also cause epididymitis (inflammation of the epididymis). Symptoms and signs of orchitis include testicular pain, swelling, and constitutional symptoms (e.g., fever, malaise). The causative organism can be cultured from urinalysis. Viral orchitis resolves spontaneously, but oral antibiotics are used for bacterial causes. Testicular pain can be treated with ice, bed rest, and analgesic therapy.

Torsion

Torsion is the twisting of the spermatic cord, causing compromised flow through the testicular artery and ischemia. This can be caused by trauma, exercise, or from predisposition secondary to undescended testes or a congenital "bell clapper" deformity (which allows for extra ease of rotation of the spermatic cord). Testicular torsion is most common in men under 30. Symptoms and signs include severe scrotal pain, swelling and erythema of the scrotum, abdominal pain, and/or nausea/vomiting. The abdominal pain is referred pain; the testes descend from the abdomen during development and thus can refer pain there. Prompt surgical repair is necessary to prevent loss of the testicle secondary to infarction.

Testicular Cancer

Testicular cancer can be completely asymptomatic, or it can present as a testicular mass, infertility, pain, and/or a sensation of testicular "fullness." It is more common in relatively young men (usually younger than 40). Failure of testicular descent at birth (*cryptorchidism*) is a risk factor for development of testicular cancer. The most common sites of metastasis are the retroperitoneal lymph nodes and the mediastinum. AFP (alpha fetoprotein), beta-hCG (human chorionic gonadotropin), and LDH (lactate dehydrogenase) may be elevated in the serum as tumor markers; diagnosis is made by ultrasound. Treatment involves surgical removal of the affected testicle combined with radiation and/or chemotherapy.

Erectile Dysfunction

Achievement of erection is as dependent on neurologic and vascular function as it is on psychological factors. Thus, any medications (e.g., antidepressants, antihypertensives), trauma/surgery, or diseases that affect the vasculature (e.g., atherosclerosis, hypertension, diabetes) or the nervous system (depression, diabetes, stroke) can lead to erectile dysfunction, as can any psychological issues in the man or between the man and his partner. Erection occurs via vasodilation, causing entry of blood into the penis. This is accomplished when paraysmpathetic nerves innervating the penile vasculature release nitric oxide, which stimulates production of cGMP, which causes vasodilation. cGMP is broken down by PDE-5. Viagra (*sildenafil*), a common treatment for impotence, works by inhibiting PDE-5. This decreases breakdown of cGMP, which prolongs erection.

FEMALE REPRODUCTIVE ORGAN PATHOPHYSIOLOGY

The Menstrual Cycle, Oral Contraceptives, and Amenorrhea

The Menstrual Cycle

Fig. 9-1. The menstrual cycle. Approximately every 28 days from puberty until menopause, a woman releases an ovum and prepares the uterine wall for implantation. If the ovum is not fertilized, the prepared endometrium is sloughed during menstruation. These processes are mediated by LH (leuteinizing hormone), FSH (follicle stimulating hormone), estrogen, and progesterone.

Day 1 of the menstrual cycle corresponds to menstruation, at which time a new ovum-containing *follicle* begins to grow under the influence of FSH (follicle stimulating hormone) from the pituitary. FSH stimulates the follicle to secrete estrogen, which causes the *proliferation* of the endometrial lining, preparing it for implantation in the event of pregnancy (ovum: *follicular* phase; endometrial lining: *proliferative* phase). In what is a rare physiologic instance of a positive feedback loop, estrogen secretion from the follicle stimulates an increase in LH and FSH secretion from the pituitary. This feedback loop leads to an LH surge, which, around Day 14 in the cycle, causes the ovum to be released (*ovulation*) and the follicle to become the *corpus luteum*, which secretes estrogen and progesterone. The estrogen and progesterone stimulate development of *secretory* glands in the endometrium (ovum: *luteal* phase; endometrial lining: *secretory* phase).

If the ovum is not fertilized, the continued estrogen and progesterone secretion will inhibit FSH and LH, leading to their decreased secretion. The fall in LH and FSH leads to the degeneration of the corpus luteum, resulting in a decrease in estrogen and progesterone secretion, causing sloughing of the endometrium (menstruation), returning the cycle to the beginning. The now low estrogen and progesterone allow for FSH and LH secretion to rise again, beginning the cycle anew. Note that estrogen can function both to increase LH/FSH secretion (leading to ovulation) *and* to inhibit it (at the end of the luteal phase). Birth control pills (oral contraceptives or OCPs) are combination estrogen/progesterone pills that serve to suppress LH/FSH, preventing ovulation.

Amenorrhea

The distinction between primary amenorrhea and secondary amenorrhea does *not* refer to the localization of the problem as in other endocrine disorders. *Primary amenorrhea* refers to the situation in which a woman

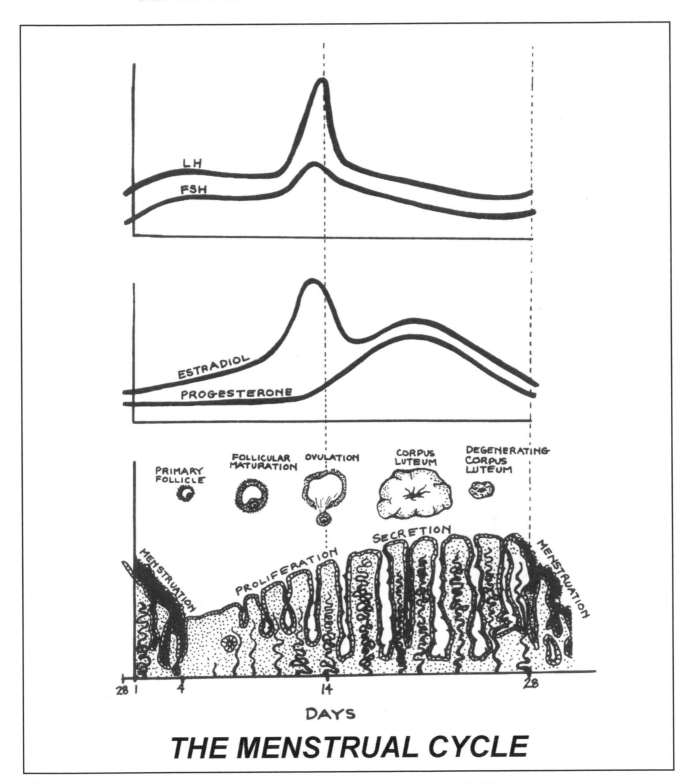

Figure 9-1. From Goldberg: *Clinical Physiology Made Ridiculously Simple*, MedMaster 2004

has *never* menstruated. *Secondary amenorrhea* refers to the situation in which a woman has *ceased* menstruating. In any case of amenorrhea, a pregnancy test (hCG) needs to be ordered to rule pregnancy in or out. Assuming the woman is not pregnant, primary and secondary amenorrhea have overlapping but slightly different differential diagnoses.

Fig. 9-2. Causes of amenorrhea. Pathology can occur anywhere along this axis. Starting from the bottom, anatomical anomalies can occur that block the passage of menses. Examples include imperforate hymen, vaginal agenesis, or disorders such as testicular femi-

nization or androgen insensitivity. The latter two conditions cause XY individuals to appear female externally despite lacking functional female internal genitalia.

Working our way up, the ovaries can be nonfunctional in Turner's syndrome, or fail secondary to drugs (e.g., cancer chemotherapy) or as a result of menopause. The pituitary can fail in its FSH/LH secretion secondary to hemorrhage (e.g., *Sheehan's syndrome*) or if there is a tumor within the pituitary or nearby. The hypothalamus can fail to secrete GnRH because of a tumor, congenital deficiency (e.g., *Kallmann's syn-*

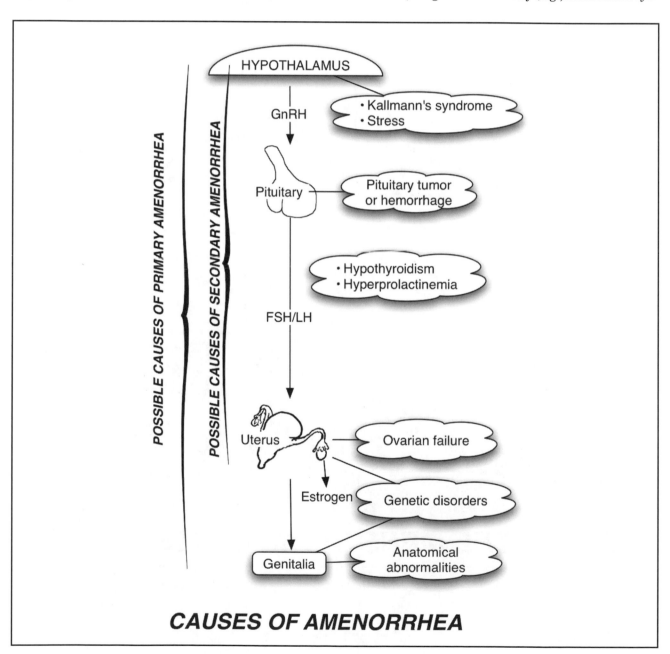

CAUSES OF AMENORRHEA

Figure 9-2

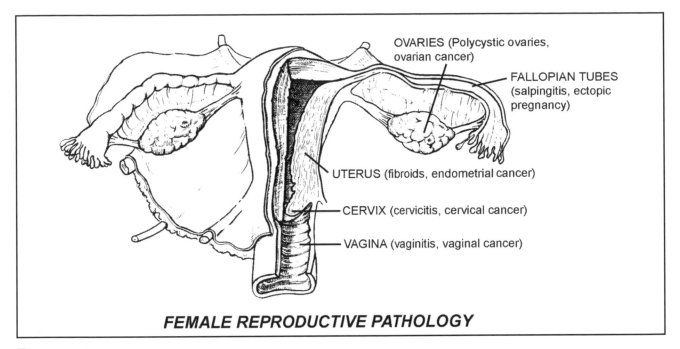

FEMALE REPRODUCTIVE PATHOLOGY

OVARIES (Polycystic ovaries, ovarian cancer)

FALLOPIAN TUBES (salpingitis, ectopic pregnancy)

UTERUS (fibroids, endometrial cancer)

CERVIX (cervicitis, cervical cancer)

VAGINA (vaginitis, vaginal cancer)

Figure 9-3

drome: loss of GnRH secreting-cells and olfactory neurons), or because of stresses such as excessive weight loss or exercise. Hypothyroidism and hyperprolactinemia can also lead to amenorrhea.

Anything from the ovaries and up (pituitary, thyroid, hypothalamus) can present as primary *or* secondary amenorrhea. Alternatively, *structural abnormalities of the uterus and vagina can only present as primary amenorrhea*, since the anatomy must be intact if periods have occurred in the past. So in primary amenorrhea it is important to rule out anatomical abnormalities by careful physical exam, and if warranted, imaging and karyotyping. Serum FSH can be measured to localize the site of pathology. If FSH is high, this suggests *ovarian failure*. Why? If the ovaries fail, the level of estrogen they secrete decreases, reducing the negative feedback on FSH secretion from the pituitary. This causes the pituitary to increase FSH release to try to increase estrogen secretion from the failing ovaries. Other important lab tests in amenorrhea are prolactin (to rule in/out hyperprolactinemia), TSH (to rule in/out hypothyroidism), and a

beta-hCG level to rule in/out pregnancy. History and physical should also assess the possibility of anorexia, excessive exercise, and/or severe stress.

Inflammation of the Female Genital Tract

Fig. 9-3. Female reproductive pathology.

Vaginitis

Vaginitis, inflammation of the vagina, can lead to itching/burning and an increase or change in vaginal discharge and/or odor. Inflammation/irritation can be caused by intercourse (and/or its associated products: lubricants, latex), hygiene products, atrophy of the vaginal wall in post-menopausal women, vulvar or vaginal cancer in rare cases, and infection.

Fig. 9-4. Infectious causes of vaginitis. Common infectious culprits include *Trichomonas vaginalis* (a protozoan), *Candida albicans* (yeast infection), *Gardnerella vaginalis* (bacterial vaginosis).

Figure 9-4 Vaginitis

ORGANISM	DISCHARGE	WET MOUNT	KOH/WHIFF TEST	TREATMENT
Trichomonas	Yellow, "frothy"	Protozoans	(no reaction)	Metronidazole (oral)
Candida	White, thick, "curds"	Branching yeast	(no reaction)	Topical antifungals
Gardnerella (Bacterial vaginosis)	Gray, thin	"Clue cells" (cells with many small bacteria attached to the surface)	Gives fishy odor (positive "whiff test")	Metronidazole (oral or vaginal cream)

Fig. 9-5. Vaginal lesions.

Men can also get any of the infections in Fig. 9-5. HPV infection in men usually leads to an asymptomatic carrier state. These men do not develop symptoms but can transmit the virus to sexual partners.

Cervicitis

Inflammation of the cervix can be caused by trauma, radiation, malignancy, or infection, e.g., *Chlamydia, gonorrhea*, herpes simplex virus (HSV), and human papilloma virus (HPV). HSV and HPV cervicitis generally co-exist with vaginitis, causing the symptoms discussed in Fig. 9-5. A classic symptom of cervical disease (including malignancy) is post-coital bleeding (bleeding immediately following intercourse). *Chlamydia* and *gonorrhea* infections of the lower genital tract tend to be asymptomatic, but these agents can spread past the cervix to the endometrium (myometritis/endometritis) and fallopian tubes (salpingitis), and even out into the abdominal cavity, causing pelvic inflammatory disease (PID).

Pelvic Inflammatory Disease (PID)

Pelvic inflammatory disease (PID) presents as acute abdominal pain, sometimes with nausea/vomiting. Abdominal exam reveals tenderness and can also show signs of peritonitis (rebound, guarding). Vaginal exam often demonstrates purulent cervical discharge and cervical motion tenderness (pain on movement of the cervix). This cervical discharge can be cultured for *Chlamydia* and *gonorrhea*. Treatment involves antibiotic therapy.

Complications of PID can include *Fitz-Hugh-Curtis syndrome* (inflammation/fibrosis surrounding the liver from intra-abdominal spread), tubo-ovarian abscess, infertility, and ectopic pregnancy. The latter two are results of scarring of the uterus/tubes from the infection.

Neoplasia of the Female Genital Tract

Vulvar, Vaginal, Cervical, Uterine, and Ovarian Neoplasia

Fig. 9-6. Neoplasia of the Female Genital Tract.

Gestational Trophoblastic Disease (GTD)

Gestational trophoblastic disease (GTD) occurs when a sperm fertilizes an "empty" ovum, i.e., an ovum with no maternal chromosomes in it. Such an egg can result from maternal nondisjunction, leaving one ovum with twice as much genetic material as normal and the other with none. This empty, so-called "blighted ovum" can be fertilized by one sperm, which then duplicates, creating a *complete mole*. Less commonly, an ovum with one set of maternal chromosomes can be fertilized by two sperm causing the formation of a *partial*

mole and abnormal triploid fetal tissue. A mole can present as pregnancy: enlarged uterus, nausea/vomiting, positive pregnancy test. Early bleeding may occur, and the uterus may be too large or too small for the presumed stage of pregnancy. Patients may notice vesicle-like material in vaginal bleeding. Diagnosis is confirmed by extreme elevation of beta-hCG and a "snowstorm" appearance on ultrasound. Immediate surgical removal is necessary, and beta-hCG is monitored to observe expected decrease after removal. Failure of beta-hCG to decrease indicates either incomplete removal of mole or possible malignant transformation (*choriocarcinoma*). Choriocarcinoma can invade blood vessels and metastasize to any organ, with the lungs being a common site. Fortunately, choriocarcinoma is very responsive to chemotherapy (usually involving methotrexate).

Other Diseases of the Female Genital Tract

Endometriosis

Endometriosis is the presence of endometrial tissue outside of the endometrium (inner uterine wall), e.g., on the ovaries, on the outer surface of the uterus or rectum, or elsewhere in the pelvis or abdominal cavity. Sites of endometriosis may be small or can be larger tumor-like endometriomas (also known as "chocolate cysts" because of the appearance of the thick dark liquid they contain). It is not known for sure how the endometriosis arises (or arrives) at these sites. Theories of endometriosis include retrograde menstruation, metaplasia of other tissues into endometrial tissue, and vascular/lymphatic dissemination of endometrial tissue. Symptoms of endometriosis can include pain during menstruation (*dysmenorrhea*) and intercourse (*dyspareunia*), abdominal and/or pelvic pain, and/or infertility. Although occasionally a mass may be palpable on bimanual example, laparoscopic exam with biopsy is necessary to confirm the diagnosis. Since sites of endometriosis contain functional endometrial tissue, they are stimulated by estrogen just as the uterine lining is. Thus, blocking this estrogen stimulation reduces symptoms caused by the ectopic endometrial tissue. This can be accomplished with oral contraceptives, danazol (inhibitor of LH/FSH), and GnRH agonists. The GnRH agonist might at first sound illogical, since GnRH stimulates LH and FSH release. GnRH agonists do indeed stimulate the receptors of LH- and FSH-secreting cells of the anterior pituitary, but continuous stimulation leads to a down-regulation of these receptors, resulting in decrease in FSH/LH secretion. If medical therapy is unsuccessful, endometriosis tissue can be removed surgically.

Polycystic Ovary Syndrome (PCOS)

Polcystic ovary syndrome (PCOS) is characterized by increased androgens, leading to amenorrhea, hirsutism

Figure 9-5 Vaginal Lesions

ORGANISM	SYMPTOMS	SIGNS	DIAGNOSIS	TREATMENT
Herpes simplex virus (HSV)	Painful; dysuria, can be accompanied by constitutional symptoms	Vesicles (that can coalesce)	Viral culture (Tzanck Prep: multinucleated giant cells)	Acyclovir
Human papilloma virus (HPV) (genital warts, condyloma acuminata)	Painless; increased risk for cervical cancer	Papules	Biopsy	Topical creams, cryotherapy
Treponema pallidum (Syphilis)	• Chancre: painless ulcer • Primary: Lesion • Secondary: Systemic symptoms (constitutional + rash) • Tertiary: Abscesses (gummas), CNS effects, cardiac effects	Ulcerated papule	VDRL, RPR (false positives possible), FTA-ABS (treponemal antibody screen)	Penicillin
H. Ducreyi (Chancroid)	Painful chancre	Ulcerated papule	Gram stain (gram negative anaerobic)	Erythromycin or ceftriaxone

Figure 9-6 Neoplasia of the Female Genital Tract

PATHOLOGY	HISTOLOGY	SYMPTOMS/SIGNS	DIAGNOSIS	OTHER	TREATMENT
Vulvar cancer	Squamous (most common); melanoma	Itching, noticeable lesion	Biopsy	Rare	Surgery/radiation/chemo
Vaginal cancer	Squamous (most common); clear cell	Vaginal bleeding	Biopsy	Rare; clear cell associated w/ in utero DES* exposure	Surgery/radiation/chemo
Cervical cancer	Squamous	Post-coital bleeding	Pap smear screens for cervical metaplasia	Associated w/HPV	Surgery/radiation/chemo
Uterine fibroids	Benign leiomyomas	Bleeding, pain, urinary symptoms, infertility, palpable mass (can be asymptomatic)	Scan, biopsy		Surgery, embolization
Endometrial cancer	Adenocarcinoma most common (also leiomyosarcoma, stromal sarcoma)	Post-menopausal bleeding	Endometrial sampling/biopsy		Surgery/radiation/chemo
Ovarian cysts	Follicular or corpus luteum	Asymptomatic or abdominal/pelvic bloating/pain. Torsion possible ? acute pain; mass may be palpable	Ultrasound/ laparoscopy		Observation—most resolve spontaneously
Benign ovarian neoplasia	Epithelial (serous, mucinous adenomas), Sex cord/Stromal (Sertoli-Leydig cell, Granulosa-theca cell) Germ cell (teratoma, dysgerminoma)	(same as cysts)	Ultrasound/ laparoscopy/biopsy		Surgical removal
Ovarian cancer	Epithelial, germ cell, or stromal cell (metastasis to ovary also possible)	Often asymptomatic leading to diagnosis at advanced stage and poor prognosis. When present: Vague abdominal/pelvic pain/bloating; pelvic mass	Tumor markers CA-125, LDH, aFP, b-hCG can be elevated in the serum with certain tumors. Ultrasound, CT scan		Surgery/chemo/radiation

* DES= Diethylstilbestrol. DES is a synthetic estrogen that was once used during pregnancy in women who were at high risk for miscarriage. Female fetuses exposed to DES in utero are at higher risk for clear cell carcinoma of the vagina.

Figure 9-7 Inflammatory and Neoplastic Diseases of the Breast

PATHOLOGY	EPIDEMIOLOGY	PRESENTATION	DIAGNOSIS	TREATMENT
INFLAMMATORY DISEASES				
Mastitis	Nursing women; most commonly *Staph. aureus*	Acute breast pain, fever, and a warm and erythematous region of the breast	Clinical	Antibiotics, analgesics
Fat necrosis	Secondary to trauma or surgery	Firm, tender mass	Biopsy	None/excision
NEOPLASTIC DISEASES				
Fibrocystic changes	Very common in women of all ages	Cyclic diffuse pain (usually right before period), lumpiness of breasts on exam	Biopsy	None needed
Fibroadenoma	Very common in younger women (20s-40)	Mass: firm, well-circumscribed, painless, movable	Biopsy	None needed
Intraductal papilloma	Women ages 35-55	Bloody discharge from nipple	Biopsy	Removal
Breast cancer	Risk increases with age	Lump noticed by woman or physician; more rarely, pain or skin changes	Biopsy	Surgery, radiation, chemotherapy

(abnormally increased body hair), acne, infertility, obesity, and, in some cases, type II diabetes mellitus and *acanthosis nigricans* (velvety darkened areas of skin, most commonly in the axillae, on the back of the neck, and/or in the genital region). The syndrome most commonly emerges in late adolescence. The underlying cause of the increased androgens is unknown. Diagnosis is confirmed by increased serum androgens (e.g., testosterone, androstenedione) and increased LH with normal FSH. Glucose tolerance may be impaired. Most cases, but not all, will also have polycystic ovaries on ultrasound examination. Oral contraceptives can restore a regular menstrual cycle. OCPs also decrease LH, thus decreasing androgen production and reducing hirsutism and acne. If diabetes is present, it is treated with weight loss/exercise and metformin (See Fig. 5-9).

Diseases of the Breasts

Diseases of the breasts can be classified as inflammatory or neoplastic. Inflammatory diseases include mastitis and fat necrosis, while neoplastic diseases include a variety of benign lesions and breast cancer.

Fig. 9-7. Inflammatory and neoplastic diseases of the breasts.

Mastitis is an infection of the breast that most commonly occurs in women who are nursing a newborn. Mastitis presents as acute breast pain, fever, and a warm and erythematous region of the breast. *Staph. aureus* is the most common causative agent. Treatment involves antibiotics. If an abscess forms, this must be treated with surgical drainage.

Fat necrosis can occur secondary to trauma or surgery. This can result in a firm mass that may mimic breast cancer.

Note: Fibrocystic changes, mastitis, and fat necrosis all cause pain, but the pain in fibrocystic changes is cyclic and usually bilateral. In mastitis, pain is acute and usually unilateral (and generally accompanied by fever and erythema). Fat necrosis presents as tenderness when the area is touched.

Most breast masses are benign, but they should always be biopsied to rule out breast cancer.

Breast Cancer

Risk factors for breast cancer include prolonged estrogen exposure (i.e., from early menarche or late menopause), nulliparity (no pregnancy), family history, and increasing age. Although breast cancer can present as a breast mass or, rarely, as breast pain or inflammatory changes of the overlying skin, it is most often asymptomatic; thus, screening is essential. Women should be advised to do self breast exams monthly, and to have annual breast exams by a physician and mammograms after age 40.

A palpable mass or suggestive mammography findings are indications for biopsy. Biopsy can be accomplished by fine needle aspiration or surgical excision.

Treatment of breast cancer involves a combination of surgery, radiation, and chemotherapy, depending on the extent of disease.

Infertility

In order for a successful pregnancy to occur, the male must produce an adequate number of viable sperm, the sperm must be able to exit the male upon ejaculation, and the sperm must be able to make it to and fertilize the ova. The female must produce viable ova, and the ova must be able to successfully implant in the uterus. Problems with any of these steps can lead to infertility.

Problems in males leading to a low sperm count or malformed/malfunctioning sperm include chromosomal abnormalities, hormonal abnormalities (e.g., LH/FSH deficiency), testicular disease (cancer, orchitis), or blockage of the vas deferens or seminiferous tubules (which can occur congenitally or secondary to cystic fibrosis or prior surgery).

Problems in the female can be divided into those affecting ovulation and those affecting the anatomy. Problems affecting ovulation are any that can cause menstrual cycle disturbances (see Fig. 9-2). Anatomical problems can be congenital (see Fig. 9-2) or acquired (e.g., uterine fibroids, endometriosis, scarring from pelvic inflammatory disease). Anatomical problems can lead either to failure of sperm to arrive at the ovum and fertilize it, or failure of implantation of the fertilized ovum.

Diagnosis is made by semen analysis, amenorrhea workup (if applicable) and examination of the female anatomy (by hysterosalpingogram, ultrasound, and/or laparoscopy).

While anatomical abnormalities are generally treated with surgery, ovulatory problems may be treated with hormonal therapy. If no therapy is possible, use of a sperm donor, in vitro fertilization, and adoption are possible alternatives for couples seeking a child.

CHAPTER 10. CASES

Normal Serum Values:
Na+ 136-145 mEq/L
K+ 3.5-5.0 mEq/L
HCO_3^- 22-28 mEq/L
Cl- 95-105 mEq/L
pH 7.35-7.45
pCO_2 33-45 mm Hg
BUN 7-18 mg/dl
Creatinine 0.6-1.2 mg/dl

CASE 1

On routine exam of an otherwise healthy 78-year-old man, you note a systolic murmur. What are the possible etiologies of this murmur? What can help you determine the cause?

What happens normally during systole? The ventricles pump blood out through the aortic and pulmonic valves, and the shut mitral and tricuspid valves prevent back-flow into the atria. So what could cause a murmur during systole? Stenosis of either the aortic or pulmonic valves could cause a murmur, because the blood would pass through narrowed openings during systole. Regurgitant mitral or tricuspid valves could also cause systolic murmurs since the backflow through these regurgitant valves would occur during systole as well. A VSD could also cause a systolic murmur. Finally, a systolic "flow murmur" can be either normal, a sign of anemia, or it can occur with fever.

How can you distinguish among these causes? Associated symptoms, quality of the murmur, location of the murmur, radiation, associated signs, and maneuvers.

Associated symptoms may or may not be present depending on the severity of the valvular pathology. Severe aortic stenosis can lead to syncope and "decreased forward flow" symptoms (weakness, fatigue, shortness of breath) and/or ischemic symptoms (e.g., angina). Mitral regurgitation can cause "backup of flow" symptoms (shortness of breath, edema).

Quality of the murmur. Recall that stenotic valves take a little time to open and *then* the blood flows through and creates a murmur. On the other hand, regurgitant valves just flop right open with the slightest push. So aortic stenosis would be a systolic ejection murmur with a *crescendo-decrescendo* pattern, whereas mitral regurgitation would be *holosystolic*.

Location of the murmur. Is it over the aortic area or the pulmonic area? The tricuspid or the mitral? Recall that the aortic area is to the patient's right of the sternum and the pulmonic area is to the left. Mitral murmurs are best heard near the cardiac apex (Fig. 1-10).

Radiation. The murmur of aortic stenosis radiates straight up...to the carotids. Mitral regurgitation radiates to the left axilla.

Associated signs. What happens "downstream" when there is aortic stenosis? Because of the stenotic valve, the blood to the carotids arrives more weakly and late (*parvus et tardus*). What happens "upstream" (i.e., in the left ventricle) in aortic stenosis? The increased resistance faced by the left ventricle can lead to left ventricular hypertrophy. Left ventricular hypertrophy can cause a laterally displaced PMI (point of maximal impulse) and possibly an S4. Mitral regurgitation causes increased *volume* demand on the left ventricle, which can result in left ventricular dilatation. A dilated left ventricle can also laterally displace the PMI and could cause an S3. Both ventricular hypertrophy and ventricular dilatation can be seen as ventricular enlargement on chest X-ray. Since mitral regurgitation also increases the volume demands on the left atrium, an enlarged left atrium can be seen on chest X-ray if mitral regurgitation is present. Mitral regurgitation can also cause atrial fibrillation, which can be seen on EKG.

Finally, the two systolic murmurs can be distinguished by *maneuvers*. Maneuvers that increase peripheral resistance (e.g., clenching the fists) will increase the intensity of mitral regurgitation and have no effect on aortic stenosis.

Echocardiography can confirm the diagnosis. It can also measure the severity of the valvular lesion. This can help to determine whether surgery is necessary.

CASE 2

A 65-year-old woman with a history of diabetes, hypertension, and hypercholesterolemia presents to the ER with chest pain. What is the differential diagnosis?

Starting simply, what is in the chest, and how can these entities cause pain? In the chest: the lungs, the heart, the esophagus, aorta, and ribs/muscles. Possible causes of pain of these organs: injury, ischemia, infection, inflammation, neoplasia, obstruction (of the esophagus), muscle strain, and costochondritis.

What can make the heart hurt? Chest pain can be a sign of angina or myocardial infarction, both of which are manifestations of ischemia. Myocarditis, endocarditis, and pericarditis are examples of cardiac infection/inflammation, though out of these, typically only pericarditis causes chest pain.

What can make the esophagus hurt? Acid reflux (GERD), esophageal cancer, esophageal rupture, and esophagitis.

What can make the lungs hurt? Infection (pneumonia), inflammation of the lungs (or pleura), and pulmonary embolus.

What can make the aorta hurt? Dissection.

What can make the ribs/muscles hurt? Costochondritis, muscle strain.

Any time you deal with pain, your clinical history should elicit characteristics of the pain (e.g., timing, palliation, quality, region) that can help to refine your differential diagnosis: What does the pain feel like? Where does it hurt? Did it begin suddenly or gradually? How long has the pain been there? Has anything like this ever happened before? What makes it better or worse?

Timing. It is useful to distinguish between acute onset and more protracted onset of pain. For example, ischemia or rupture of an organ are acute events. More specific examples of such acute events include myocardial infarction, pulmonary embolus, esophageal rupture, and aortic dissection. Alternatively, the pain of GERD or pneumonia can come about less suddenly. If the "same chest pain has happened before," this could be angina or GERD.

Palliation. How would you distinguish between the pain of GERD and the pain of a heart attack and/or angina? Remember the pathophysiology: GERD occurs secondary to reflux of acid from the stomach to esophagus, cardiac ischemia occurs from a mismatch of oxygen demand and supply in the myocardium. In what situations would you expect the patient to have pain from either of these pathophysiological bases? Cardiac pain would most likely occur when the difference between the supply and demand of oxygen is exacerbated, i.e., in a time of increased demand such as increased physical activity/exercise. This would cause shortness of breath, a symptom we would *not* expect to find in GERD. GERD will be relieved by antacids and can be exacerbated by lying horizontally or bending over, since these positions increase reflux. Exercise should have no effect on GERD's symptoms. Pericarditis pain can also get worse when a patient lies down, but it is characteristically relieved when the patient leans forward.

When in doubt, an EKG can assess the possibility of a cardiac-related cause of chest pain.

Quality. The quality of the pain may also give clues to its origin: "pressure" in ischemia, "tearing" in dissection, "burning" in GERD, stabbing upon breathing in if the pain is pleuritic.

Region / Radiation. Aortic dissection is an acute cause of chest pain that should always be considered, since it can be fatal if not immediately repaired. The patient may report "tearing, ripping pain" radiating through to the back. The pain of myocardial infarction can radiate to the chest, jaw, and/or arm.

Associated findings / diagnostic tests:

Infections such as endocarditis or pneumonia will often cause fever and an increased WBC count.

Pericarditis can cause a *pericardial rub* to be heard on auscultation.

Endocarditis can present with a new cardiac murmur.

In aortic dissection, blood pressures in the arms may differ, and there may be a widened mediastinum on chest X-ray.

A pulmonary embolus can also present acutely as chest pain and/or shortness of breath. An EKG can show signs of right heart strain and a chest X-ray can reveal signs of infarction, but these are not present in all cases; the chest X-ray is often completely normal in patients with pulmonary embolism. When suspecting pulmonary embolism, spiral CT scanning or ventilation perfusion scanning is often necessary. D-dimer level in the serum is a diagnostic marker that can also help to rule in or out the diagnosis of pulmonary embolism.

A detailed discussion of the predictive value and timing of the presence of various *cardiac enzymes* is beyond the scope of this text. Let it suffice to say that when cardiac tissue dies (i.e., when it is infarcted) some of the cardiac enzymes, e.g., creatine kinase (CK) and troponin, are released into the bloodstream, and high levels of these enzymes can be indicative of cardiac injury (e.g., myocardial infarction).

CASE 3

A newborn baby looks blue. What is the differential diagnosis?

If the baby is blue, deoxygenated blood is somehow making it into the circulation. What are the possible etiologies? We have seen various cardiac causes of cyanosis in Chapter 1 (e.g., tetralogy of Fallot, transposition of the great arteries). However, the heart could be fine, and the *lungs* may not be doing their job of oxygenating the blood. Examples include meconium aspiration, tracheoesophageal fistula, congenital diaphragmatic hernia, etc.

Can you think of any other organ systems whose dysfunction could lead to cyanosis? The lungs may bring the oxygen to the blood and the heart may bring the blood to the lungs, but the *blood itself* may be incapable of receiving the oxygen. What part of the blood is necessary for oxygen uptake? Hemoglobin. So hemoglobinopathy is one possible cause of neonatal cyanosis. *Methemoglobinemia* is one cause of hemoglobinopathy in the newborn. Methemoglobinemia can be induced by toxin ingestion or an inborn error of metabolism. Finally, CNS dysfunction can lead to respiratory depression, and neuromuscular disorders can lead to impairment of respiratory muscle function.

With any symptom or sign, think of *all* of the possible physiologic mechanisms that could lead to its appearance. Pathology in the blood, lungs, heart, and/or neuromuscular system can lead to cyanosis.

CASE 4

A 60-year-old man is found to have a pulse of 40 beats per minute on physical exam. What are the possible pathophysiologic mechanisms underlying this slow heart rate?

A heart rate below 60 is defined as bradycardia. First, just because there is bradycardia does not necessarily mean that there is pathology. Some elderly patients, conditioned athletes, and children can have asymptomatic bradycardia.

What are the potential pathological causes of bradycardia? Either the pacemaker (the SA node) is firing slowly, or the SA node is firing normally, but the signal is getting blocked somewhere (heart block). Causes include ischemia of the SA node (e.g., atherosclerosis), previous myocardial infarction (i.e., infarction of the conduction system), drugs (e.g., beta blockers, calcium channel blockers, anti-arrhythmics), hypothyroidism, or infiltrative diseases.

CASE 5

Ten days after an acute myocardial infarction, a 67-year-old woman suddenly complains of chest pain. She is confused, short of breath, pale, and weak. What are the possible etiologies of these symptoms?

There are a variety of post-myocardial infarction complications that could cause these symptoms: a second myocardial infarction, arrhythmia (e.g., conduction block, ventricular fibrillation, or any other arrhythmia), papillary muscle rupture leading to acute mitral regurgitation, ventricular wall rupture leading to tamponade, and ventricular septal rupture.

Let's say that on examination this patient has increased JVP, hypotension, and distant heart sounds. Now what do you think?

If the blood pressure is *down* but the JVP is *up,* what does that tell you? It must mean that forward flow is decreased (hypotension), and flow is backing up (elevated JVP). Arrhythmia or acute mitral regurgitation are possible, *but* there is *no new murmur* here. If there were acute mitral regurgitation, there

would be a new *systolic* murmur. Rather than a new murmur, in this case there are *distant heart sounds.* How could that be? There must be something *between* the heart and the stethoscope that was not there before. This triad of symptoms (increased JVP, decreased blood pressure, and distant heart sounds) is known as *Beck's triad* and is associated with cardiac tamponade. Tamponade can be caused by ventricular rupture after a myocardial infarction as in this case. The diagnosis can be confirmed with an echocardiogram or by pericardiocentesis, and urgent surgical repair is essential. Unfortunately, many of these patients do not survive.

CASE 6

A 45-year-old woman complains of shortness of breath when she climbs stairs or runs. What is your differential diagnosis?

When a patient presents with shortness of breath on exertion, the cause can be cardiac (e.g., angina, heart failure), pulmonary (e.g., when pulmonary function is impaired), or hematological (i.e., anemia). How could you distinguish among these by history and physical exam?

On history: does the patient have a history of cardiac or pulmonary disease or of predisposing factors to either (e.g., hypertension for cardiac disease or smoking for pulmonary disease)? Are there additional symptoms of cardiac disease (e.g., orthopnea, paroxysmal nocturnal dyspnea) or pulmonary disease (e.g., wheezing) or anemia (e.g., seeking strange foods such as ice in iron deficiency or peripheral numbness/tingling in B12 deficiency)? Are there episodic exacerbations in response to cold, allergens, or exercise (e.g., asthma), or has the course been more chronic and indolent (e.g., progressive interstitial lung disease, emphysema, or cardiac disease)?

On physical exam: is there a displaced point of maximal impulse/impact (PMI), which could indicate a hypertrophied or dilated heart)? Is there a murmur, or an S3 or S4, that would indicate cardiac disease? Does lung percussion yield dullness (e.g., consolidation or edema) or increased resonance (e.g., hyperexpansion, pneumothorax)? Is there tachycardia and pallor (which could indicate anemia)? Is there fever and sputum production (e.g., pneumonia or COPD flare)?

Cardiac function can be assessed with EKG, exercise stress testing and/or coronary angiography. Anemia can be ruled in or out by looking at hemoglobin, hematocrit, and blood smear. A chest X-ray could indicate whether there is cardiac enlargement, pulmonary congestion, hyperexpansion, tumor, interstitial disease, etc. Pulmonary function can be assessed with pulmonary function tests (PFTs).

In this patient, PFTs revealed a *normal* FEV1/FVC ratio with *decreased* DLCO. A normal FEV1/FVC ratio tells us that this is probably *not* obstructive lung disease, but does not rule out lung disease. Restrictive lung disease can still have a normal FEV1/FVC ratio. The decreased DLCO tells us that the membrane is somehow thickened, preventing optimal diffusion. The combination of normal FEV1/FVC ratio and decreased DLCO is most consistent with restrictive lung disease secondary to pulmonary fibrosis. When you go back for a closer look at this patient, you notice some dilated capillaries in the nail beds, some telangectasia, and some minor tightening of the skin of the hands and forehead. You suspect that this patient has scleroderma with pulmonary fibrosis. A test for anti-centromere antibodies comes back positive, confirming your diagnosis.

CASE 7

A 65-year-old man with a long history of smoking presents with acute onset of shortness of breath, wheezing, and fever. A chest x-ray shows hyperexpansion of the lungs. What is the most likely diagnosis and how would you treat the patient?

With acute onset of shortness of breath, life-threatening causes must be ruled out, e.g., cardiac (myocardial infarction, arrhythmia), pulmonary embolus, tension pneumothorax, etc. In this patient, the smoking history and signs of obstruction (wheezing, hyperexpansion on chest X-ray) point to obstructive lung disease. The accompanying fever and acute onset seem most consistent with a COPD flare, perhaps secondary to infection. Treatment would involve antibiotics to fight the infection, anti-inflammatories to combat the inflammation (e.g., prednisone), and beta-agonists to activate the sympathetic nervous system to *open* the airways (e.g., albuterol, as long as the patient does not have cardiac disease).

CASE 8

A 7-year-old boy complains of "getting tired" in gym class. Further history reveals that the tiredness seems to be a difficulty with breathing. What is the differential diagnosis?

Again, with exertional dyspnea, cardiac causes must be ruled out. Congenital defects must be considered in children and could be suggested by murmurs on physical exam and confirmed by echocardiography. EKG could assess the possibility of arrhythmia. Chest X-ray could indicate anatomical abnormalities, hyperexpansion in pulmonary obstructive disease, and/or consolidation in pneumonia. With this child, further history reveals that the child only has trouble breathing during heavy exercise, and his mother notices that he seems to be making a funny whistling sound when

he tries to catch his breath. The diagnosis is exercise-induced asthma. One can give the child an inhaler of albuterol (to activate beta receptors and open the airways), ipratropium (to block acetylcholine receptors, thus blocking the parasympathetic system's closure of the airways), or steroids and/or drugs like cromolyn (which block the inflammatory response).

CASE 9

An obese 55-year-old man complains of dozing off at work and even once while driving. His wife reports that he snores quite loudly. What is the most likely diagnosis?

This patient may have sleep apnea. The snoring indicates some narrowing of the airway at night. This may be accompanied by episodes of complete upper airway obstruction during sleep that result in repetitive hypoxemic events and arousals from sleep. The frequent interruptions in normal sleep can result in extreme fatigue during the day. The diagnosis could be confirmed by doing a sleep study, during which the patient's sleep is observed overnight in a sleep lab. During the study, breathing patterns, sleep stages, and oxygen saturation are examined for signs of apneic events. Patients diagnosed with sleep apnea benefit from weight loss and/or a nasal continuous positive airway pressure (CPAP) mask at night. The CPAP keeps the airway open, thus preventing apnea secondary to upper airway collapse.

CASE 10

A 75-year-old man with long-standing pulmonary fibrosis from extensive asbestos exposure now presents with edema, elevated JVP, and ascites. What is the most likely pathophysiology underlying these symptoms?

The edema, elevated JVP, and ascites indicate right heart failure. The history of long-standing pulmonary fibrosis should lead you to expect that pulmonary hypertension has given rise to these symptoms. Pulmonary fibrosis leads to distortion of the architecture of the pulmonary vasculature, which increases the vascular resistance, causing pulmonary hypertension. This pulmonary hypertension leads to increased work for the side of the heart that is pumping into it: the right heart. This increased workload eventually causes failure of the thin-walled right heart (*cor pulmonale*). When the right heart fails, its forward pumping ability is reduced, and blood backs up into its input, which is the venous system. This backup is manifested in edema, elevated JVP, and ascites.

CASE 11

A mother brings in her 4-year-old daughter because she says the child's urine looks dark. She says this is the first time it has ever looked dark. What is the differential diagnosis?

Dark urine could signify hematuria, but what *outside* the genitourinary system could lead to dark urine? Any hemolytic anemia (e.g., sickle cell) can cause hemoglobinuria. Dark urine can be a sign of jaundice from conjugated bilirubin. Why is it important that this was the first time the urine was dark? If the child were younger (or the urine has always been dark) you would want to consider inborn errors of metabolism (e.g., alkaptonuria).

In hematuria, it is necessary to distinguish an upper genitourinary tract (i.e., glomerular) source of bleeding from a lower GU tract (i.e., bladder, urethra, genitals) source. To distinguish the two by history, ask whether there is frank blood or if the urine is rather "cola-colored." If the blood is coming from the genitals or urethra it is more likely to be visible as red, whereas blood from a glomerulopathy tends to turn the urine "cola-colored." It is important to rule out genital or urethral trauma (e.g., abuse) as a cause of hematuria. If the urine is cola-colored and there is no history or evidence of trauma, why would a child have glomerulonephritis? What is one question you should definitely ask? Ask the mother "did the child just recently get over a sore throat?" Post-infectious (often streptococcal) glomerulonephritis can cause hematuria in a child.

What about the urinalysis could help you distinguish whether the bleeding is up at the level of the glomeruli or coming from lower in the genitourinary tract? Red cells that come from bleeding in the glomeruli would appear squished and damaged in urinalysis. Red cell *casts* always signify glomerular disease. Damaged glomeruli in glomerulonephritis can also lead to elevated protein leaking through into the urine (proteinuria). Infection (i.e., UTI) can also cause hematuria and would present with the complaint of pain on urination and WBCs in the urinalysis. You know hematuria in adults should raise suspicion for stones (especially when accompanied by flank pain), but can children have stones? They can if they have genetic disorders of metabolism or medications that cause hypercalciuria or hyperuricosuria. Crystals in urinalysis can be present in such instances.

CASE 12

Three days after resection of a pituitary tumor, a patient develops confusion, lethargy, and increased dilute urine output. Serum sodium is measured at 160. What is the differential diagnosis?

An elevated serum sodium with an *increased* urine output means one of three possibilities:

- *Hypovolemic hypernatremia* (i.e., massive loss of urine fluid leaves behind a hypernatremic serum)

- *Euvolemic hypernatremia* (i.e., less drastic urine fluid loss leaves behind a hypernatremic serum)

- *Hypervolemic hypernatremia* (i.e., massive hypertonic intake leading to hypernatremia and increased urine output in an attempt to get rid of the excess volume. This could occur from an IV solution).

Any association of sodium/volume abnormalities and neurosurgical procedures should make you think of some problem with ADH. Is ADH elevated or decreased in this case? ADH causes an increase in water absorption from the collecting duct. So if we have an increased urine output and increased serum sodium, is ADH increased or decreased?

The increased serum sodium here suggests concentration of the serum (i.e., the opposite of dilution), which could mean fluid loss...and the urine volume is increased. So it looks like there is a *failure* of ADH. Fluid is not being appropriately retained but rather *lost,* leading to an increased dilute urine output and hypernatremia in the serum secondary to this water loss. This is diabetes insipidus. Diabetes insipidus can be central or nephrogenic. Here, given the history of pituitary surgery, central is most likely. How can you check? You can give an injection of ddAVP (synthetic ADH). How will this help make the diagnosis? If the kidneys respond to the ddAVP by retaining water, the urine will become more concentrated. This will only occur if the kidneys *can* respond, thus indicating central diabetes insipidus. If there is no response to ddAVP, the urine will remain dilute; this occurs in nephrogenic diabetes insipidus (Fig. 3-9).

CASE 13

A patient is brought to the emergency room unconscious. The labs show $Na^+ = 145$, $K^+ = 5$, $Cl^- = 114$, pH = 7.2, $HCO_3^- = 9$ $CO_2 = 22$. Urinalysis shows calcium oxalate crystals. Choose from one of the following, give a differential diagnosis, and suggest the most likely diagnosis.

- ▶ R espiratory acidosis
- ▶ Respiratory alkalosis
- ▶ Metabolic acidosis
- ▶ Metabolic alkalosis

With a pH of 7.2, we are dealing with acidosis. The next question then is whether it is respiratory or metabolic acidosis. Here, HCO_3^- and CO_2 are both decreased. What does this suggest? First, a low HCO_3^- with acidosis suggests metabolic acidosis. Second, you know that respiratory acidosis comes from *increased* CO_2, so a decreased CO_2 could not *cause* an acidosis. So this must be *metabolic acidosis with respiratory com-*

pensation. Now what's causing it? In metabolic acidosis, the first step is to determine whether there is an anion gap or not. How do you calculate an anion gap?

$Na^+ - Cl^- - HCO_3^-$. In this case 145 - (9+114) = 22, so we *do* have an anion gap. What does an anion gap tell us? It tells us that there is some extra acid in the serum accounting for the gap...and the possibilities are the MUDPILES (Methanol, uric acid, diabetic ketoacidosis, paraldehyde, isoniazid/iron, lactic acid, ethylene glycol, salicylates). The presence of calcium oxalate crystals in the urine is most consistent with *ethylene glycol ingestion*.

CASE 14

After a long day outside at a family picnic in mid-July, an 85-year-old woman is brought to the ER after her family found her acting "weird." They say she had just been getting over a bad bout of food poisoning from which she had diarrhea and vomiting. The labs show BUN = 75, Cr = 2.5. How do you explain the labs? What would you expect to see on physical exam? How would you treat the abnormality?

From the history of disorientation following heat exposure, diarrhea, and vomiting, this has something to do with dehydration. But what does dehydration have to do with the abnormal BUN and creatinine? An elevated creatinine signifies renal failure, so the question is whether this is prerenal, renal, or postrenal failure. Postrenal failure occurs from obstruction and if this is an acute event (i.e., nephrolithiasis) one would expect complaints of flank pain, hematuria, etc. How can we distinguish between prerenal and intrinsic renal failure? BUN/Cr ratio holds a clue. Here the BUN/Cr ratio is 75/2.5 = 30. Remember that a BUN/Cr ratio greater than 20:1 generally indicates *prerenal failure* (Fig. 3-2). Is prerenal failure a logical diagnosis for this patient? Yes; dehydration leads to decreased perfusion of the kidneys, which is the definition of prerenal failure.

What would you expect to find on exam as signs of dehydration? Dry mucous membranes, tenting of the skin, tachycardia. What would the labs show? Remember the physiology underlying prerenal failure: the kidneys are not being adequately perfused. In an effort to counteract this, the kidneys go on a reabsorbing spree via the renin-angiotensin-aldosterone and ADH systems. This leads to reabsorption of sodium and water respectively from the filtrate in the collecting tubule. Thus, we would expect the urine to be very concentrated (since the water was pulled out by ADH) and also for FENa to be *decreased* (because aldosterone stimulates sodium reabsorption).

The treatment: volume expansion with IV fluids. How do you expand intravascular volume? That is, do you want hypertonic, hypotonic, or isotonic saline? If you put hypotonic solution in the veins, water would flow out of the vasculature into cells, but we want to increase the *intravascular* volume. If you give isotonic saline, this will expand volume and be at equilibrium with cellular fluid, so it would be effective in causing a net increase in intravascular volume without losing much fluid to the cells. Finally, if you give hypertonic saline, this would expand the volume *and* pull in more volume due to its higher tonicity. Hypertonic saline is generally used only in extreme cases of hypovolemia, e.g., shock. In this case, *isotonic* saline would be appropriate for volume expansion (Fig. 3-7). As always, remember that volume expansion needs to be done gradually to prevent central pontine myelinolysis (also known as osmotic demyelination syndrome).

CASE 15

On work-up of a hypertensive patient, you notice that sodium is 155 and potassium 2.9. What is your first thought?

When sodium and potassium are aberrant *in opposite directions*, think of aldosterone. Aldosterone causes reabsorption of Na^+ (sodium) and secretion of potassium. So elevated sodium and decreased potassium could indicate that aldosterone is elevated. Hyperaldosteronism is one cause of hypertension. Hyperaldosteronism can be primary or secondary (see Chapter 5). The point here is just to remind you that when sodium is up and potassium is down, think of elevated aldosterone; when potassium is up and sodium is down, think of decreased aldosterone (e.g., adrenal insufficiency).

CASE 16

A 59-year-old patient notices that his eyes and skin seem to be turning yellow. What is the differential diagnosis?

What causes jaundice? Elevated bilirubin. Why does that happen? Bilirubin comes from breakdown of red blood cells (RBCs) and is then taken up into the liver, conjugated, and secreted into the bile. So increased RBC breakdown (hemolysis), or problems with any of the steps just listed can lead to jaundice. Genetic diseases can also cause jaundice: **G**ilbert's (problem **g**etting bilirubin into the liver and conjugating it), Crigler-Najjar (**C**-N patients **c**annot **c**onjugate), and Dubin-Johnson (cannot secrete) (Fig. 4-10). Alternatively, liver pathology of any sort and biliary tract obstruction can both lead to a backup in the process and hence jaundice. *Un*conjugated bilirubin is *in*soluble in water. Conjugated bilirubin is water-soluble, so elevated *conjugated* bilirubin can end up turning the urine dark, and its absence from the stool (e.g., secondary to obstruction) can make the stool light. What other questions can you ask? Does the person have a history of alcohol abuse (which could cause cirrhosis)? How about a family history of liver disease (e.g., hemochromatosis, Wilson's, autoimmune liver disease)? Risk factors for viral hepatitis (e.g., tattoos, risky sexual behavior)? Pain (which could indicate some kind of inflammation)? Recent drug or toxic ingestion of some sort?

On physical exam, is the liver enlarged? This could indicate congestion (right heart failure or portal hypertension), cirrhosis, infection, tumor, etc. Is the liver tender? This could indicate inflammation or biliary obstruction. Are there any signs of portal hypertension (caput medusa, varicose veins, hemorrhoids, ascites)?

Labs. AST/ALT elevation, elevated prothrombin time, and decreased serum albumin can indicate liver disease. Is alk ph**os** (**o** for **o**bstruction) also elevated? Is bilirubin elevation predominantly conjugated or unconjugated (Fig. 4-10)?

Imaging. Ultrasound: Are stones visible? Dilated bile ducts that indicate obstruction (e.g., from primary sclerosing cholangitis, primary biliary cirrhosis, stones, or tumor—pancreatic, biliary, and small bowel tumors are all potentially close by)? Percutaneous transhepatic cholangiography (PTC) and endoscopic retrograde cholangiopancreatography (ERCP) can be used to assess intrahepatic ductal dilatation (e.g., secondary to primary biliary cirrhosis, liver tumor, etc.).

CASE 17

A 56-year-old male patient tells you that he has been having abdominal pain about 3 hours after he eats. It feels like burning and is mostly in the upper abdomen. He gets some relief with over-the-counter antacids. What is the differential diagnosis?

This could be simple heartburn/indigestion, but an ulcer should also be considered. Duodenal or gastric? When one eats, the stomach starts releasing acid right away, so gastric ulcers tend to cause pain *with eating* since the acid irritates the ulcer. Alternatively, duodenal ulcers typically hurt *later* when the acid passes from the stomach to the duodenum, as in this case (Fig. 4-5).

You order an endoscopy on this patient, and he is found to have multiple scattered duodenal ulcers. Now what do you think? This patient must have lots of acid. So you ask yourself, "How does acid end up getting secreted in the first place?" One hormone that causes acid secretion is_____.[1] If this hormone is really high, it could be coming from some tumor that is producing it. Multiple duodenal ulcers require checking serum gastrin level to explore the possibil-

_____
[1] Gastrin

ity of gastrinoma (Zollinger-Ellison syndrome). Suppose you find a high serum gastrin. How can you confirm the diagnosis of Zollinger-Ellison syndrome? The secretin test (Fig. 4-4).

CASE 18

A 46-year-old patient tells you he's been vomiting blood, but he does not bring any in for you to see. What is the differential diagnosis?

With bleeding, one must first determine whether the patient is stable; if the patient seems to have waning consciousness or is hypotensive, s/he must be emergently stabilized. Let's say the patient is stable. Your next task is to find out the source of the GI bleed. Red blood in the vomit usually means a source above the gastroesophageal junction, because the blood would be fresh, i.e., not digested. This could be from the esophagus (e.g., bleeding varices). Dark coffee grounds vomit generally means a source below the gastroesophageal junction, e.g., a bleeding gastric or duodenal ulcer. A very rapid-onset bleed from below the gastroesophageal junction can also cause red blood to appear in the vomit. See Fig. 4-9.

CASE 19

A 67-year-old patient says he saw blood in his stools. What is the differential diagnosis?

As in Case 18, first establish whether the patient has bled a lot and needs immediate IV fluids and stabilization. Next, same task: Where is the blood coming from? Again, remember the principle that close to the source of bleeding generally = *red*. So in the stools, red blood (hematochezia) could be from a hemorrhoid, anal fissure, colon cancer, or ulcerative colitis. The presence of black tarry stools (melena) generally means the blood has traveled in the GI tract for a significant distance (e.g., bleeding gastric or duodenal ulcer), however, right-sided colon cancer can also cause melena. See Fig. 4-9.

CASE 20

A 45-year-old woman schedules an appointment with you for what she calls "panic attacks." She says she feels suddenly extremely anxious, hot, and like her heart is beating very fast. What is your differential diagnosis, and how will you proceed?

A psychological disorder is certainly a possible cause of panic attacks, but ruling out physiological causes is essential, e.g., a tachyarrhythmia, hypoglycemia, etc. An EKG and blood sugar during symptoms could help give clues as to whether either of these etiologies is present. What else could cause these symptoms? A pheochromocytoma can produce paroxysmal symptoms when the blood pressure and heart rate rise. Urine metanephrines (catecholamine breakdown products) can be measured to look for evidence of pheochromocytoma. Additionally, hyperthyroidism can cause such symptoms, so you would want to examine the thyroid and order a TSH. What will that tell you? If the TSH is abnormally low, that would indicate increased negative feedback, i.e., primary hyperthyroidism (e.g., Grave's disease). If it is normal or high, it would be helpful to check thyroid hormone level. If TSH and thyroid hormone are *both* high, that would be most consistent with secondary hyperthyroidism (e.g., pituitary TSH-secreting tumor).

CASE 21

A 50-year-old man complains of weakness, fatigue, and weight loss. On exam you notice darkened areas of skin on his elbows. His blood pressure is 90/65, and his labs show a sodium of 130 and a potassium of 5.2. What is the most likely diagnosis?

In any case of weakness/fatigue/weight loss, your history should include an assessment of cancer risk (family history, blood in the stools, shortness of breath, night sweats, etc.), and you should do a complete workup for malignancy (looking for evidence of hematologic malignancy on blood work and evidence for other tumors on imaging studies). You also want to consider depression. In this case, a few things should jump out at you: Na^+ and K^+ being aberrant *in opposite directions,* hyperpigmentation, and hypotension. The Na^+ and K^+ abnormalities tell you that this has something to do with *aldosterone.* Increased potassium and decreased sodium suggest that aldosterone is _____.[2] Why would aldosterone be decreased? Aldosterone is secreted from the adrenal cortex (specifically, from the zona glomerulosa of the adrenal gland). Remember that aldosterone secretion is under the influence of potassium concentration and renin (which is secreted in response to decreased sodium concentration). So decreased aldosterone can occur from hypokalemia (not the case here), decreased renin (hyporeninemic hypoaldosteronism), or a problem with the adrenal cortex. What would make you suspect the adrenal gland in this case? The above features *plus* the hyperpigmentation. Remember that if the adrenal gland fails in *primary adrenal insufficiency,* ACTH secretion from the pituitary increases in an effort to stimulate the failing gland. ACTH and MSH share a common precursor, POMC, so that when ACTH levels are increased, MSH also becomes increased, leading to hyperpigmentation. This is a case of primary adrenal insufficiency. Review the labora-

tory distinction of primary from secondary adrenal insufficiency in Fig. 5-6.

CASE 22

A 60-year-old male patient's routine blood work comes back showing elevated calcium. He is otherwise healthy and all other labs are normal. What is the differential diagnosis?

Calcium is regulated by PTH, vitamin D, and calcitonin. Calcium is stored in the bones and excreted by the kidneys. So *increased PTH* (e.g., primary hyperparathyroidism or secondary hyperparathyroidism in renal failure), *increased vitamin D* (increased consumption or increased ectopic conversion, e.g., lymphomas, granulomas), *increased bone breakdown* (e.g., Paget's disease, primary bone tumor, or bone metastases), or *decreased renal excretion of calcium* can all lead to hypercalcemia. If this patient is otherwise healthy with otherwise normal labs (i.e., you do not expect lymphoma or renal disease), you should also check a PTH and a urine cAMP. The urine cAMP offers a window into whether the hypercalcemia is PTH-induced or not. Urine cAMP increases in PTH-related disorders, while it should *not increase* in vitamin D-induced hypercalcemia or bone breakdown. One can also check PTH level. If PTH is elevated, this is most likely a case of hyperparathyroidism. If PTH is decreased, this could be a case of vitamin D excess (Fig. 5-12), bone breakdown, or PTHrP-related hypercalcemia. See Fig. 5-13. If this is primary hyperparathyroidism, the origin can be a parathyroid adenoma, parathyroid cancer, or parathyroid hyperplasia. Imaging can help distinguish among these.

CASE 23

A 37-year-old man comes for a physical for work. His history and physical are completely normal. When his routine blood work comes back, you note that his hematocrit is lower than normal. How will you work him up?

Why is this patient anemic? From the routine blood work you should also have an MCV (mean cell volume) and a reticulocyte count. Why are these important? The MCV tells you whether this is a macrocytic or microcytic anemia, and the reticulocyte count tells you whether this is a problem with blood loss (hemolysis or bleeding in which case the reticulocyte would be *high)* or a problem with production (in which case the reticulocyte count would be *low*). In this case the MCV was slightly elevated and the reticulocyte count was normal. The elevated MCV tells you that this is a macrocytic anemia. Is the normal reticulocyte count normal? No. Since there is anemia, *the reticulocyte count should be elevated,* so if it is normal, it is "too low" given the scenario. So we are dealing with a macrocytic anemia due to a problem with RBC production. Macrocytic

---

[2] Decreased

anemias caused by problems with RBC production include B12 deficiency and folate deficiency.

In this case, the B12 level was found to be low. B12 is absorbed in the terminal ileum by being bound to intrinsic factor, which is made in the parietal cells of the stomach. Either terminal ileum disease, loss of intrinsic factor, or decreased dietary intake (e.g., a vegan diet) can lead to B12 deficiency. What is the name of the disease in which there is loss of intrinsic factor, and what antibodies underlie its pathophysiology?[3] What diagnostic test can make the distinction between decreased intrinsic factor and terminal ileum disease?[4] You run this test (Fig. 6-4) and find that in phase 1 there is no radioactivity in the urine. This indicates that B12 was not absorbed, so can you make a diagnosis? Not yet. You must run phase 2: Give the patient radioactive B12 and intrinsic factor to see if that corrects the problem. In this case it does *not*. This means there is terminal ileum disease. The diagnosis in this patient turned out to be Crohn's disease.

CASE 24

Ten days after removal of a benign osteoma from his tibia, a 47-year-old man develops acute onset shortness of breath and chest pain with deep inspiration. What is the differential diagnosis?

Acute onset shortness of breath should make you think of a number of potentially lethal etiologies such as pulmonary embolus, myocardial infarction, pneumothorax, etc., so you want to assess the patient's oxygen saturation and probably get a chest X-ray stat. In this patient, the fact that he has had orthopedic surgery on his leg means he is probably not moving around very much. This stasis can lead to deep venous thrombosis, which can embolize via the right heart to the pulmonary artery, leading to pulmonary embolism.

CASE 25

A parent brings her 2-year-old son to your office because she says he seems to "bleed a lot and bruise easily even from the smallest injuries." PT is normal, but PTT is elevated. What is the differential diagnosis?

If the patient has a bleeding disorder, it must be a problem with either platelets or coagulation factors. Coagulation defects can be assessed by checking the PT and PTT. If one of them is abnormal, there is something wrong with the clotting cascade. Here PT is normal and PTT is elevated. This tells you that the intrinsic pathway is affected. Thus, the problem is with one of the following: XII, XI, IX, VIII. Hemophilia

[3] Pernicious anemia; anti-parietal cell antibodies
[4] The Schilling test

is the most likely diagnosis (Hemophilia A is the diagnosis if an assay tells you that factor VIII is decreased; Hemophilia B if factor IX is decreased). Factor VIII can also be decreased in von Willebrand's disease.

CASE 26

A parent brings her 4-year-old daughter to your office because she says she seems to "bleed a lot and bruise easily even from the smallest injuries." PT and PTT are both normal. What is the differential diagnosis?

If both PT and PTT are normal, yet a bleeding disorder clearly exists, the problem must be with the platelets. This can either be decreased number (thrombocytopenia) or decreased function (e.g., von Willebrand's disease, Bernard-Soulier syndrome, Glanzmann thrombasthenia, storage pool diseases). This can be further assessed by looking at platelet number and function. Realize that a normal PTT does not exclude von Willebrand's disease, since the alteration of factor VIII level may be minimal, depending on the severity of the disease. See Fig. 6-11.

CASE 27

A 75-year-old man awakens to find that he is unable to move his right arm and barely able to move his right leg. His left side is completely normal. There is decreased sensation on the right side. His wife says that he is not making any sense when he talks and does not seem to understand what she says to him. You notice at first glance that his face seems to be drooping on the right side but that he raises his eyebrows symmetrically. He is unable to follow simple commands such as "Raise your left hand." Where is the lesion?

Loss of both motor and sensory function over a large region on the *same* side suggests that this lesion is higher than the spinal cord. That is, the lesion is in the brainstem or cerebral hemispheres. How can we distinguish between the two? The fact that he is having trouble with speech could indicate Broca's or Wernicke's aphasia (left cerebral hemisphere) but could also be a problem with CN XII leading to difficulty with tongue movements. The difficulty comprehending commands, however, suggests a true problem with language as opposed to just articulation of speech. This is a *receptive* aphasia. This suggests a lesion in Wernicke's area. In Wernicke's aphasia, words themselves are clearly articulated, but sentences do not make any sense. Comprehension is also impaired in Wernicke's aphasia. Regarding the pattern of deficits in the face, remember that lesions of the cranial nerve VII pathway that allow forehead sparing result from *upper motor neuron lesions* of nerve VII (Fig. 7-11). This lesion thus localizes to somewhere above the brainstem, i.e., in the cerebral hemispheres or internal capsule. Which side? Right-sided findings = left-sided cerebral lesion. What about the arm weakness greater than the leg weakness? This indicates a lesion affecting the lateral surface of the left hemisphere more so than the medial surface. This patient is having a left MCA stroke, specifically involving its posterior branch. See Figs. 7-18, 7-19.

CASE 28

A patient with known multiple sclerosis complains of double vision when looking to the left and some stiffness in her left leg. On exam you notice that on leftward gaze, her left eye abducts but her right eye does not adduct, though her right eye adducts on convergence. Her left leg is indeed stiff with hyperactive reflexes and a positive Babinski's sign. You also notice difficulty with finger-to-nose and heel-shin testing in both limbs. Where are her multiple sclerosis lesions?

The ocular movement problem is internuclear ophthalmoplegia (Fig. 7-10), which localizes to the *right* medial longitudinal fasciculus. Would you classify the left leg problems as upper or lower motor neuron deficits? Spasticity, increased reflexes, and Babinski's sign indicate an *upper motor neuron lesion.* Recall that multiple sclerosis *only* affects the central nervous system (i.e., not the peripheral nervous system), and thus can only affect the *brain and spinal cord* (and thus only *upper* motor neurons). The upper motor neuron lesion here could be anywhere from the motor cortex to the brainstem to the spinal cord. The difficulty with coordinating movements localizes to the cerebellum.

CASE 29

A 45-year-old lab technician complains of pain and "electrical shock" sensations in his left hand at night. He also notices increasing clumsiness and weakness of his left hand. On physical exam you note decreased sensation to light touch, pinprick, and temperature, on the palmar surfaces of the thumb and first two fingers on the left hand. The thumb is weak and its muscle is atrophied. Tapping the palmar surface of the left wrist sends "electrical shocks" through the first two fingers. The right hand is entirely normal in function and sensation. The patient is otherwise healthy. What is the diagnosis?

There are motor *and* sensory (including pain perception) deficits in the same place, so we know this lesion is *not* in the spinal cord (since the pain fibers in the spinothalamic tract *cross*). A spinal cord lesion would give loss of motor/proprioception/discrimination ipsilateral to the lesion and loss of pain and temperature contralateral to the lesion. The loss of motor and sensory function in the territory of one nerve, in this case, the median nerve, points to a problem with

the *nerve.* This is classic *carpal tunnel syndrome.* Swelling of the tendons in the carpal tunnel are thought to put pressure on the median nerve, leading to sensory and motor dysfunction in the distribution of this nerve. The reproduction of symptoms by tapping on the wrist is known as "Tinel's sign."

CASE 30

After attempting to lift a heavy bookcase, a 55-year-old man notices tingling pain down the back of his left leg all the way down to the foot. On physical exam you note an absence of the ankle reflex on the left. Where is the lesion?

This is classic disc herniation, but which nerve root and which disc? First we must determine the nerve root; the prolapsed disc is usually at the spinal level directly above this nerve root. We have a little help here: the absent ankle reflex. Remember (S)1-2; (L)3-4; (C)5-6;(C)7-8 = ankle-knee-biceps-triceps. Loss of the ankle reflex along with these sensory findings indicates an S1 nerve root lesion. Thus, this is most likely a prolapse of the *L5 disc* impinging upon the S1 root. Note that L4 disc prolapse hitting the L5 nerve root is also common, but this would have different sensory signs (namely on the lateral thigh and anterior/lateral calf). Also, since L5 is not part of any reflexes, an L4 prolapse (hitting the L5 root) would *not* affect any reflexes. Lateral disc herniation (e.g., L5 disc affecting L5 root or S1 disc affecting the S1 root) is also possible, but it is less common.

CASE 31

A 45-year-old female patient whom you have not seen in awhile comes in for a physical. You notice she has gained lots of weight, has acne, and has purple striae on her abdomen. She tells you she got into a car accident last week because she tried to change lanes and didn't see that there was a car next to her. What is the differential diagnosis?

This sounds like Cushing's syndrome: an elevation of blood cortisol either due to adrenal hyperactivity, increased ACTH from the pituitary (i.e., Cushing's *disease*), or ectopic ACTH (e.g., small cell lung cancer). Concerned about the car accident, you check her visual fields and notice a deficit in peripheral vision on both sides. Where is this lesion? This is a *bitemporal hemianopsia,* which means a midline chiasmatic lesion. Cushing's syndrome plus symptoms of a chiasm lesion point to Cushing's *disease,* the special case of Cushing's syndrome that occurs *secondary to a pituitary adenoma.*

INDEX